RADIOLOGY TODAY

A Multinational Series

Radiology Today 1

Edited by M. W. Donner and F. H. W. Heuck

1981. 290 figures, 61 tables. XIX,431.
ISBN 3-540-10099-7

Radiology Today 2

Edited by F. H. W. Heuck and M. W. Donner

1983. 306 figures, 44 tables. XII,362.
ISBN 3-540-11754-7

Contents: Gastrointestinal Radiology, Swallowing Disorders, Liver Disease and Function, Renal Transplant, Obstructive Uropathy, Direct Coronal CT, Embolization, Digital Angiography, Lymphatic System, CT of Lung and Mediastinum, Bone Mineral Analysis, Soft Tissue Tumors, Interventional Neuroradiology, Nuclear Magnetic Resonance

Radiology Today 3

Edited by

M.W. Donner and F.H.W. Heuck

With 196 Figures and 45 Tables

Springer-Verlag
Berlin Heidelberg New York Tokyo

Proceedings of the Multinational Postgraduate Course,
held in Salzburg, June 21–24, 1984.

Editors

Professor Dr. Martin W. Donner
Department of Radiology and Radiological Science
The Johns Hopkins Medical Institutions
Baltimore, MA 21205, USA

Professor Dr. Friedrich H. W. Heuck
Radiologisches Institut im Zentrum Radiologie
des Katharinenhospitals der Stadt Stuttgart
7000 Stuttgart 1, FRG

ISBN-13: 978-3-642-69739-5 e-ISBN-13: 978-3-642-69737-1
DOI: 10.1007/978-3-642-69737-1

Softcover reprint of the hardcover 1st edition 1985

2121/3140-543210

Preface

Radiology Today 3 presents papers and panel discussions from a multinational faculty at the biannual Salzburg Symposium, which this time covered three important topics: critical diagnostic pathways in gastrointestinal and genitourinary radiology, interventional radiology of the abdomen, and cost containment in radiology.

The choice of these topics illustrates the changing role of the radiologist in the practice of medicine today and in the foreseeable future. He will have to serve as a consultant more than ever before, assuming increasing responsibility for sequencing of imaging procedures and participating more and more in therapeutic intervention. In order to provide meaningful assistance, the imaging consultant must be aware of the efficacy and the limitations of every procedure. In this context, cost containment is a worldwide public concern, and the most appropriate procedures must be identified.

Radiology Today 3 demonstrates how the radiologist functions as a member of diagnostic and management teams to provide optimal information and efficient, low-risk patient care at the lowest possible cost.

Martin W. Donner
Friedrich H.W. Heuck

Contents

List of Contributors

P. Alken
Institut für Klinische Strahlenkunde, Urologische Klinik,
Universität Mainz, Langenbeckstrasse 1, 6500 Mainz, FRG

K. Amplatz
Department of Radiology, University of Minnesota, Box 292,
420 Delaware Street, Minneapolis, MN 55455, USA

A. L. Baert
Department of Radiology, University Hospitals K.U.L.,
3000 Leuven, Belgium

K. H. Barth
Department of Radiology, Georgetown University Hospital,
3800 Reservoir Road, N.W. Washington, DC 20007, USA

K. Becker
Institut für Allgemeine Pathologie und Pathologische Anatomie,
Klinikum Rechts der Isar, Technische Universität München,
Ismaninger Strasse 22, 8000 München 80, FRG

M. A. Bosniak
Department of Radiology, New York University Medical Center,
550–560 First Avenue, New York, NY 10016, USA

E. Bücheler
Radiologische Klinik, Universitätskrankenhaus Eppendorf,
Martinistrasse 52, 2000 Hamburg 20, FRG

H. J. Burhenne
Department of Radiology, University of British Columbia,
Vancouver General Hospital, 855 West, 12th Avenue, Vancouver,
British Columbia, V5Z 1M9, Canada

P. Carl
Hauptkrankenhaus, Perlasberger Strasse 41, 8360 Deggendorf, FRG

W. P. Cockshott
Harward Medical School, Department of Radiology, Brigham and
Women's Hospital, Dana-Farber Cancer Institute, 25 Shattuck Street,
Boston, MA 02115, USA

H. Czembirek
Röntgenstation, I. Medizinische Universitätsklinik, 1090 Wien, Austria

G. Egender
Universitätskliniken, Ordinariat für Strahlentherapie, Anichstrasse 35,
6020 Innsbruck, Austria

F. Eisenberger
Urologische Klinik, Katharinenhospital, Kriegsbergstrasse 60,
7000 Stuttgart 1, FRG

L. Ekelund
Department of Diagnostic Radiology, University of Lund,
22185 Lund, Sweden

R. Felix
Abteilung Radiologie mit Poliklinik, Strahlenklinik und Poliklinik (WE 07), Universitätsklinikum Charlottenburg, Freie Universität Berlin, Spandauer Damm 130, 1000 Berlin 19, FRG

G. Fenzl
Radiologische Klinik und Poliklinik, Klinikum Grosshadern, Ludwig-Maximilians-Universität München, Marchioninistrasse 15, 8000 München 70, FRG

J. T. Ferrucci, Jr.
Department of Radiology, Massachusetts General Hospital,
Fruit Street, Boston, MA 02114, USA

S. Feuerbach
Institut für Röntgendiagnostik, Klinikum rechts der Isar, Technische Universität München, Ismaninger Strasse 22, 8000 München 80, FRG

J. Fevery
Department of Internal Medicine, University Hospitals K.U.L.,
3000 Leuven, Belgium

W. Frank
Röntgenstation, I. Chirurgische Universitätsklinik Wien,
Alser Strasse 4, 1090 Wien, Austria

H. Frommhold
Universitätskliniken, Ordinariat für Strahlentherapie, Anichstrasse 35,
6020 Innsbruck, Austria

W. Frommhold
Medizinisches Strahleninstitut, Eberhard-Karls-Universität Tübingen,
Röntgenweg 11, 7400 Tübingen, FRG

G. Fuchs
Division of Urology UCLA, School of Medicine, Center for Health Sciences, 18033 Le Conte Avenue, Los Angeles, CA 90024, USA

W. A. Fuchs
Institut für Diagnostische Radiologie, Inselspital,
3010 Bern, Switzerland

A. Furtschegger
Universitätskliniken, Ordinariat für Strahlentherapie, Anichstrasse 35,
6020 Innsbruck, Austria

K. Geboes
Department of Pathology, University Hospitals K.U.L.,
3000 Leuven, Belgium

E. Grabbe
Radiologische Klinik, Universitätskrankenhaus Eppendorf,
Martinistrasse 52, 2000 Hamburg 20, FRG

R. Günther
Abteilung Radiologische Diagnostik, Neuklinikum,
Pauwelsstrasse, 5100 Aachen, FRG

P. Hajek
Zentrales Institut für Radiodiagnostik, Universität Wien,
Alser Strasse 4, 1090 Wien, Austria

H. Hötzinger
Abteilung für Radiologie, Städtisches Krankenhaus Passau,
Bischof-Pilgrim-Strasse 1, 8390 Passau, FRG

H. Hricak
Department of Radiology, School of Medicine,
University of California, San Francisco, CA 94143, USA

H. Imhof
Zentrales Institut für Radiodiagnostik, Universität Wien,
Alser Strasse 4, 1090 Wien, Austria

T. Irnberger
Röntgendiagnostisches Zentralinstitut der Landeskrankenanstalten,
Müllner Hauptstrasse 48, 5020 Salzburg, Austria

S. L. Kaufman
Department of Radiology, The Johns Hopkins Hospital,
Baltimore, MD 21205, USA

J. A. Kirkpatrick, Jr.
Department of Radiology, The Children's Hospital,
300 Longwood Avenue, Boston, MA 02115, USA

R. Kloss
Röntgendiagnostisches Zentralinstitut der Landeskrankenanstalten,
Müllner Hauptstrasse 48, 5020 Salzburg, Austria

M. Kormano
Department of Diagnostic Radiology, University Central Hospital,
20520 Turku, Finland

J. Kuikka
Department of Clinical Physiology, University Central Hospital,
Kuopio, Finland

W. Kumpan
Zentrales Institut für Radiodiagnostik, Universität Wien,
Alser Strasse 4, 1090 Wien, Austria

E. K. Lang
Department of Radiology, School of Medicine,
Louisiana State University, Medical Center,
1542 Tulane Avenue, New Orleans, LA, USA

I. Laufer
Hospital of the University of Pennsylvania, 3400 Spruce Street/G1,
Philadelphia, PA 19104, USA

G. Lechner
Röntgenstation, I. Chirurgische Universitätsklinik Wien,
Alser Strasse 4, 1090 Wien, Austria

J. Lissner
Radiologische Klinik und Poliklinik, Klinikum Grosshadern,
Ludwig-Maximilians-Universität München, Marchioninistrasse 15,
8000 München 70, FRG

E. Löhr
Röntgendiagnostisches Zentralinstitut, Universitätsklinikum der Gesamthochschule Essen, Hufelandstrasse 55, 4300 Essen, FRG

G. Marchal
Department of Radiology, University Hospitals K.U.L., 3000 Leuven, Belgium

A. R. Margulis
Department of Radiology, University of California, School of Medicine, San Francisco, CA 94143, USA

S. McCarthy
Department of Radiology, University of California, San Francisco, CA 94143, USA

K. Miller
Urologische Klinik, Katharinenhospital, Kriegsbergstrasse 60, 7000 Stuttgart 1, FRG

N. Muzika
Röntgenstation, 1. Chirurgische Abteilung, Krankenhaus der Stadt Wien-Lainz, Wolkersbergenstrasse 1, 1130 Wien, Austria

F. Olbert
Röntgenstation, 1. Chirurgische Abteilung, Krankenhaus der Stadt Wien-Lainz, Wolkersbergenstrasse 1, 1130 Wien, Austria

K. Partanen
Department of Diagnostic Radiology, University Central Hospital, Kuopio, Finland

P. E. Peters
Institut für Klinische Radiologie, Westfälische-Wilhelms-Universität Münster, Albert Schweitzer-Strasse 33, 4400 Münster, FRG

J. Pirschel
Medizinisches Strahleninstitut, Eberhard-Karls-Universität Tübingen, Röntgenweg 11, 7400 Tübingen, FRG

H. Pokieser
Zentrales Institut für Radiodiagnostik, Universität Wien, Alser Strasse 4, 1090 Wien, Austria

E. Ponette
Department of Radiology, University Hospitals K.U.L., 3000 Leuven, Belgium

J. Rassweiler
Urologische Klinik, Katharinenhospital, Kriegsbergstrasse 60, 7000 Stuttgart 1, FRG

W. Reichardt
Seelbergstrasse 9, 7000 Stuttgart 50, FRG

P. Reindl
Hauptkrankenhaus, Perlasberger Strasse 41, 8360 Deggendorf, FRG

M. Reiser
Institut für Röntgendiagnostik, Klinikum rechts der Isar, Technische Universität München, Ismaninger Strasse 22, 8000 München 80, FRG

N. Rupp
Institut für Röntgendiagnostik, Klinikum rechts der Isar, Technische Universität München, Ismaninger Strasse 22, 8000 München 80, FRG

E. Salomonowitz
Röntgenstation, I. Medizinische Universitätsklinik Wien, Lazarettgasse 14, 1090 Wien, Austria

H. M. Saxton
Department of Diagnostic Radiology, Guy's Hospital, St. Thomas Street, London SE1 9RT, Great Britain

A. Schekatz
Institut für Röntgendiagnostik, Klinikum rechts der Isar, Technische Universität München, Ismaninger Strasse 22, 8000 München 80, FRG

A. Schlegl
Röntgenstation, 1. Chirurgische Abteilung, Krankenhaus der Stadt Wien-Lainz, Wolkersbergenstrasse 1, 1130 Wien, Austria

H. Schmoller
Röntgendiagnostisches Zentralinstitut der Landeskrankenanstalten, Müllner Hauptstrasse 48, 5020 Salzburg, Austria

G. H. Schneider
Universitätsklinik für Radiologie, Landeskrankenhaus, 8036 Graz, Austria

H. Schreyer
Abteilung für spezielle Röntgendiagnostik, Universitätsklinik für Radiologie, Landeskrankenhaus, 8036 Graz, Austria

U. Speck
Schering Aktiengesellschaft, Postfach 65 03 11, 1000 Berlin 65, FRG

E. Tölly
Universitätsklinik für Radiologie, Landeskrankenhaus, 8036 Graz, Austria

H. Treugut
Radiologisches Institut, Katharinenhospital, Kriegsbergstrasse 60, 7000 Stuttgart 1, FRG

K. N. Vizy
Eastman Kodak Company, Health Sciences Markets Division, 343 State Street, Rochester, NY 14650, USA

M. Zieger
Olgahospital, Pädiatrisches Zentrum, Radiologisches Institut, Bismarckstrasse 8, 7000 Stuttgart 1, FRG

Critical Diagnostic Pathways

The Diagnosis of Pancreatic Cancer

G. Marchal, A.L. Baert, K. Geboes, E. Ponette, and J. Fevery

The incidence of cancer of the pancreas increases each year, particularly in the industrial countries. The disease is now considered the fifth most common cause of cancer death in the USA [1]. According to Japanese statistics, mortality from pancreatic carcinoma increased about 6 times during the last 25 years [2]. The overall 5-year survival rate of pancreatic cancer is about 1% [1], one of the lowest for all cancers, reflecting the ineffectiveness of our diagnostic modalities for early detection and the inefficiency of currently available treatment, which has mainly been surgical.

Considering the different radiologic diagnostic modalities, one has to face the question: Do we consider pancreatic cancer as a curable disease or does its diagnosis represent a death sentence? Unfortunately the latter is the case in most patients. The choice of diagnostic techniques should therefore be made on these considerations. The failures of both diagnostic modalities and surgical treatment are related to the particular topographic location of the pancreas, the anatomy of the gland, and the aggressivity of pancreatic cancer.

Although from the histologic point of view, different types of malignant tumors of the exocrine pancreas can be recognized [3], this differentiation is not really of clinical significance, since they have all the same clinical course and fatal outcome. Cystadenocarcinoma, in which better survivals have been reported [4], is probably the only exception to this rule.

Of all pancreatic cancers, duct cell adenocarcinoma, with an incidence of nearly 90%, can be considered the prototype.

Pancreatic adenocarcinoma probably arises from the epithelium of the large main pancreatic ducts or secondary branches, not from the ductules. According to Cubilla and Fitzgerald [3] different arguments favor this hypothesis:

1. Pancreatic ductular adenocarcinoma is a mucin-producing tumor. In the normal pancreas, mucin is a constituent of duct cell epithelium of the primary and secondary branches, but absent in the ductules.
2. In about 25% of resected specimens of pancreatic cancer, histology reveals cancer in situ in the large ducts adjacent to the tumor.
3. Some cases of cancer in situ have been reported which involve the whole pancreatic duct but do not extend into the secondary branches.

If this hypothesis is verified, it has various clinical implications. It suggests not only the possibility of a multicentric origin of pancreatic carcinoma, but also that there may be a latent period between the appearance of carcinoma in situ in the duct epithelium and the development of grossly identifiable pancreatic adenocarcinoma. It explains the success rate of ERCP, even when only the primary and secondary ducts are opacified, the peripheral growing tumors being rather uncommon. On the other hand, although frequently associated with macroscopic adenocarcinoma, carcinoma in situ has never been demonstrated by ERCP.

Most growing ductal adenocarcinomas show important desmoplastic reaction (Fig. 1) as well as areas of necrosis. On contrast-enhanced CT the hypodense areas during the early phase after bolus injection reflect heavy fibrosis, necrosis, or both (Fig. 2). Nonenhancing areas on the delayed scans suggest necrosis. By ultrasound (US), necrosis (Fig. 3) is more seldom identifiable as such, since liquefaction necrosis is rather uncommon.

Although about 65% of all pancreatic cancers originate in the pancreatic head, in only about 30% of these are bile duct obstruction and jaundice presenting symptoms [5]. Pancreatic duct obstruction is more frequent and can be associated with acute pancreatitis, as well as pressure atrophy of the proximal pancreatic tissue (Fig. 4) [6]. Although histologic signs of acute pancreatitis are found in about 10% of the patients, clinically evident acute pancreatitis is uncommon [7, 8, 9].

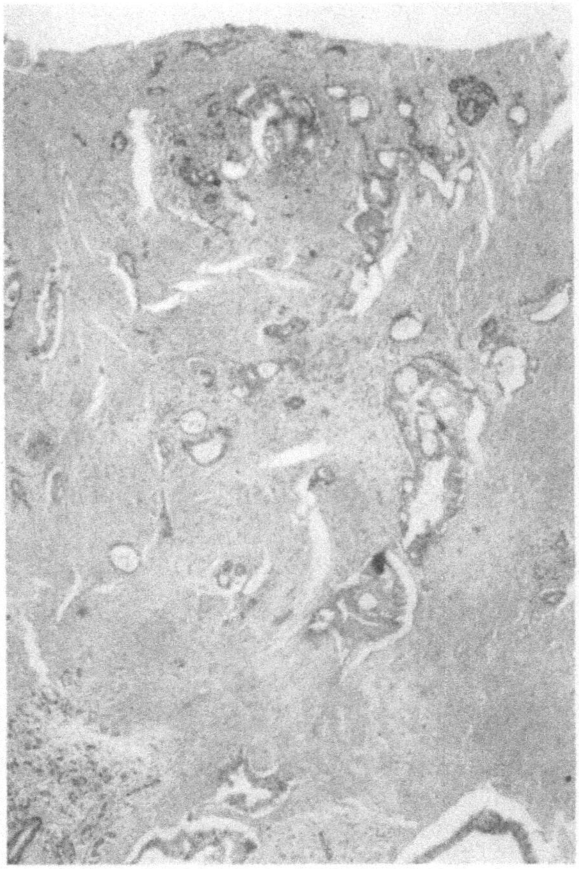

Fig. 1. Duct cell adenocarcinoma of the pancreas, biliary pancreatic duct type, with considerable fibrosis

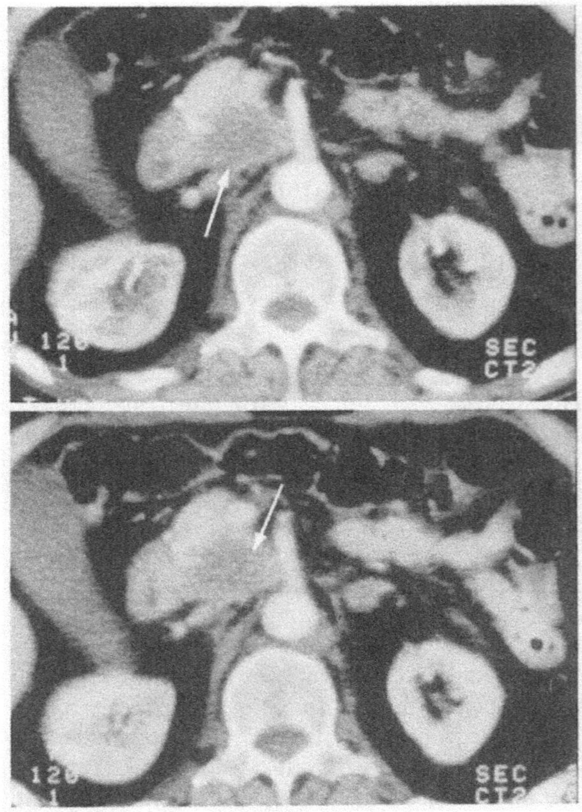

Fig. 2. Pancreatic cancer of the uncinate process: contrast-enhanced CT, early phase. The tumor is seen as a nonenhancing mass dorsal to the superior mesenteric vein. The fat planes (*arrows*) between the tumor and the superior mesenteric artery and inferior caval veins are no longer visible, pointing to local infiltration by the tumor

Adenocarcinoma of the pancreas is a particularly aggressive neoplasm which tends to spread along different pathways. Seeding occurs along paths of least resistance, such as the intrapancreatic nerve sheaths (Fig. 5), in which clusters of tumor cells can be found at quite a distance from the primary tumor.

Lymphatic and venous involvement are responsible for nodal and hepatic metastases.

Direct visualization of intravascular tumor growth is difficult with both US and CT. In general, venous obstruction is suggested by the presence of peripancreatic collaterals (Fig. 4).

The location of the pancreas near vital vascular structures and the aggressivity of the cancer make early diagnosis, at a stage when curative resection can still be considered, very difficult. Without surgical resection or other treatment, the mean survival rate varies between 5 and 6 months. After curative surgery, survival for up to 5 years has been reported [10].

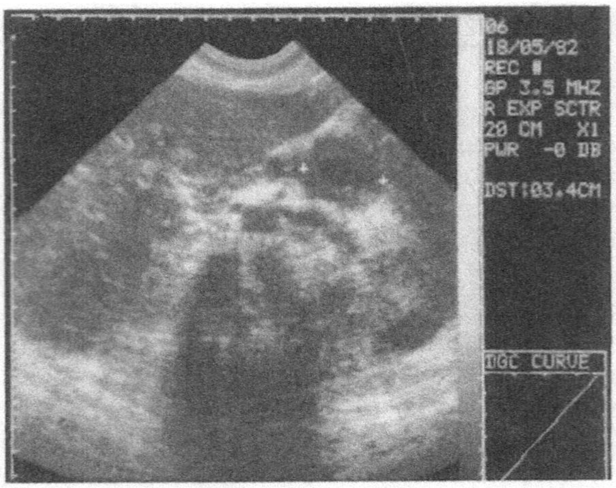

Fig. 3. Adenocarcinoma of the body of the pancreas: transverse sonogram. Hypoechoic mass in the body of the pancreas; the areflective center of this mass supports central necrosis

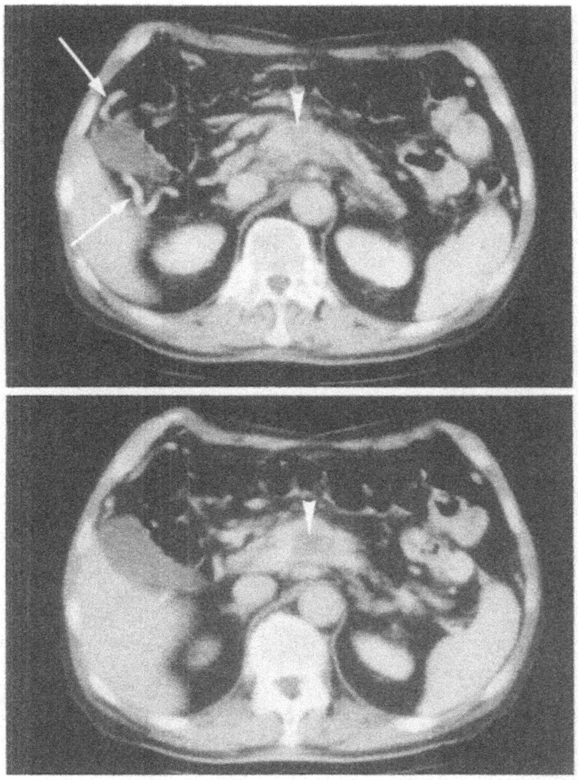

Fig. 4. Adenocarcinoma of the body of the pancreas: contrast-enhanced CT. The tumor is visible as a small hypodense area (*arrowheads*) ventral to the mesenteric vessels. The tail of the pancreas is atrophic and the common pancreatic duct slightly dilated. Obstruction of the splenic vein is suggested by the extensive collateral network at the level of the gallbladder (*arrows*)

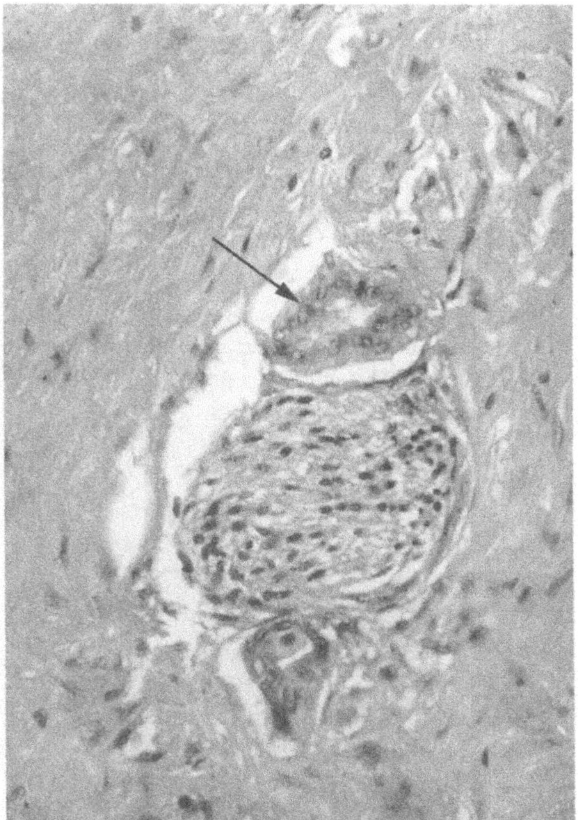

Fig. 5. Perineural metastases of duct cell adenocarcinoma of the pancreas. Transverse section of a small intrapancreatic nerve. Small clusters of tumoral cells (*arrow*) are seen in the fibrous perineural sheath

No diagnostic measures will be taken before the patient starts complaining – of pain, jaundice, or more general symptoms. At this stage most cancers are no longer curable. In this context, the diagnostic work-up should start with the less invasive techniques such as US and CT. In general, CT will yield slightly better results because it is less prone to technical failure and less dependent on patient habitus and the skill of the examiner [11]. Very frequently, incurability will already have been proven by the demonstration of local tumor extension (Fig. 2), adenopathies, or distant metastases [2, 6]. When problems arise in differentiating chronic pancreatitis from carcinoma, ERCP is indicated. In incurable patients with carcinoma, palliation with endoprothesis is very promising, avoiding the morbidity and mortality of palliative surgery [12].

Confirmation of the malignant nature can also easily be obtained by cytologic aspiration biopsy under sonographic CT or ERCP control [13, 14]. Finally, angiography should be limited to the small number of patients in whom a curative resection can still be attempted [15].

References

1. Silverberg E (1977) Cancer Statistics 1977. CA 27: 26–41
2. Ariyama J et al. (1977) The diagnosis of small resectable pancreatic carcinoma. Clin Radiol 28: 437–444
3. Cubilla AL, Fitzgerald PJ (1980) Cancer (nonendocrine) of the pancreas. A suggested classification in the pancreas, chapter 6. Williams and Wilkins, Baltimore, pp 82–110
4. Hodgkinson DJ et al. (1978) A clinicopathologic study of 21 cases of pancreatic cystadenocarcinoma. Ann Surg 188:679–684
5. Braganza JM, Howat HT (1972) Cancer of the pancreas. Clin Gastroenterol 1:219–237

6. Itai Y et al. (1982) Computed tomographic appearance of resectable pancreatic carcinoma. Radiology 143:715–726
7. Miccolini DG et al. (1976) Tumor-induced acute pancreatitis. Gastroenterology 71:442–445
8. Gambill E (1971) Pancreatitis associated with pancreatic carcinoma. Mayo Clin Proc 46:174–177
9. Itai Y et al. (1982) Pancreatic cysts induced by carcinoma of the pancreas, a pitfall in the diagnosis of pancreatic carcinoma. J Comput Assist Tomogr 6:772–776
10. Shapiro TM (1975) Adenocarcinoma of the pancreas. A statistical analysis of biliary bypass vs Whipple resection in good risk patients. Ann Surg 1982:715–721
11. Hessel SJ et al. (1982) A prospective study of computed tomography and ultrasound of the pancreas. Radiology 143:129–133
12. Huibregtse K, Tytgat GN (1982) Palliative treatment of obstructive jaundice by a transpapillary introduced large bore bile duct endoprothesis. Experience in 45 patients. Gut 23:371–375
13. Frable WJ (1983) Fine needle aspiration biopsy. Hum Pathol 14(1):9–28
14. Isler JJ et al. (1981) Tissue care biopsy of abdominal tumors with a 22 Gauge Cutting needle. AJR 136:725–728
15. Stanley RJ (1980) The impact of new imaging methods on pancreatic angiography. Radiology 136:251–253

Localization Techniques for Hormonally Active Pancreatic Tumors

W. Reichardt

The diagnosis of functioning endocrine pancreatic tumors has usually already been established by case history and laboratory findings by the time the patient is referred to the radiologist.

Today there are four methods for preoperative localization of endocrine tumors of the pancreas. Angiography was the method of choice after Olsson, in 1963, first reported the angiographic findings in an islet cell tumor [8]. In the 1970s three other methods were added: selective catheterization of the pancreatic veins for blood sampling and hormone assay, CT, and ultrasound.

All kinds of islet cell tumors show the same radiologic features with the various methods, independent of the cell group from which they arise. However, the tumor size when diagnosed, the probability of multiplicity and malignancy, and the therapeutic course are different in different syndromes, and therefore the use of the localization procedures differs.

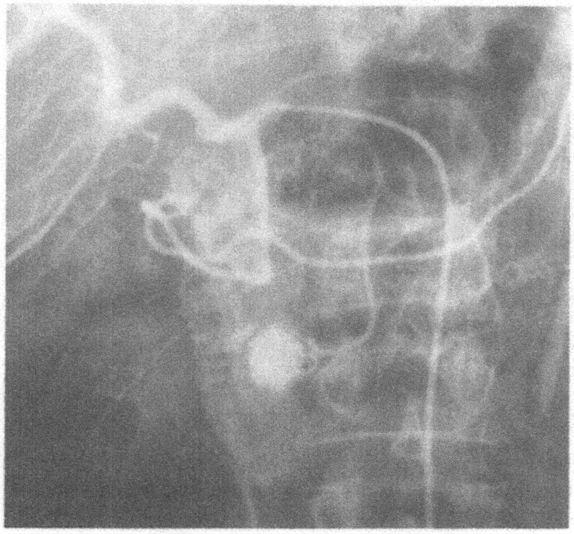

Fig. 1. Insulinoma of the head of the pancreas: intense accumulation of contrast medium within the tumor in the arterial phase of angiography

Techniques

Angiography

When islet cell tumors are less than 2 cm in size – usually insulinomas and gastrinomas – arteriography shows intense accumulation of contrast medium within the tumor in the early arterial phase, persisting to the late venous phase (Fig. 1). Usually no pathologic vessels can be recognized and no early venous filling is to be seen [1]. Tumors larger than 5 cm when diagnosed are often malignant and usually belong to the group of rarely observed tumors producing somatostatin, VIP, GIP, HPP, or other polypeptides, or they are nonfunctioning tumors.

Even if it is true that larger tumors with marked neovascularity (Fig. 2a) and early venous filling often are malignant these are no reliable criteria for differentiation of malignant and benign islet cell tumors. The only reliable sign of malignancy is metastases, which are characterized by the same intense staining as the primary tumor.

Angiographic examinations for localization of islet cell tumors should, as a rule, always include selective injection of the splenic and gastroduodenal arteries, even when a tumor is demonstrated on celiac trunk angiograms. False-positive identification can be caused by accessory spleen, hemangioma of the pancreas, enlarged lymph nodes, duodenal ulcers – especially in Zollinger-Ellison syndrome – and orthograde projected normal body of the pancreas [6].

The reported success rate varies widely, between 10% and 100%; about 60% should be realistic.

Computed Tomography

The results with older CT machines were poor, only about 30% positive identification of en-

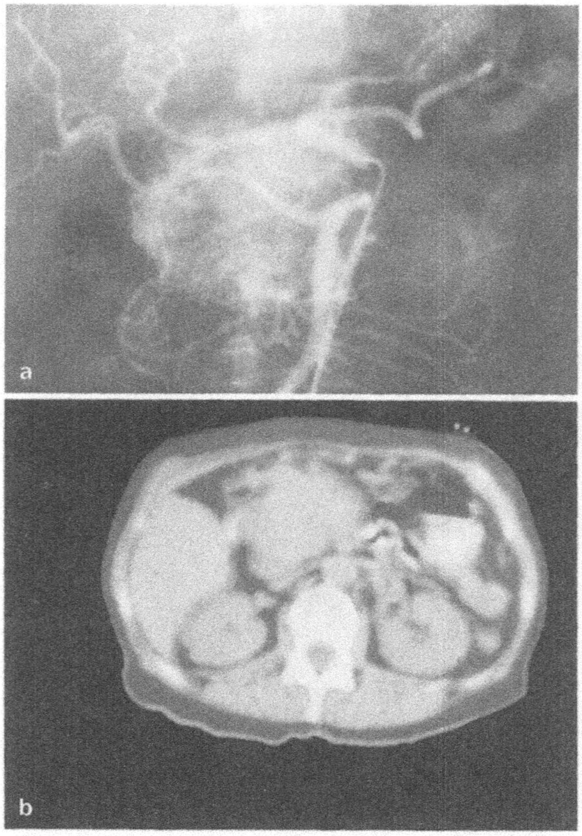

Fig. 2 a, b. Large glucagonoma of the head of the pancreas in a 62-year-old woman. **a** Marked neovascularity is found in the arterial phase of angiography. **b** An isodense tumor mass is demonstrated by CT

docrine tumors. Using up-to-date techniques, CT results are improved, especially in tumors larger than 2 cm in size (Fig. 2b). Recently, D. Stark et al. [14] reported their results in localization of pancreatic islet cell tumors. In 21 of 27 tumors proved at surgery the tumor site was correctly demonstrated by CT (sensitivity 78%), and in 14 of 14 patients the diagnosis was correctly excluded. In the group of tumors less than 2 cm in size six of 12 were missed by CT (50%). Other authors report the same results in tumors less than 2 cm in size [4].

As a rule the islet cell tumors are isodense with the normal pancreatic tissue and cannot be identified without contrast medium (Fig. 3). After bolus injection of 50 ml contrast medium there is a difference of 10 – 20 HU between the tumor and the surrounding pancreatic tissue for about 60 s. With a fast scan sequence you are often able to examine the entire pancreas in this time; if not, the bolus injection should be repeated.

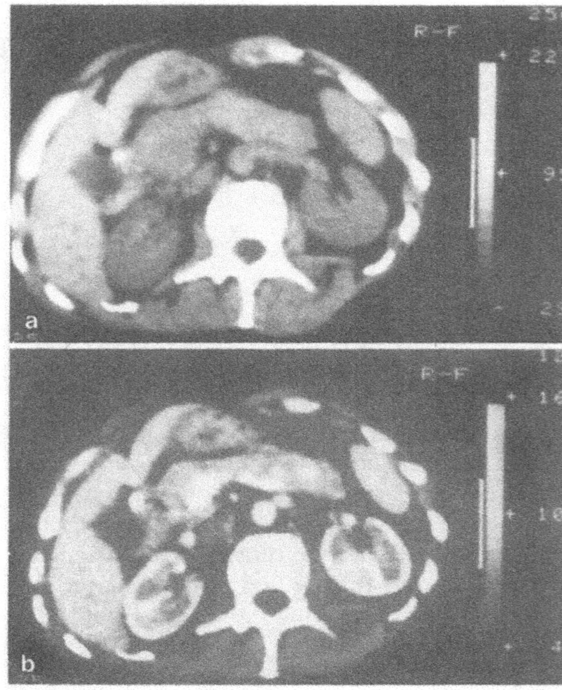

Fig. 3 a, b. Insulinoma of the tail of the pancreas. **a** The isodense tumor is not visualized. **b** After bolus injection of 50 ml of contrast medium the tumor can be demonstrated during the 60 s after injection

Ultrasound

Günther et al. [4] have demonstrated that ultrasound localization of endocrine pancreatic tumors as small as 7 mm in size is possible. The tumor has a lower echogenicity than the surrounding pancreatic tissue. However, the number of reported cases is too small to judge the usefulness of the method.

Selective Catheterization of Pancreatic Veins for Hormone Assay

The localization of endocrine pancreatic tumors by venous sampling is demonstrated in insulinomas, glucagonomas, gastrinomas and tumors producing HPP, 5-HT, and somatostatin [3, 9, 11, 12].

In insulin- and gastrin-producing tumors the accuracy has been 80% – 97%, making this by far the most accurate method, especially in small tumors. Venous sampling has the disadvantage of being invasive, sometimes painful, and time consuming. The rate of major complications, such as bile leakage and intra-abdominal bleeding, is 1% – 3%

[5]. The complications are due to the transhepatic puncture of the portal vein. Major complications caused by selective catheterization of the pancreatic veins are not known.

In endocrine tumors of the pancreas no morphologic changes of the veins are seen. In occasional tumors larger than 3 cm in size, displacement of the major veins is the only tumor sign [11]. If blood sampling for tumor localization is performed, selective catheterization of the pancreatic veins is essential. Some authors have discussed preoperative venous sampling only in the large portal vein tributaries and reported successful localization in some cases. All recent papers stress that sampling in the main portal vein tributaries often fails [9, 11, 12]. One reason is the variation in the venous anatomy of the pancreas. The head of the pancreas is usually drained by two arcades, a dorsal one and a ventral one. As a rule, one or two parts of the arcades dominate [10]. The body of the pancreas is often drained by a transverse pancreatic vein to the superior mesenteric vein (Fig. 4). The transverse vein may even drain the tail of the pancreas. Thus a peak value of hormone concentration in the superior mesenteric vein can be caused by a tumor in the tail, the body, or the head of the pancreas, depending on the individual venous anatomy.

After blood sampling the venous drainage should be documented by phlebograms to chart the individual anatomy. Sometimes the hormone concentration in the main portal vein tributary at the tumor level is within the range of hormone concentrations of the portal venous system, which further stresses the importance of selective catheterization (Fig. 5a, b) [11].

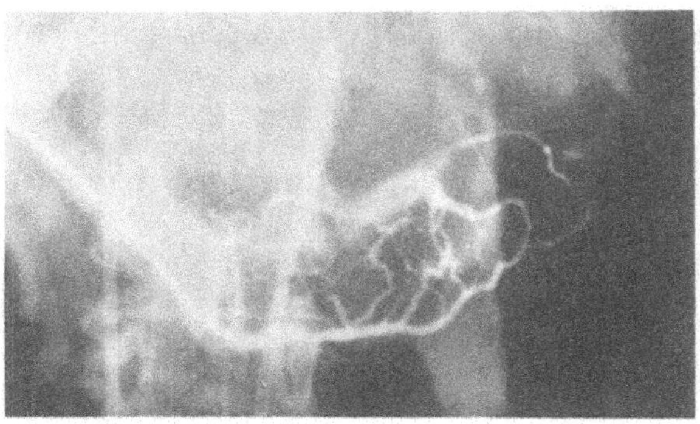

Fig. 4. Selective injection of the transverse pancreatic vein, which in this unusual case is draining the main part of the body of the pancreas and even parts of the tail of the pancreas

Tumors

Insulinoma

Insulinomas arise from B cells in the pancreatic islets and are the most common endocrine pancreatic tumors. In more than 90% of patients the hyperinsulinism results from single adenomas. Most of the tumors are less than 3 cm, about 65% less

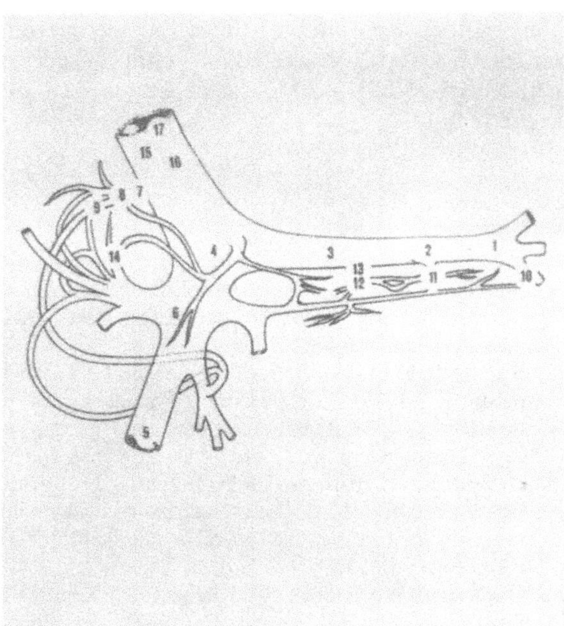

◂ **Fig. 5.** Hormone concentrations in a 32-year-old woman with B-cell hyperplasia in the tail of the pancreas. The lesion cannot be localized by samples obtained in the splenic vein only

			IRI μU/ml
1	v. lienalis	=	13
2	v. lienalis	=	missed
3	v. lienalis	=	45
4	portal confluens	=	56
5	v. mes. sup.	=	11
6	v. mes. sup. (outside GCT)	=	63
7	v. PSPD	=	13
8	v. PSPD	=	71
9	v. PSPD	=	90
10	v. lienalis (anastomosis to distal pancreatic vein)	=	165
11	pancreatic vein	=	950
12	pancreatic vein	=	1130
13	pancreatic vein	=	280
14	v. ASPD	=	14
15	v. porta centr.	=	58
16	v. porta centr.	=	62
17	v. porta centr.	=	59

than 1.5 cm in size. According to Stefanini et al. [13] who summarized the findings in 1067 cases reported in the literature, the tumors are spread almost evenly throughout the head, body, and tail of the pancreas. Today there is no longer any place for blind resection of the pancreas.

Ultrasound and CT should be the first examinations in patients with suspected insulinomas. If the tumor cannot be localized, angiography and if necessary venous sampling should be the next steps. In patients previously operated on without success venous sampling has to be done. We examined two patients with persistent symptoms after previous resection and were able to localize the tumor correctly by venous sampling in both of them.

We had previously successfully localized eight of nine insulin-producing islet cell tumors. In one patient with an insulinoma in the dorsocranial part of the head of the pancreas the tumor could not be located by hormone analyses, but selective phlebography revealed an anomalous venous connection between the head of the pancreas and the left lobe of the liver. The tumor was not palpable at operation and was only found because of the anomalous venous drainage.

Gastrinoma

Gastrinoma are tumors of the G cells and are a feature of Zollinger-Ellison syndrome, which is characterized by ulcer diathesis, excessive gastric hypersecretion, and presence of an islet cell tumor. In approximately 60% of cases the tumor is malignant, and in more than half the benign cases there are multiple tumors. The treatment of Zollinger-Ellison syndrome used to be total gastrectomy but this has changed recently due to the efficient control of the symptoms with histamine H_2-receptor antagonists. But as most gastrinomas are malignant, extirpation of the tumor is desirable. If accurate preoperative localization of gastrinomas can be obtained, curative surgery is possible, as reported by Burcharth et al. [2]. In all patients with suspected gastrinomas undergoing localization procedures, angiography, CT, and venous sampling should be performed, even if one of the methods has already localized a tumor. Venous catheterization is necessary because multiple tumors are common. As a rule, angiography and CT only demonstrate one or some of multiple tumors [11, 12].

A single gastrinoma can also be localized by vein catheterization and hormone assay. Generally, elevated gastrin concentrations cannot localize the tumor but suggest multiplicity.

Glucagonoma

The clinical syndrome associated with a tumor of the A-cells of the pancreatic islets is the glucagonoma syndrome, first described by McGavran et al. in 1966 [7]. The syndrome is characterized by intolerance for glucose, necrolytic migratory erythema, glossitis, anemia, and weight loss. The necrolytic migratory erythema has led to diagnosis in most of the recent cases reported.

More than 50% of the tumors have metastases and most of the tumors are more than 4 cm in diameter, often huge, when diagnosed.

However, our smallest glucagonoma with successful preoperative localization was only 8 mm in size and malignant. We have examined three glucagon-producing tumors in Lund, and all were correctly localized. In one patient, a tumor in the head of the pancreas also contained insulin and serotonin.

Summary

Ultrasound and CT should be done in all patients with suspected endocrine pancreatic tumors. If both methods are successful, no further work-up is necessary; otherwise angiography and in rare cases venous sampling should be performed. Exceptions are patients with multiple endocrine adenomatosis or Zollinger-Ellison syndrome and patients previously operated on without success. In these cases all localization procedures should be carried out.

References

1. Boijsen E (1970) Angiographic diagnosis of tumours arising from the pancreatic islets. Acta Radiol [Diagn] 10:161
2. Burcharth F, Stage JG, Stadil F, Jensen LJ, Fischermann K (1979) Localization of gastrinomas by transhepatic portal catheterization and gastrin assay. Gastroenterology 77:444
3. Doppmann JL, Brennan MF, Dunnick NR, Kahn CR, Gorden P (1981) The role of pancreatic venous sampling in the localization of occult insulinomas. Radiology 138:557
4. Günther RW, Klose KJ, Rückert K, Kuhn FP, Beyer J, Klotter HJ, Cordes U (1983) Islet-cell tu-

mors; detection of small lesions with computed tomography and ultrasound. Radiology 148:485

5. Hoevels J, Lunderquist A, Tylén U (1978) Percutaneous transhepatic portography. Acta Radiol [Diagn] 19:643
6. Korobkin MT, Palubinskas AJ, Glickman MG (1971) Pitfalls in arteriography of islet cell tumors of the pancreas. Radiology 100:319
7. McGavran MH, Unger RH, Recant L, Polk HC, Kilo C, Levin MF (1966) A glucagon-secreting alpha-cell carcinoma of the pancreas. N Engl J Med 274:1408
8. Olsson O (1963) Angiographic diagnosis of an islet cell tumour of the pancreas. Acta Chir Scand 126:346
9. Pasariello R, Feltrin GP, Miotto D, Pedrazzoli S, Rossi P, Simonetti G (1981) Transhepatic portal catheterization with pancreatic venous sampling versus angiography in the localization of pancreatic functioning tumours. European Journal of Radiology
10. Reichardt W, Cameron R (1980) Anatomy of the pancreatic veins. Acta Radiol [Diagn] 21:33
11. Reichardt W, Ingemannson S (1980) Selective vein catheterization for hormone assay in endocrine tumours of the pancreas. Acta Radiol [Diagn] 21:177
12. Roche A, Raisonnier A, Gillon-Savouret MC (1982) Pancreatic venous sampling and arteriography in localizing insulinomas and gastrinomas – procedure and results in 55 cases. Radiology 145:621
13. Stefanini P, Carboni M, Patrassi N, Basoli A (1974) Beta-islet cell tumors of the pancreas. Results of a study on 1067 cases. Surgery 75:597
14. Stark DD, Moss AA, Goldberg HI, Deveney CW (1984) CT of pancreatic islet cell tumors. Radiology 150:491

Hepatic Mass Lesions

A. R. Margulis and S. McCarthy

Since the introduction of roentgen rays, the identification of hepatic mass lesions have been one of the great challenges to diagnostic imaging. For many years, the diagnosis was based on the presence of calcification and/or displacement of the contrast-filled stomach, duodenum, and colonic hepatic flexure. Attempts to visualize the liver directly by introducing contrast media, such as Thorotrast, ended in failure. Later, this was followed by equally unsuccessful attempts at visualization by means of the intravenous injection of emulsified lipids.

Nuclear medicine techniques to visualize liver masses were introduced at approximately the same time as selective angiography. Tumors could be demonstrated either as relatively radiolucent defects within the contrast-opacified hepatic parenchyma or as causing abnormal angioarchitecture within the liver. The advent of ultrasound radically changed the imaging approach to liver masses since this was the first cross-sectional technique that directly viewed hepatic pathology. Recently, however, CT has become the method of choice due to its greater sensitivity and specificity than ultrasound or scintigraphy in the diagnosis of focal hepatic lesions [1]. Currently, magnetic resonance imaging (MRI) demonstrates great capability as a hepatic imaging modality [2, 3] and may eventually replace the preeminence of CT in cross-sectional imaging.

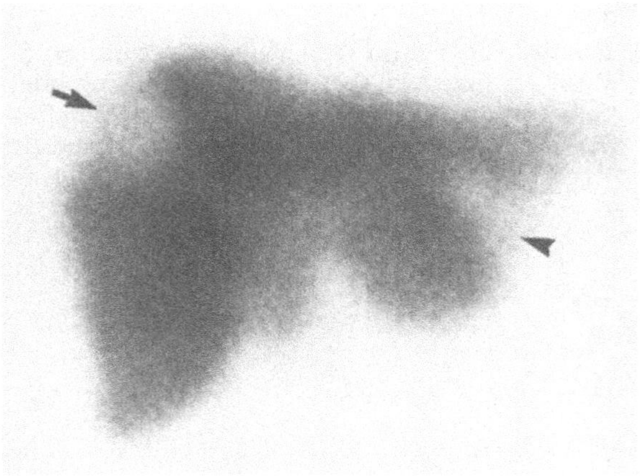

Fig. 1. Technetium-99m liver spleen scan demonstrates large metastasis (*arrow*) in right lobe; however, smaller peripheral metastasis in lateral segment of left lobe (*arrowhead*) could easily be missed

The Comparative Value of the Various Imaging Modalities

Nuclear Medicine

Scintigraphy is rarely used today as the sole technique for the detection of liver masses. The main reasons are as follows: (a) the spatial resolution is much lower than that of ultrasound, CT, or MRI; (b) intravenous radioactive contrast materials must be used; (c) the rate of false positives is too high, due to normal variants such as prominent porta hepatis, costal or renal impression; (d) the rate of false negatives is also high, caused by small (≤ 2 cm) or peripheral lesions (Fig. 1) [4]; (e) the full extent of disease cannot be determined, e.g., biliary dilatation, adenopathy; (f) the specificity is very low, i.e., tissue characterization of a photopenic defect is not possible.

Ultrasound

This modality has excellent spatial resolution, although the contrast resolution is less than that of CT or MRI. It is safe, inexpensive, fast, and portable. Thus, bedside needle-guided biopsy is possible. Since any plane of imaging is possible, particularly with real time, the location of a lesion can be depicted relative to hepatic blood vessels, thus delineating the involved hepatic segment(s) (Fig. 2). Disadvantages of the method are the following: (a) absence of a contrast medium to im-

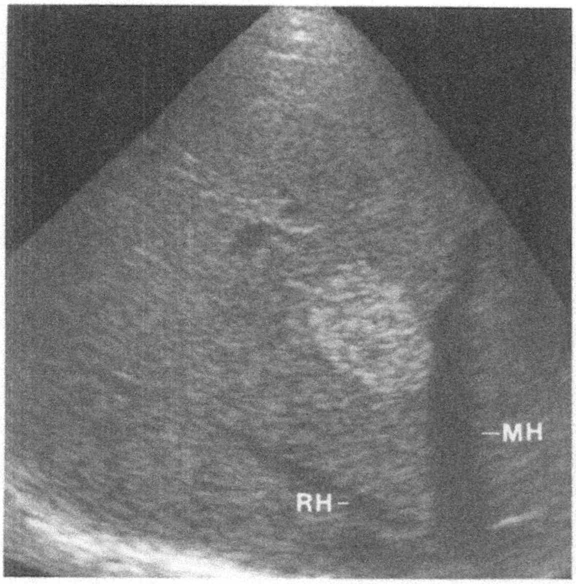

Fig. 2. Transverse sonogram revealing hemangioma in anterior segment of right lobe. *MH*, middle hepatic vein; *RH*, right hepatic vein

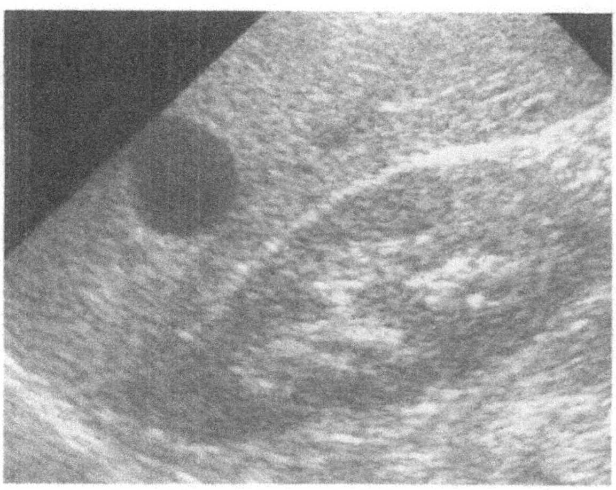

Fig. 3. Longitudinal sonogram through right lobe and kidney is diagnostic of a simple cyst, since there is acoustic enhancement and no internal structure or perceptible wall

prove contrast resolution, (b) significant operator dependence, and (c) large number of technically inadequate scans due to body habitus (e.g., high subcostal liver, obesity, bowel gas, and surgical incisions or tubes).

Nonetheless, sonography is very successful as a complementary tool to characterize a known lesion. Cystic masses detected by CT can be further classified according to their internal morphology. Benign cystic disease is recognizable with CT, but wall thickness, septations, and mural nodules are better appreciated by sonography (Fig. 3) [5]. Analogously, an isodense metastasis suspected on CT can be confirmed with ultrasound. Additionally, sonography can be used to find a cleavage plane between the right hepatic lobe and retroperitoneum, thus ascertaining the intrahepatic vs extrahepatic origin of a right upper quadrant mass [6].

Computed Tomography

CT is today the method of choice for the diagnosis of hepatic mass lesions [7]. Although relatively expensive, it is accurate and has a favorable signal-to-noise ratio, as well as excellent spatial and acceptable contrast resolution. When used with and without intraveneous contrast media, particularly bolus injection, lesion detectability is optimal [8, 9]. Although cysts and solid lesions are easily differentiated, abscesses have no characteristic appearance. The ability to reformat images in a variety of planes and determine relative tissue attenuation values increases the specificity of this method. Furthermore, CT-guided biopsy enables detection and diagnosis in one setting (Fig. 4). Extrahepatic involvement, and thus staging, is readily assessed with CT.

The main disadvantage of CT is the need for iodinated intravascular contrast media. Contrast is essential not only for detection of primary hepatocellular carcinomas and metastases but also for determination of extent of involvement (Fig. 5). Since it is unpredictable whether the lesion will be better seen with or without contrast media, both scans must be performed, aggravating time constraints and posing major problems in patients with contrast allergies or renal dysfunction. Furthermore, visualization of the hepatic vasculature to identify segmental anatomy, thrombosis, or a dilated biliary system necessitates that ample contrast be given in a very precisely timed fashion [10]. Another drawback of CT is the image degradation which occurs in patients with surgical hardware or a bowel containing barium.

Magnetic Resonance Imaging

The advantages of MRI are (a) superb contrast resolution, close to 80 times better than that of CT, with a spatial resolution that is only slightly

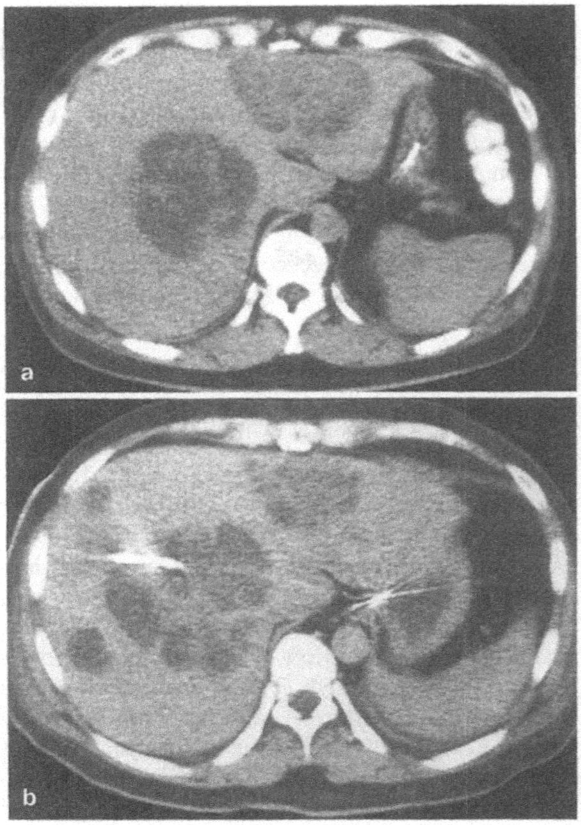

Fig. 4. a CT scan demonstrating two large lesions that could represent tumor or abscess. **b** Following CT-guided aspiration, which revealed abscess, a catheter was placed into larger lesion for drainage

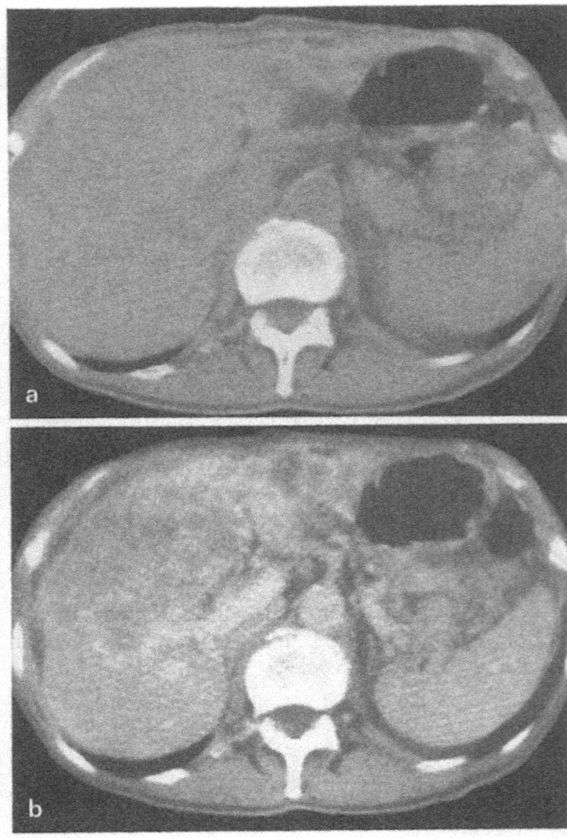

Fig. 5. a Noncontrast CT scan exhibits vague heterogenicity of left lobe. **b** Following intravenous contrast, hepatoma can be seen to involve both left and right lobes

worse; (b) the ability to image in any plane directly, without reformatting; (c) vascular involvement, i.e., thrombosis can be directly assessed due to the natural contrast of flowing blood (Fig. 6); (d) patient throughput is faster than for CT since it is possible to obtain multiple simultaneous slices with minimal gaps; and (e) freedom from clip or barium artifact (Fig. 7). Advantages unique to MRI are based on the fact that it utilizes not only one imaging parameter, such as the tissue-attenuation coefficient in CT, but is dependent on at least four:

1. Proton spin density (the amount of hydrogen protons in any location in the liver).
2. The tissue relaxation parameter, T1 (spin lattice), which depends on contributions from atoms other than protons that surround hydrogen in the liver tissue.
3. The T2 (spin-spin) parameter, which depends on the relative locations of protons and their influence on each other, hence resulting in loss of signal synchronicity.
4. Proton bulk motion, which contributes information about blood flow.

Thus, there are a multiplicity of techniques available for the acquisition and display of data. Both quantitative and qualitative information is available. At UCSF we use predominantly spin-echo techniques with variable recovery time (TR) and multiple echoes. Usually only two echoes are used with an echo delay (TE) of 28 and 56 ms. The other technique frequently used at UCSF is inversion recovery, in which the time of inversion (TI; time between the 180° and 90° pulses) can be adjusted according to the lesion examined (Fig. 8). MRI therefore has multiple advantages. Not only is it possible to visualize lesions in the liver with considerably improved contrast resolution, but it is also possible to locate them accurately in any plane, using the direct visualization of blood

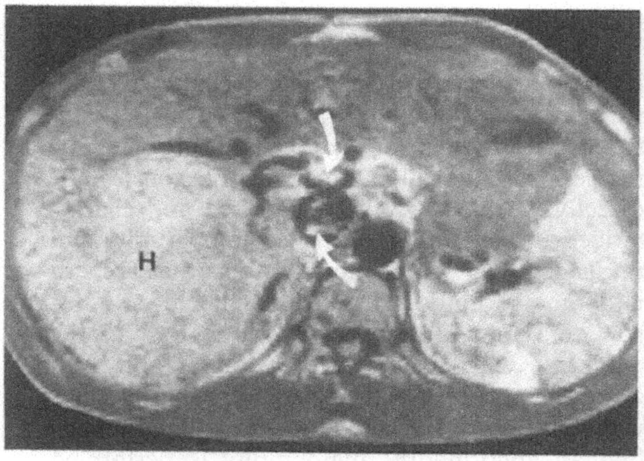

Fig. 6. MRI, spin-echo technique (TR 2.0 s, TE 28 ms) demonstrates a high-intensity hepatoma (*H*), in right lobe. Signal in inferior vena cava and portal vein (*arrows*) is representative of thrombosis

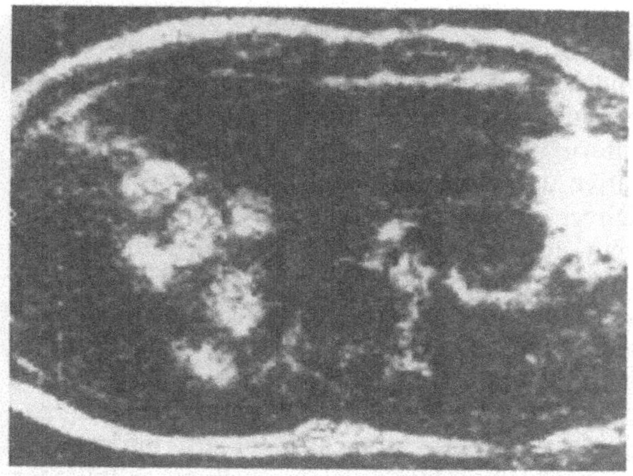

Fig. 8. MRI, inversion-recovery technique (TR 1.9 s, TE 56 ms, TI 210 ms) demonstrates high contrast between hepatic abscesses and parenchyma but a poor signal-to-noise ratio

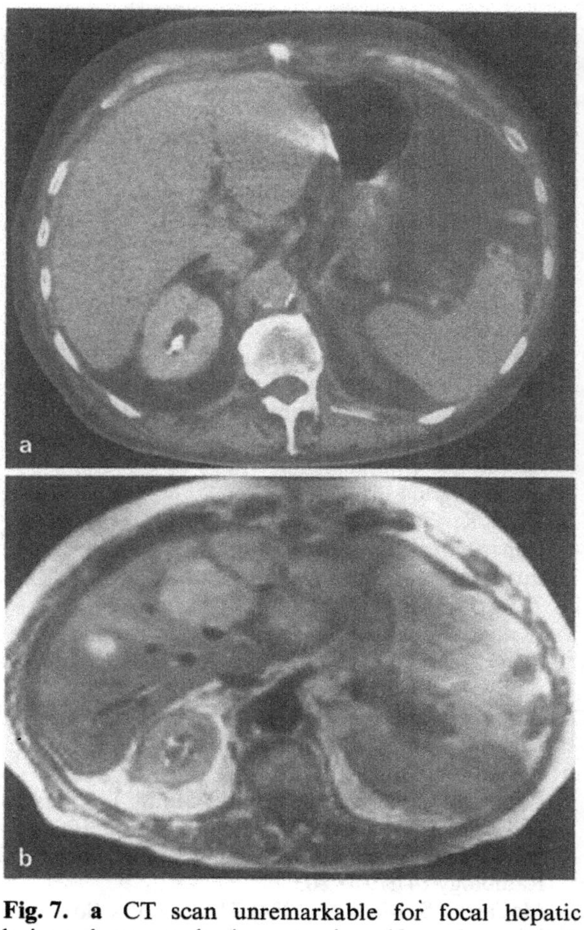

Fig. 7. **a** CT scan unremarkable for focal hepatic lesions; however, barium streak artifact obscures left lobe. **b** MRI, spin-echo technique (TE 2.0 s, TE 28 ms) reveals several carcinoid metastases

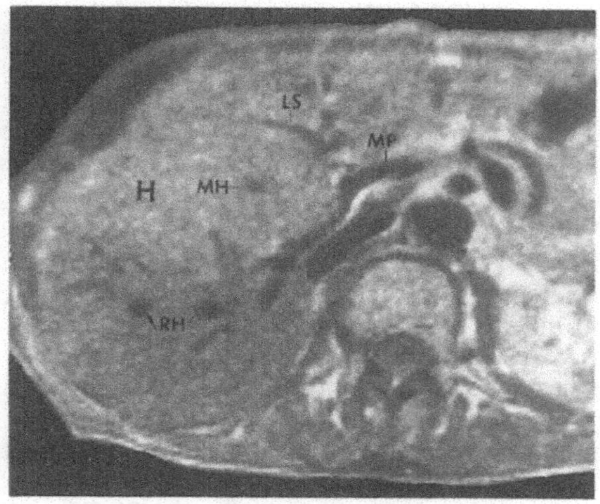

Fig. 9. MRI, spin-echo technique (TR 2.0 s, TE 28 ms) of same patient as in Fig. 4 shows that hepatoma (*H*) involves left lobe and anterior segment of right lobe. Middle hepatic vein (*MH*), which lies in interlobar fissure, is surrounded by tumor. *MP,* main portal vein; *LS,* lateral segmental branch of left portal vein; *RH,* right hepatic vein branches

vessels as anatomical orientation markers (Fig. 9). The examination can be performed fast, safely, and without using ionizing radiation, a particular advantage for the pediatric patient. Qualitative information such as biliary dilatation or quantitative data such as blood flow can be obtained. Direct noninvasive visualization of the portal vein, attenuated intrahepatic portal radicals, and varices permits the diagnosis of portal hypertension. Macroscopic areas of fibrosis, as in cholangiocarcinoma, can also be discerned. Furthermore, it is possible to ascertain the relative concentration of bile in the gallbladder in fasting patients, thus providing physiologic information about normal bile flow as well as gallbladder function.

The disadvantages of the method are: (1) it is expensive; (2) it is difficult to examine patients on life support systems; (3) respiratory gating is necessary in patients that breath rapidly, thus lengthening imaging time; (4) the spatial resolution of MRI is still inferior to that of the best CT devices, such as the General Electric 9800 or the latest Siemens or Picker systems; and (5) calcifications are not well seen, thus limiting the ability to differentially diagnose such entities as echinococcal cysts, embryonal hepatomas, and/or adenomas.

A potential advantage, but currently also a serious drawback, is the availability of a multiplicity of techniques to gather and display data. It is thus possible to miss lesions if the wrong technique is used. Partial-saturation or spin-echo techniques with short TRs have in the past led to obscuration of liver lesions. The advantage of multiple techniques, however, is that it is possible to design an individualized approach that enhances specificity. As long as the proton spin density, T1, T2, and proton motion are different between lesion and normal tissue, the lesion should be demonstrable by MRI. With the use of contrast media like chelated gadolinium or monoclonal antibodies with chelated metals, most techniques will be capable of demonstrating lesions as the margin of error in specificity and sensitivity is narrowed. Such contrast materials are currently being investigated in Europe and are soon to be evaluated in several centers in the United States, including UCSF. It is very likely, however, that even without contrast media, computed artificial intelligence will be developed for MRI, thus enabling the computer to select the appropriate technique once the pertinent clinical data are introduced.

Conclusion

In the past decade, tremendous technological advances in cross-sectional imaging have produced several techniques for the evaluation of hepatic masses. Both benign and malignant lesions can be directly, yet noninvasively, detected and characterized by MRI. Computerized tomography and ultrasound are complementary tools that are still undergoing rapid instrumental changes. Radionuclide scintigraphy has waned as a screening modality, whereas the role of angiography has changed from purely diagnostic to primarily interventional. Once the above methods have identified an abnormality, angiography is performed therapeutically via catheter placement for drainage, chemotherapy, and/or embolization.

References

1. Alderson P, Adams D, McNeil B, Sanders R, Siegelman S, Finberg H, Hessel S, Abrams H (1983) Computed tomography, ultrasound and scintigraphy of the liver in patients with colon or breast carcinoma: a prospective comparison. Radiology 149:225–230
2. Moss AA, Goldberg HI, Stark D et al. (1984) Hepatic tumors: magnetic resonance and CT appearance. Radiology 150:141–147
3. Doyle F, Pennock J, Banks L et al. (1982) Nuclear magnetic resonance imaging of the liver: initial experience. AJR 138:193–200
4. Knopf D, Torres W, Fajman W, Sones P (1982) Liver lesions: comparative accuracy of scintigraphy and computed tomography. AJR 138:623–627
5. Federle M, Filly R, Moss A (1981) Cystic hepatic neoplasms: complementary roles of CT and sonography. AJR 136:345–348
6. Gore K, Callen P, Filly R (1982) Displaced retroperitoneal fat: sonographic guide to right upper quadrant mass localization. Radiology 142:701–705
7. Berland K (1984) Screening for diffuse and focal liver disease: the case for hepatic computed tomography. J Clin Ultrasound 12:83–89
8. Berland L, Lawson T, Foley W et al. (1982) A comparison of pre- and post-contrast CT in hepatic masses. AJR 138:853–858
9. Foley W, Berland L, Lawson T, Smith T, Thorson M (1983) Contrast enhancement technique for dynamic hepatic computed tomographic scanning. Radiology 147:797–803
10. McCarthy S, Moss A (1984) The use of a flow rate injector for contrast enhanced computed tomography. Radiology 151:800

Dynamic Liver CT and New Contrast Agents *

M. Kormano, K. Partanen, and J. Kuikka

Introduction

The technique of performing rapid sequential CT scans after a bolus of contrast medium (CM) is commonly called dynamic CT scanning. The ability of dynamic CT to produce images at the time of maximal contrast enhancement (CE), which occurs at varying times in the normal liver, in hepatic lesions, and in adjoining organs, has brought an improvement in imaging and diagnosis of localized liver lesions as reported by several authors [1, 4, 5, 14, 15, 16, 21, 22, 23]. Intra-arterial injection of CM would improve the diagnostic ability of dynamic liver CT [16], but for practical reasons intravenous injections are the common method in dynamic CT.

While the size of the liver makes it easily accessible for dynamic CT studies and partial volume effects are readily avoided, several other factors limit the usefulness of dynamic CT in liver disease:

1. Peak aortic CE, is attained 10–30 s after the beginning of intravenous bolus injection, depending on the patient's circulation time [12]. Peak liver CE occurs 20–40 s after peak CE of the aorta, because of the portal venous component of the hepatic circulation. Proper timing of the dynamic CT series therefore involves a certain amount of guesswork, unless rapid sequence series lasting over a minute are used. Both the ascending and the descending part of the CE curve should be available.
2. Patients are not able to hold their breath for the whole duration of the dynamic series. This produces a problem of scan slice registration and motion artifacts. Differences in slice registration produce inconsistency in both visual and curve-fitting analysis of localized lesions. The volume of liver which is consistently free of artifacts throughout the study is limited anteriorly by the streak artifact produced by the moving air fluid level of the stomach [20] and superiorly by the moving interface of the diaphragm and the right lung. Good dynamic CE vs time curves are rarely obtained in the left lobe of the liver or in the liver tissue immediately beneath the dome of the diaphragm.
3. The present dynamic studies are restricted to one slice level per scan and a dynamic study is meaningful only after identification of a localized lesion or in diffuse liver disease.

Diagnostic Potential of Dynamic CT in Liver Disease

The interest in the clinical use of dynamic CT scanning of the liver has been focused on localized liver lesions. Careful analysis of the time-density curves of such lesions can demonstrate the predominantly arterial blood supply of most hepatic lesions [9, 16]. Dynamic series also effectively demonstrate variations of the vascularization of the hepatic lesion which may result in various patterns [11]. The only lesion which can enhance characteristically enough to provide histologic diagnosis is cavernous hemangioma of the liver [3, 7, 10]. No consistent difference in the pattern of CE has been found between other hepatic lesions. Multiple lesions of similar pathology may present a spectrum of CE patterns [16].

Diffuse liver diseases present more suitable anatomic conditions for dynamic CT, since minor inaccuracy in slice registration may not be as critical as in localized lesions. Despite the more favorable anatomic prerequisites, only few authors have described the time-density curves of a normal liver after intravenous bolus injection of CM, and only few remarks in the literature are found on the changes of time-density curves of the liver

* The financial support of the Sigrid Jusélius Foundation, Helsinki and the Finnish Academy is gratefully acknowledged

and spleen in portal hypertension and liver cirrhosis [8, 18]. The normal CE curve of the liver consists of the arterial component and a later portal venous component. The sum of these attains maximum value about 20–40 s after the aortic peak CE. The maximum CE of the spleen, an important reference in the evaluation of the liver disease, occurs 10–20 s after the aortic peak CE. The mean peak CE of the liver is approximately 30 HU lower than that of the spleen. The downward slope of the hepatic and splenic time-density curves consists of two components, the fast disposition phase with T½ of about 20 s and a slow one with T½ of about 300–400 s [18]. The fast disposition phase consists of the extravascular diffusion of CM, while the slow one appears to be dominated by the renal excretion of CM.

In liver cirrhosis the peak CE of both liver and spleen are delayed and lower than in the normal patient, and the fast disposition phase is longer [18]. With a more advanced mathematical analysis of the dynamic CE curves of the liver and spleen, the mean transit time can be calculated from the deconvolved impulse-response curves [13]. The mean transit time of the liver in cirrhosis is significantly longer (0.75 ± 0.12 min) than in controls (0.63 ± 0.1 min). Computer analysis of the dynamic CT curves can be extended to the estimation of liver blood flow, which was lower in cirrhotic patients (0.50 ± 0.16 ml/min/g) than in the controls (0.76 ± 0.25 ml/min/g) [13]. With this approximation an error is introduced in the flow values, as the diffusion of the CM to the extravascular space is not instantaneous and the combined arterial/portal system disturbs the descending part of the impulse response curve of the CE. Although the blood flow estimates will be inherently too low, both the mean transit time and liver blood flow, as calculated from the deconvolved impulse response curves, are reproducible and suitable for diagnostic purposes, as also suggested by Axel et al. [2]. Dynamic CT may even provide a new method of estimating organ blood flow.

New Contrast Media in Dynamic CT

The radiologic contrast obtained in clinical intravenous use of different CM is difficult to evaluate quantitatively. There is experimental [6] and clinical [12] evidence that the early pharmacokinetics of different ionic and nonionic CM differ to some extent. In rat experiments, the liver uptake of metrizamide, with relatively low hydrophilicity,

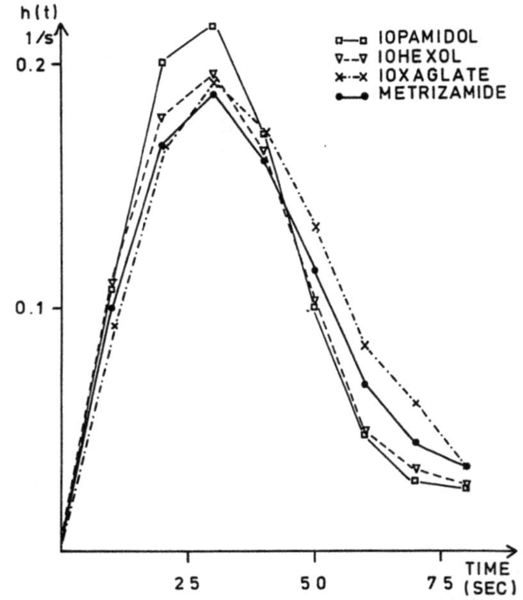

Fig. 1. Means of the deconvolved impulse-response curves [$h(t)$] of liver CE after administration of four new CM, calculated from dynamic CT scans

was markedly higher than of the more hydrophilic iohexol [6]. In clinical dynamic CT, hydrophilic/lipophilic properties did not have any significant bearing on the CE of the liver [19]. Iopamidol resulted in somewhat higher peak CE of the aorta, liver, and spleen than did ioxaglate, ioxitalamate, diatrizoate, metrizamide, and iohexol [12, 19].

The mathematical modelling of time-density curves as described by Kuikka and Partanen [13] also gives some insight into the clinical pharmacokinetic properties of different CM. The impulse-response curves resulting from equal doses of different new CM (Fig. 1) shows that the transfer function [h (t)] in the liver does not differ much from one CM to another. Table 1 presents calculated mean liver transit times and liver blood flows for patients studied similarly using different CM. The iohexol and metrizamide groups are large and homogeneous enough to allow conclusions to be made. From this data it appears that iohexol, a more hydrophilic agent, diffuses more readily than metrizamide into the extravascular space of the liver. Minor differences between CM such as those shown in Table 1 should, however, be evaluated with caution, as they may represent interindividual variation, differences in the tissue-blood partition coefficient, or even different effects of CM on intra-organ blood flow. The last-named can be suspected from the different metabolic effects of different CM [17].

Table 1. Mean transit times and liver blood flows as calculated from dynamic liver CT of normal patients using different contrast media

Contrast medium	Number of patients	Mean transit time (s)	Liver blood flow (ml/min/g)
Iohexol	18	39± 9	0.88±0.22
Iopamidol	9	37± 5	0.92±0.23
Metrizamide	14	43±12	0.81±0.23
Ioxaglate	7	40± 9	0.85±0.26
Diatrizoate	14	37± 5	0.84±0.38
Ioxitalamate	9	41± 8	0.70±0.10

Summary

Dynamic CT of the liver can improve the detectability of localized liver lesions. The specificity of contrast enhancement curves of such lesions is poor and visual patterns are nondiagnostic, except for a few entities like cavernous hemangioma. In diffuse liver diseases, computer analysis of time-density curves is promising and may provide new physiologic information not available to the naked eye, e.g., mean transit time and tissue blood flow. Characteristic changes in these parameters have been found in liver cirrhosis. New contrast media provide little help in improving the diagnostic potential of dynamic CT of the liver. Computer analysis of contrast enhancement curves of the liver shows only slight, clinically insignificant differences between different ionic and nonionic contrast media.

References

1. Araki T, Itai Y, Furni S, Tasaka A (1980) Dynamic CT densitometry of hepatic tumors. AJR 135:1037–1043
2. Axel L, Dean PB, Moss AA, Stansberry D (1984) Functional imaging of the liver. New information from dynamic CT. Invest Radiol 19:23–29
3. Barnett PH, Zerhouni EA, White RI Jr, Siegelman SS (1980) Computed tomography in the diagnosis of cavernous hemangioma of the liver. AJR 134: 439–447
4. Burgener FA, Hamlin DJ (1983) Contrast enhancement of hepatic tumors in CT: comparison between bolus and infusion techniques. AJR 140:291–295
5. Burgener FA, Hamlin DJ (1983) Contrast enhancement of focal lesions in CT: effect of size and histology. AJR 140:297–301
6. Dean PB, Kivisaari L, Kormano M (1983) Contrast enhancement pharmacokinetics of six ionic and nonionic contrast media. Invest Radiol 18:368–374
7. Hartel M (1980) Das kavernöse Leberhämangiom im Computertomogramm. ROFO 133:379–381
8. Hübener K-H, Klott KJ (1980) „Statisches" und dynamisches Kontrastmittelenhancement der Körperstamm-Computertomographie. ROFO 133:347–354
9. Hübener K-H, Kurtz B (1984) Sequentielle Computertomographie bei fokalen und diffusen Lebererkrankungen. Paper presented at congress on computed tomography, May 23–25, East Berlin
10. Itai Y, Furvi S, Araki T, Yashiro N, Tasaka A (1980) Computed tomography of cavernous hemangioma of the liver. Radiology 137:149–155
11. Kormano M (1981) Kinetics of contrast media after bolus injection and infusion. In: Felix R, Kazner E, Wegener OH (eds) Contrast media in computed tomography. Excerpta Medica International Congress Series 561, pp 38–45
12. Kormano M, Partanen K, Soimakallio S, Kivimäki T (1983) Dynamic contrast enhancement of the upper abdomen: effect of contrast medium and body weight. Invest Radiol 18:364–367
13. Kuikka J, Partanen K (1984) Mathematical modelling of time-density curves. The application to the diagnosis of liver cirrhosis. Invest Radiol (submitted)
14. Kunstlinger F, Federle MP, Moss AA, Marks W (1980) Computed tomography of hepatocellular carcinoma. AJR 134:431–437
15. Marchal GJ, Baert AL, Wilms GE (1980) CT of noncystic liver lesions: bolus enhancement. AJR 135:57–65
16. Moss AA, Dean PB, Axel L, Goldberg HI, Glazer GM, Friedman MA (1982) Dynamic CT of hepatic masses with intravenous and intra-arterial contrast material. AJR 138:847–852
17. Paajanen H, Uotila P, Kormano M (1983) Different effect of diatrizoate and iopamidol on prostaglandin synthesis in perfused hamster lungs. Invest Radiol 18:375–381
18. Partanen KPL (1984) Dynamic CT of liver cirrhosis. Invest Radiol (in press)
19. Partanen KPL, Kormano M, Kivimäki T, Soimakallio S (1984) Comparison of iohexol and metrizamide in dynamic CT of the upper abdomen. Eur J Radiol (in press)
20. Partanen KPL, Kormano M (1984) Streak artifacts in dynamic CT. A phantom study of anterior upper abdomen. Acta Radiol (in press)
21. Tala S, Fukuda K, Aoyagi Y, Harada J (1980) CT of abdominal malignancies: dynamic approach. AJR 135:455–461
22. Tschakert H (1980) Zeitlicher Ablauf des Dichteverhaltens von Lebermetastasen nach Kontrastmittelgabe. ROFO 133:171–176
23. Young SW, Turner RJ, Castellino RA (1980) A strategy for the contrast enhancement of malignant tumors using dynamic computed tomography and intravascular pharmacokinetics. Radiology 137: 137–147

Gallbladder Diseases: Imaging Sequences

W. Frommhold and J. Pirschel

Introduction

At the first Radiology Today symposium in June 1980, I stated that radiologic diagnostics of the biliary tract system provides a classic example of an unexpected dynamic advancement in the field of diagnostic radiology which has been decisively influenced by the technical development of new imaging modalities. I would like now to make a few basic comments which, in my opinion, should not be left out of any discussion about the rational sequence of diagnostic radiologic methods. We must call for honesty in establishing indications, particularly when complicated and sophisticated diagnostic procedures are involved, and we must be courageous enough to review them and, if necessary, to call them into question. The guiding principle should be to use any method that ensures fast, reliable, accurate, complication-free diagnosis so that effective therapy can be started as early as possible [8].

Today, ultrasound investigation is unquestionably of paramount importance in the diagnosis of gallbladder and biliary tract diseases, having surpassed oral and particularly intravenous cholegraphy, the previously leading method for diagnosing diseases of the right upper abdomen. The performance of oral and intravenous cholecystangiography is currently justified in only a few, very special cases. Sonography is of outstanding importance particularly in the diagnosis of gallstones, cholecystitis, empyema of the gallbladder, and differential diagnosis of jaundice. It is rationally supplemented by CT, also a noninvasive method, in patients with biliary tract obstruction.

Functional bile flow phenomena are detectable with nuclear medical techniques, which, by the way, also provide essential morphologic information on basic changes. Direct and morphologically exact demonstration of pathologic changes in the biliary tract is provided only by endoscopic retrograde cholangiography (ERC) and percutaneous transhepatic cholangiography (PTC), both of which are invasive methods. PTC, offering the possibility of percutaneous transhepatic biliary drainage, has crossed the line separating diagnostic from therapeutic radiology.

There is good reason to expect that endoscopic sonography, one of the newest methods, will provide additional information on the cause of biliary tract obstruction. Preliminary experience with intraoperative sonography has shown it to be superior to intraoperative cholangiography for the detection of gallstones in the major biliary ducts. Intraoperative sonography therefore is well on its way to becoming an alternative method to intraoperative cholangiography [22, 29]. Ultrasound examination is the first diagnostic method for diseases of the gallbladder and biliary tract after the clinical examination. Its many indications include the following three important disease complexes.

Cholelithiasis and Cholangiolithiasis

Sonography is unquestionably the diagnostic method of choice for *gallstones.* In the hands of an experienced examiner, it is extremely accurate, with a specificity and sensitivity as high as 99% [30]. False-negative findings are possible with smaller stones for the real-time units routinely used today; the lower limit of detection for stones in an echo-free gallbladder lumen should be set at 2 mm. The infrequent false-positive findings are caused by misinterpretation of acoustic shadows behind gas-filled, topographically adjacent organs such as the transverse colon and particularly, in the case of suspected stones near the papilla, the duodenal bulb [25]. Obviously, the chemical composition of the stones cannot be determined with sonography [7, 9, 33]. The stones with the lowest acoustic impedance, namely bilirubin stones, are less apt to cast acoustic shadows [7]; cholesterol stones, however, cannot be definitively identified. Oral cholecystography unquestionably

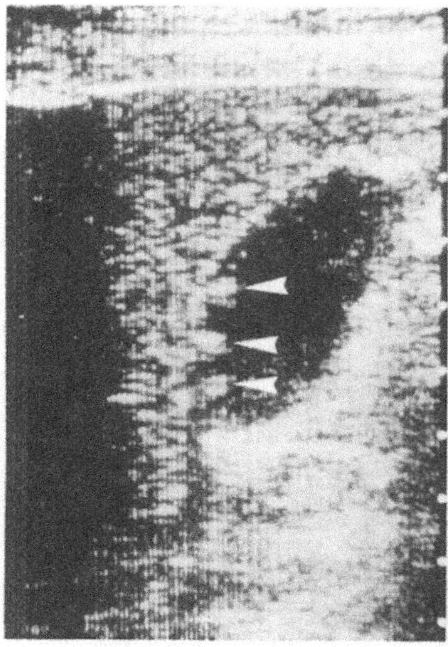

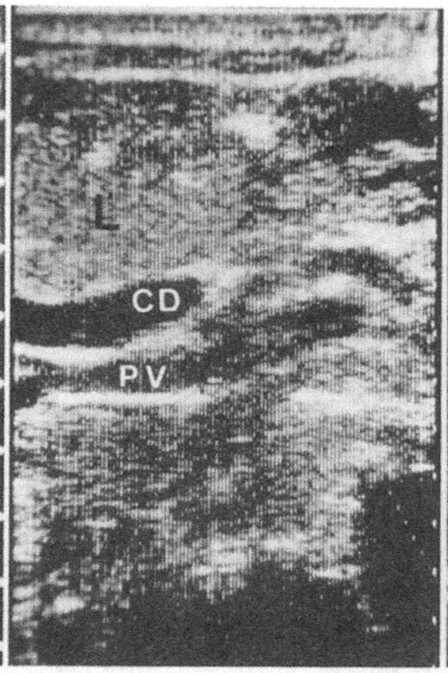

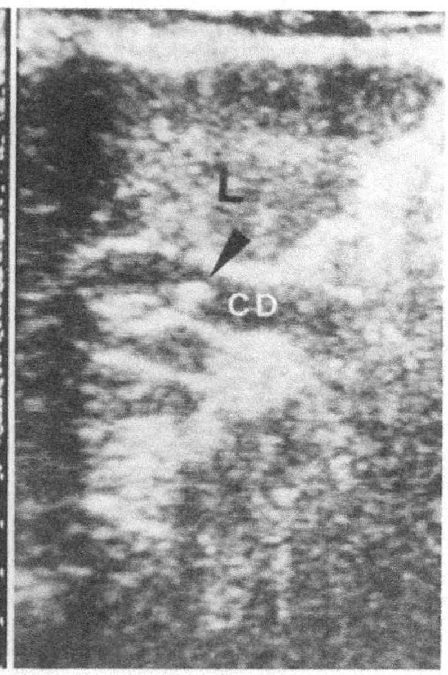

Fig. 1 (*Left*). Cholesterosis of the gallbladder. The *arrowheads* show cholesterol polyps adherent to the gallbladder wall

Fig. 2 (*Middle*). Shotgun phenomenon: sign of intrahepatic stasis. *L*, liver; *CD*, dilated choledochal duct; *PV*, portal vein

Fig. 3 (*Right*). Choledocholithiasis. The *arrowhead* indicates a small concrement in the choledochal duct (*CD*), floating in bile fluid. *L*, liver. Note the acoustic shadow behind the small stone

retains its importance in the selection of patients for drug litholysis, which, by the way, is successful only with non-calcium-containing stones in a gallbladder with preserved contractility [33]. Thus, for example, pure, young "floating" cholesterol stones in patients with no signs of calcium incrustation on plain films of the gallbladder region respond to litholysis only when the fundus too is free of sedimented calcium-containing concrements [33, 34]. On the other hand, it should not be forgotten that 10%−15% of the calcifications escape detection with conventional radiographic techniques [9]. As potential crystallizing material [33], they are apparently the reason for both the failure of chemical litholysis and the differing frequencies of stone recurrence [9, 34].

The contractility of the gallbladder necessary for litholysis can, of course, be tested by sonography before and after a "stimulating meal" or the injection of substances similar to cholecystokinin [2, 26]. In this context, it should be noted that cholesterosis is equally well diagnosed with sonography or conventional procedures (Fig. 1) [12]; circumscribed or generalized intramural diverticulosis (adenomyomatosis), however, is more often detected with oral cholegraphy after a stimulating meal [12, 24].

The differential diagnosis of a shrunken or stone-filled gallbladder with sonography can present problems; the accuracy of the method drops to between 75% and 85% [25]. The absent delineation of the normally fluid-filled gallbladder complicates identification of the organ and of circumscribed mural changes. In extreme cases, the curved surface reflex with dorsal acoustic shadows in a stone-filled gallbladder can even be confused with a gas-filled bowel loop.

A plain film of the right upper abdomen is always a valuable supplement in patients with inconclusive sonographic findings. It can be used to differentiate calcium-containing stones and limy bile from calcium-containing incrustations in the gallbladder wall (porcelain gallbladder) and from intrahepatic calcium calcifications of various etiologies, the definitive origin of which is, however, difficult to determine with sonography [20].

Sonography has become extremely important for the differentiation of *cholangiolithiasis or choledocholithiasis* with biliary tract obstruction from nonobstructive jaundice, its accuracy being almost 100% [16, 18, 20]. Diagnostically relevant in this context is the identification or exclusion of the so-called shotgun phenomenon [3]. This sign of intrahepatic stasis of the biliary tract, together

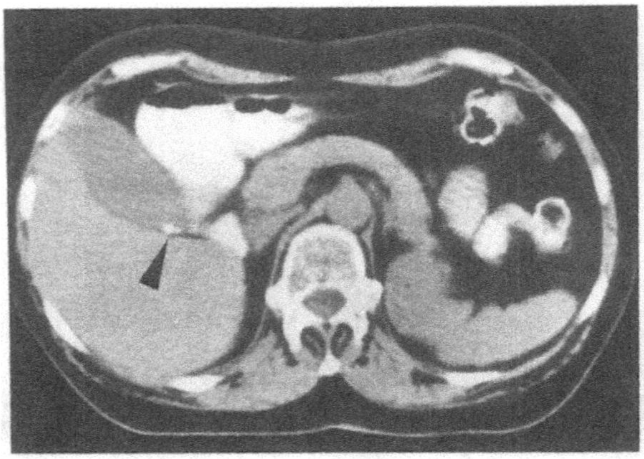

Fig. 4. Hydrops of the gallbladder in a patient with acute cholecystitis. The *arrowhead* shows occlusion of the cystic duct by a small concrement

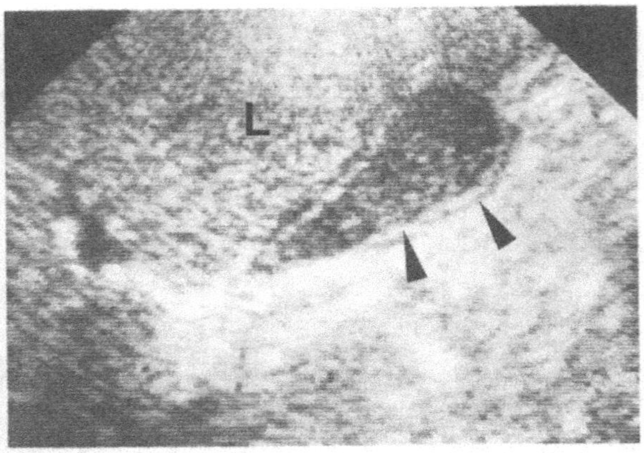

Fig. 5. Acute cholecystitis. Note the small perivesical exudate (*arrowheads*). *L*, liver

with the identification of a choledochal duct dilated to a caliber of at least 6 mm, serves as a criterion of peripheral mechanical obstruction (Fig. 2). Primary determination of the exact etiology of the obstruction with sonography, however, is successful in only approximately 60% of cases [6, 31]. Physically, bile duct stones are comparable with stones in the gallbladder; their identifiability, however, is improved by the surrounding bile. Because of the absent acoustic shadows and the minor difference in impedance against the surroundings, visualization of small bile duct stones is considerably more difficult when they are not floating in bile (Fig. 3).

Acute and Chronic Cholecystitis

Choledocholithiasis with or without jaundice, a complication of lithiasis, is a far less common clinical occurrence than cholecystitis. Stones are identifiable in 90%–95% of patients suffering from cholecystitis [17, 30]; other causes of the inflammation are found in only 5% [28].

The *acute* symptoms of cholecystitis are triggered by occlusion of the cystic duct, which, with rare exceptions, is caused by a stone. The aim of each investigation should therefore be the demonstration of this occlusion (Fig. 4). Initial hydrops of the gallbladder is of course unmistakable on the ultrasound scan [14, 20], and when the typical clinical signs are present, it presents no problems for the differential diagnosis. The initially edematous thickening of the gallbladder wall, eventually involving the entire organ equally and sometimes amounting to as much as 8 mm [4, 23], with or without concurrent detection of stones, is a typical sonographic sign [1, 17, 30], particularly when exudate in the form of a narrow perivesical band of fluid is also identifiable (Fig. 5) [1, 11].

The specificity of nuclear medical assessment of bile flow with ^{99m}Tc-labeled hepatobiliary test substances (iminodiacetic compounds, IDA derivatives), a highly specific technique for clarifying acute right upper abdominal symptoms in general, is virtually 100%, with less than 1% false-positive findings and less than 4% false-negative findings [15, 32]. In patients with free activity flow over the choledochal duct into the duodenum, no activity enrichment is detectable in the gallbladder 1 h after intravenous injection of radionuclides. Although in rare cases absence of activity uptake in the gallbladder can be due to other causes, such as alcoholism [27], this technique – as always in correlation with the clinical picture – provides extremely valuable diagnostic information. In comparison with these noninvasive diagnostic techniques, oral and particularly intravenous visualization of cystic duct occlusion in the form of the "excluded gallbladder" has totally lost its diagnostic significance.

The incidence of *chronic or chronic-recurrent cholecystitis* is far higher than that of acute cholecystitis. The inflammation-induced thickening of the gallbladder wall is, of course, easily identifiable with sonography [1, 17, 30]. Gallbladder contractility after a stimulating meal does not exclude the possibility of chronic-inflammatory mural processes, and conversely, absence of contraction does not necessarily indicate cholecystitis. Such gallbladder wall thickening is not an infrequent occurrence, and is often a secondary

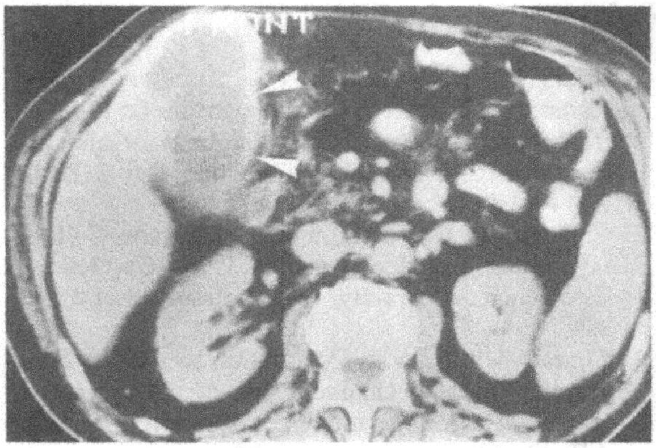

Fig. 6. Thickening of the gallbladder wall (*arrowheads*) caused by chronic recurrent cholecystitis

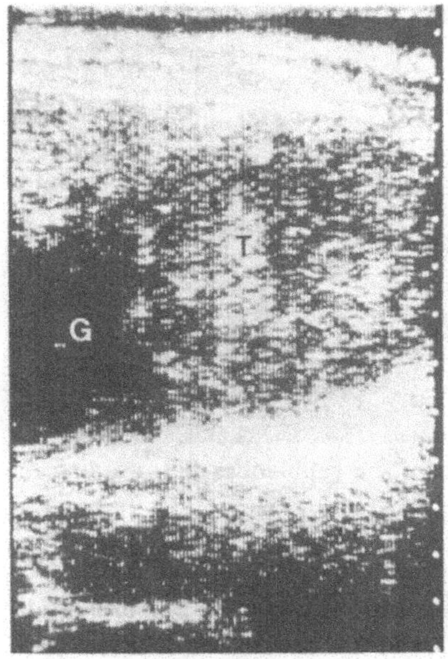

Fig. 7. Carcinoma of the gallbladder fundus. *G*, bile; *T*, tumor

finding on CT scans of the abdominal cavity made for a totally different indication (Fig. 6). We should, however, guard against the temptation of considering this expensive technique a necessary primary diagnostic investigation for every patient with suspected biliary tract disease. On the other hand, the differential diagnosis of a *shrunken gallbladder*, with its considerably thickened wall and stone-filled residual lumen does present certain problems for sonography [25].

CT is a reliable diagnostic procedure that provides additional valuable information, and is indicated in every patient with suspected tumor disease [13, 20]. Nuclear medical investigation plays no leading role in the preoperative phase of chronic cholecystitis.

Differential Diagnosis of Jaundice

In obstructive jaundice, the serum bilirubin level is always elevated, often considerably. Attempting oral or intravenous cholangiography is futile when the serum bilirubin level exceeds 4.0 mg/100 ml. The diagnostic advantages of CT are as evident with these patients as with extremely adipose patients and patients in whom diagnostic ultrasound is impossible because of overlying air in the bowel loops. This applies predominantly to assessment of the distal choledochal duct, which passes behind the duodenum and therefore cannot be definitively evaluated in approximately 20% of the cases.

This is diagnostically significant in patients with suspected secondary cholangitis of the terminal choledochal segment, the so-called papillary stenosis. When it appears as "postcholecystectomy syndrome", it can present considerable problems in differential diagnosis, particularly since it usually only leads to a moderate dilatation of the common bile duct. In cases of choledochal stenosis with prestenotic dilatation and cholestasis, one must always consider carcinoma of the gallbladder (Fig. 7), and in cases of a low-seated occlusion, papillary carcinoma of the head of the pancreas.

Exact clarification of the symptoms is also not always possible with CT; additional information is provided only when tumor invasion can be detected in adjacent tissue (Fig. 8).

Nevertheless, most seriously ill patients can still be spared unnecessary invasive diagnostic procedures [20].

If an invasive tumor cannot be detected in a patient with mechanical jaundice, the localization and cause of the stenosis must be clarified by ERC or PTC [5, 10, 19, 21], both of which are invasive procedures. Whereas the accuracy of ERC depends only on the experience and skill of the examiner, and exact diagnosis is possible in approximately 90% of the cases, the success rate for PTC is decisively influenced by the degree of biliary tract dilatation. In punctures of only slightly dilated intrahepatic bile ducts, its accuracy is of course considerably lower. It is therefore clear that ERC is the method of choice in patients with a well-founded suspicion of stone occlusion, since

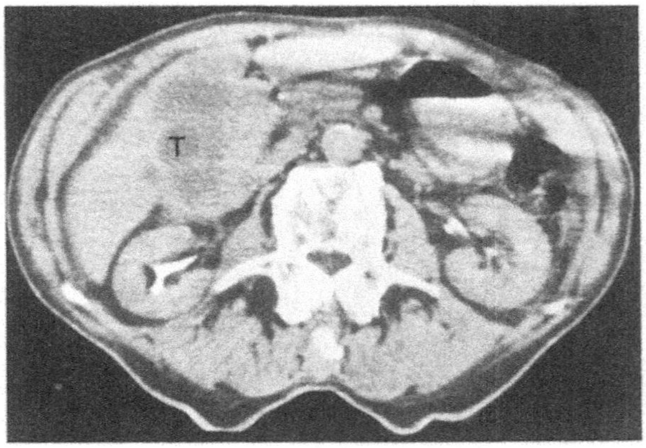

Fig. 8. Carcinoma of the gallbladder (*T*) invading the liver parenchyma

endoscopic sphincterotomy can be performed directly thereafter should stones be detected [20]. PTC is the method of choice in the case of suspected tumor obstruction because of the possibility of temporary or permanent external biliary drainage or internal catheterization [18, 29, 20]. Opinions differ as to whether lowering serum bilirubin by preoperative drainage actually simplifies surgery and minimizes postoperative complications. Many experienced surgeons still prefer immediate surgery when preliminary studies tend to indicate operability.

Summary

These three examples from the wide range of biliary diseases are characteristic, and the advice given can be applied to almost all hepatobiliary symptoms. It should be born in mind that sonography is already unparalleled in the diagnosis of biliary tract diseases and will become even more important in the future. CT should be considered a supplementary method which provides valuable diagnostic information in patients with unclarified symptoms suggesting a tumorous process, but it should never be used as a primary screening procedure. CT does, of course, take precedence over the invasive methods of ERC and PTC. Oral and particulary intravenous cholecystangiography should be limited to certain special diagnostic problems.

References

1. Brizzi F, Pozzi-Marcelli RS, Rizzatto G, Maffessanti M, Bazzocchi M, Dalla Palma L (1982) Ultrasonographic aspects of inflammatory and neoplastic diseases of the gallbladder. Eur J Radiol 2:214–220
2. Colosimo C Jr, Vecchioli A, Colagrande C (1983) Hyperplastic cholecystosis: study by Ceruletid-assisted cholecystography. Gastrointest Radiol 8:255–259
3. Conrad MR, Landay MJ, Janes JO (1978) Sonographic "parallel channel" sign of biliary tree enlargement in mild to moderate obstructive jaundice. AJR 130:279
4. Croce F, Montali G, Solbiati L, Marinoni G (1981) Ultrasonography in acute cholecystitis. Br J Radiol 54:927–931
5. Cruz FO, Barriga P, Tocornal J, Burhenne HJ (1983) Radiology of the Mirizzi syndrome: diagnostic importance of the transhepatic cholangiogram. Gastrointest Radiol 8:249–253
6. Dewbury KC, Joseph AEA, Hayes S, Murray C (1979) Ultrasound in the evaluation and diagnosis of jaundice. Br J Radiol 52:276
7. Frentzel-Beyme B, Fähndrich R, Arnan-Thiele B (1983) Kann die Sonographie Hinweise auf die chemische Zusammensetzung von Gallensteinen geben? Fortschr Röntgenstr 138:458–463
8. Frommhold W, Wolf F (1983) Clinics in gastroenterology, vol 12, no 1. Radiological and radionuclide methods for the diagnosis of biliary disorders. Saunders, London, pp 65–100
9. Gladisch R, Deininger HK (1983) Die Darstellung von Gallensteinen im Sonogramm und Radiogramm. Fortschr Röntgenstr 139:249–255
10. Gold RP, Casarella WJ, Stern G, Seaman B (1979) Transhepatic cholangiography: the radiological method of choice in suspected obstructive jaundice. Radiology 133:39–44
11. Hutton L, Lamki N, Rankin R (1982) Halo around the gallbladder: a prognostic sign? J Can Assoc Radiol 33:80–83
12. Jenett M, Dohrmann E (1984) Adenomyomatose und Cholesterinpolypen der Gallenblase. Vergleich radiologischer und sonographischer Diagnostik. Fortschr Röntgenstr 140:524–531
13. van Kaick G, König R (1982) Der Beitrag der Computertomographie zur Diagnostik von Erkrankungen der Gallenblase und der Gallenwege. Therapiewoche 32:2782–2788
14. Karp W, Herlin P, Holmin T, Owman T (1979) Infusion tomography and ultrasonography of the gallbladder in the diagnosis of acute cholecystitis. Gastrointest Radiol 4:253–261
15. Kempken K, Nitz DW, Pabst HW, Wolf F (1982) Nuklearmedizin, Sonographie und Radiologie –

Differentialindikationen in der Leber-/Gallenwegsdiagnostik. Nuklearmedizin 5:131–137
16. Koenigsberg M, Wiener SN, Walzer A (1979) The accuracy of sonography in the differential diagnosis of obstructive jaundice: a comparison with cholangiography. Radiology 133:157
17. Laing FC, Federle MP, Jeffrey RB, Brown TW (1981) Ultrasonic evaluation of patients with acute right upper quadrant pain. Radiology 140:449–455
18. Lukes PJ, Wihed A, Almersjö D (1981) Ultrasound in the differential diagnosis of jaundice. Acta Radiol [Diagn] 22:25–29
19. Makuuchi M, Bandai Y, Ito T, Watanabe G, Wada T, Abe H, Muroi T (1980) Ultrasonically guided percutaneous transhepatic bile drainage. Radiology 136:165–169
20. Malchow H, Frommhold W, Jenss H, Schindler G (1980) Diagnostik bei Erkrankungen der Gallenwege. Internist 21:565–576
21. Muhletaler CA, Gerlock AJ Jr, Fleischer AC, James AE Jr (1980) Diagnosis of obstructive jaundice with nondilated bile ducts. AJR 134:1149–1152
22. Plainfossé MC (1982) L'ultrasonographie peropératoire. Ann Radiol 25:538–542
23. Raghavendra BN, Feiner HD, Subramanyam BR, Ranson JHC, Toder SP, Horii SC, Madamba MR (1981) Acute cholecystitis: sonographic-pathologic analysis. AJR 137:327–332
24. Raghavendra BN, Subramanyam BR, Balthazar EJ, Horii SC, Megibow AJ, Hilton S (1983) Sonography of adenomyomatosis of the gallbladder: radiologic-pathologic correlation. Radiology 146:747–752
25. Raptopoulos V, D'Orsi C, Smith E, Reuter K, Moss L, Kleinman P (1982) Dynamic cholecystosonography of the contracted gallbladder: the double-arc-shadow sign. AJR 138:275–278
26. Schindler G, Pirschel J, Grehn S (1979) Optimierung der peroralen Cholezyst-Cholangiographie mit Ceruletid. Fortschr Röntgenstr 130:423–431
27. Shumann WP, Gipps P, Rudd TG, Mack LA (1982) PIPIDA scintigraphy for cholecystitis: false positives in alcoholism and total parenteral nutrition. AJR 138:1–5
28. Shuman WP, Rogers JV, Rudd TG, Mack LA, Plumley T, Larson EB (1984) Low sensitivity of sonography and cholescintigraphy in acalculous cholecystitis. AJR 142:531–534
29. Sigel B, Machi J, Beitler JC, Coelho JCU, Donahue PE, Duarte B (1982) Operative ultrasonography of pancreatic and biliary pathology. Ann Radiol 25:547–550
30. Trotteur G, Boverie J, Magotteaux P (1983) Gallbladder and ultrasound: review of a six years' experience. Limits of interpretation. J Belg Radiol 66:173–190
31. Weill F, Marmier A, Paronneau P, Zeltner F, Charton MN (1978) Diagnostic ultrasonore des ictères 199 malades. Nouv Presse Méd 7:3729
32. Weissmann HS, Badia J, Sugarman LA, Kluger L, Rossenblatt R, Freeman LM (1981) Spectrum of ^{99m}Tc-IDA cholescintigraphic patterns in acute cholecystitis. Radiology 138:167–175
33. Wolpers C (1982) Die Bedeutung der Cholegraphie für die Indikation zur Litholyse. Fortschr Röntgenstr 137:444–450
34. Wolpers C (1984) Cholelitholyse und Gallenblasendivertikel. Fortschr Röntgenstr 140: 397–407

Abdominal Masses in Children: Selection of Imaging Techniques

J. A. Kirkpatrick, Jr.

The clinician and radiologist confronted by an infant or child in whom an abdominal mass has been discovered is concerned to select those diagnostic modalities that will result in a diagnosis or differential diagnosis with relative rapidity and minimal risk. One is interested in the anatomic location of the mass, the characteristics of its tissue, its extent within or outside an organ, and its involvement of adjacent structures. Before the maturation of nuclear medicine, the sophistication of ultrasonography (particularly real-time ultrasonography), and the birth of CT, an image of the body or an organ was obtained using conventional radiographic equipment and the techniques that it permitted. Thus one utilized plain radiographs (Fig. 1); fluoroscopy; intravenous injection of contrast material to visualize the urinary tract and, in the course of these studies, to obtain total body opacification. The latter, of course, would give one an estimation of the vascularity of a structure, i.e., diminished in a cyst or an area of necrosis within a mass. In order to obtain appropriate projections, fluoroscopy could be utilized, and further proved to be of value in appreciation of pulsations and other dynamic physiologic phenomenon. Of course, fluoroscopy was made more valuable by the advent of image intensification and the subsequent ability to record the image on tape, disk, or cine film (Table 1). Contrast examination of the gastrointestinal tract most often reveals displacement by a mass, and as such can be helpful in localization of the mass itself (Fig. 2).

Before the discussion of specific techniques and tumors, one should note some of the special problems peculiar to children. The amount and nature of the tissues of the body vary with age. Perivisceral fat is small in amount and limited in its distribution in infants. Infants have more gas in the bowel than the older child or adult. Bodily proportions change with growth, and as a result the relationship of organs to external landmarks are quite different in early life than in the adult.

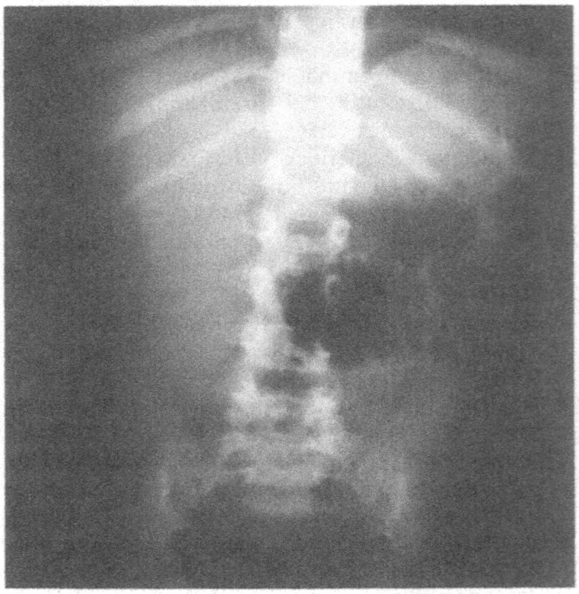

Fig. 1. Wilms tumor. The mass is evident in the right upper quadrant by virtue of its displacement of gas in the gastrointestinal tract

Growth, differentiation, and development affect anatomy. The liver, for example, tends to be relatively large in infants, comprising approximately 10% of total body weight compared to 2% in the adult. The abdomen is prominent until the 4th year of life, by which time the child has become relatively lean.

Diseases to which the infant and older child are prone have a lower incidence in the adult and in fact may not be encountered at all in later life. Intraperitoneal masses tend to be cystic and originate from the bowel; retroperitoneal non-neoplastic masses are apt to be renal in origin. The neoplasms most frequently encountered are Wilms' tumor of the kidney; neuroblastoma arising from the adrenal gland or the sympathetic chain; and teratoma arising in the root of the mesentery. Ovarian teratoma comprises 10% of ovari-

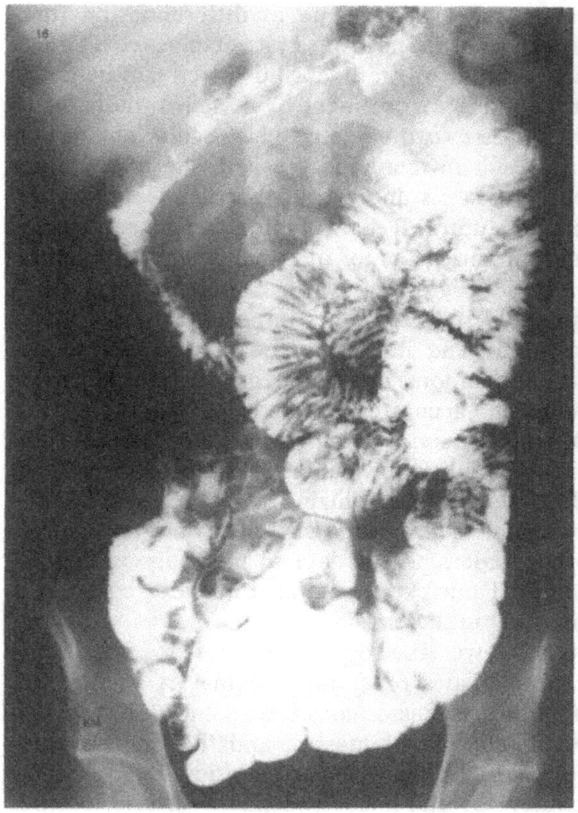

Fig. 2. A retroperitoneal lymphangioma in relation to the pancreas has displaced the duodenum, widening its loop

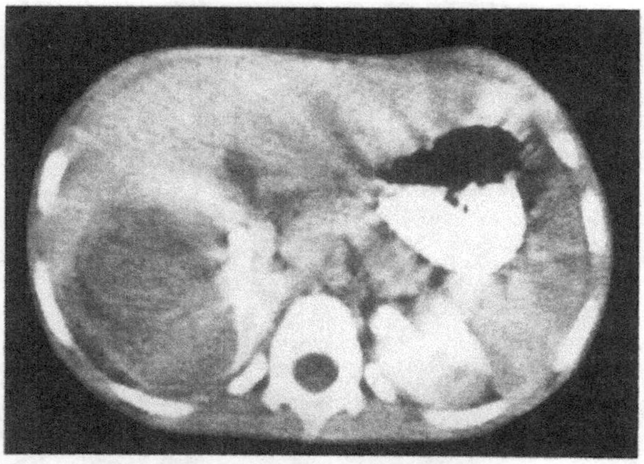

Fig. 3. CT of bilateral Wilms tumor. There is a large intrarenal mass on the right and a smaller one on the left. The latter was not seen on ultrasonography

Table 1. Abdominal masses in infants and older children: Modalities available for imaging

Plain Radiography
Fluoroscopy
Intravenous urography
Inferior vena cavography
Total body opacification
Cystourethrography
Ultrasonography
Computed tomography
Nuclear medicine
Angiography
Magnetic resonance imaging

an neoplasms in the adult but in the most common ovarian neoplasm in a child, although simple/follicular cysts are probably the most common ovarian lesion encountered in early life. Pancreatic carcinomas are rarely encountered in children, while post-traumatic or post-inflammatory pseudocysts of the pancreas are not uncommon. A large liver may of course reflect an abscess, developmental abnormality associated with cysts, a congenital vascular lesion, a primary neoplasm, or metastases from distant tumor such as neuroblastoma. However, the liver may be enlarged because of a storage disease or fatty infiltration. The gallbladder may be enlarged and palpable in patients who are suffering from sepsis; the mass of a choledochal cyst may be appreciated at any time during the pediatric years. Primary neoplasms of the intestinal tract are unusual in children. Inflammatory problems do occur; approximately 70% of children under 5 years of age with acute appendicitis have a perforation when first seen. As a result, abscesses may occur anywhere in the peritoneal cavity but particularly in the pelvis. Enlargement of the bladder may be associated with primary tumors such as rhabdomyosarcoma, and the same tumor, of course, may involve the prostate in the male and the genital tract in the female. Over the past 5 years, nuclear medicine, ultrasonography, and CT have become increasingly important to the diagnosis of abdominal masses in the infant and child; in fact, ultrasonography and CT have become readily available and particularly useful [5]. It may be worthwile considering these two modalities with respect to the characteristics of each – the characteristics, not the advantages or disadvantages.

Computed tomography responds to and quantifies differences in X-ray absorption, and therefore the images obtained conform to standard anatomic presentations (Fig. 3). Contrast enhancement will distinguish between structures of similar absorption density but different vascularity. Gas and bone cause minor artifacts; respiratory motion, metals, and barium cause major artifacts.

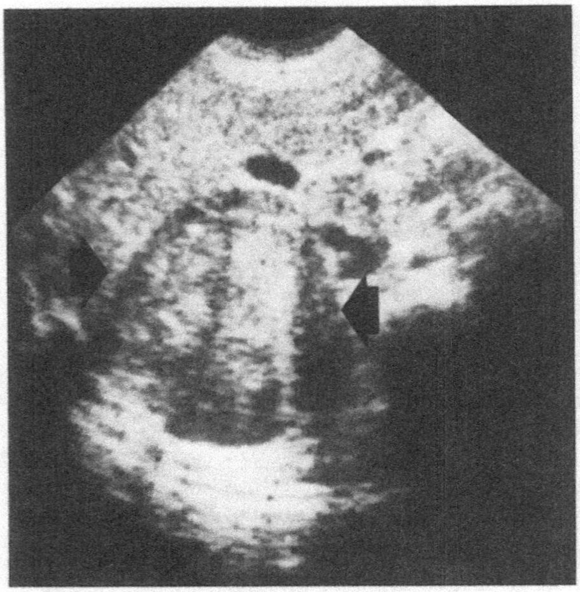

Fig. 4. Wilms tumor. The mass is complex and well visualized on ultrasonography

The quality of the image is but moderately dependent upon the skill of the operator; examination time is relatively long. Ionizing radiation is utilized. Sedation is often required, and there this modality cannot be used at the bedside. The presence of perivisceral fat is very helpful in the definition of organs.

Ultrasonography, on the other hand, is unaffected by those factors important for X-ray absorption (Fig. 4). However, the images conform less to standard anatomic presentation and are unrelated to contrast material. Major artifacts are caused by gas and bone, whereas respiration and metal cause minor artifacts; the latter is particularly true with the advent of real-time ultrasonography. Quality is heavily dependent upon the skill of the operator. The basic image is related to differences in acoustic impedance. Examination time is relatively short; ionizing radiation is not utilized; sedation is seldom required; and the modality can be used at the bedside. Unlike CT there is no dependence on fat for the definition of an organ, and in fact the leanness of the child is an advantage.

The application of *nuclear medicine* to the diagnosis of abdominal masses in infants and children has increased over the past years because of advances both in the design and capability of equipment and in radiopharmacology. Hepatobiliary agents are available that demonstrate the function of hepatocytes as well as the patency of the biliary tree. Agents that demonstrate the renal cortex have great value in differentiating functional renal tissue from cysts or masses. The size and contour of the liver and spleen can be determined, and involvement by certain tumors, cysts, or abscesses can be detected. Vascular abnormalities result in increased focal uptake of the agent on early scans and are further delineated by dynamic studies. Renal function can be ascertained and in the neonate, at a time when the intravenous urogram may be unreliable, this study may be of paramount importance. Obstructive uropathy and lesions in the kidney such as abscesses, tumors, cysts, and pseudotumors can be noted and accurately defined [1].

Magnetic resonance imaging is of course an exciting possibility for pediatric patients, because it does not require ionizing radiation and has the potential of providing chemical data of tissue in vivo. Experience to date in the diagnosis of abdominal masses in infants and older children is limited but increasing.

It may well be of significance to note some characteristics of abdominal masses in the neonate. Renal masses constitute somewhat over half of all abdominal masses, and the majority represent hydronephrosis or multicystic, dysplastic kidney. Genital masses, such as hydrometrocolpos or ovarian cyst, make up approximately 15% of the total; gastrointestinal masses such as duplication and mesenteric-omental cyst another 15%; nonrenal retroperitoneal masses 10%; and hepatosplenobiliary masses 5%. In infants and older children, renal masses make up a bit over 55%, and of these Wilms' tumor and hydronephrosis are the most significant. Nonrenal retroperitoneal masses, for the most part neuroblastomas, make up approximately 25% of the total. Gastrointestinal masses come to about 20%, a significant portion of these being abscesses related to appendiceal rupture or hepatobiliary disease. Genital masses contribute approximately 5% [1].

With the foregoing, it becomes apparent that one might look at algorithms for diagnosis in the two age groups.

In the *neonate,* the first examination should be an abdominal radiograph, followed by ultrasonography. If no abnormality of the liver, spleen, kidneys, retroperitoneum, or pelvic structures is found, one need go no further. If a mass is identified by ultrasound, and is renal in nature, the injection of contrast material with resultant total body opacification and intravenous urography may be all that is needed. If the mass is genital, appropriate genitography should be performed. If the mass is identified as adrenal, then sequential ultrasonography may differentiate hemorrhage from neuroblastoma. If hepatobiliary, one must consider the possibility of scintigraphy, angiography, and perhaps CT [2–4].

In the *infant or older child,* the abdominal radiograph is most frequently followed by ultrasonography. If the spleen, liver, or biliary tract is involved, scintigraphy and CT, in that order, are helpful; in cases of definite biliary tumors, angiography can be added for purposes of definition of the vascular supply to the liver. A pelvic mass noted by ultrasonography may be delineated by cystography and contrast studies of the distal colon; exact definition may require CT. A renal mass, after characterization by ultrasonography, may be further delineated by CT (CT plus contrast may be very significant in the diagnosis of bilateral Wilms' tumor in which one of the lesions is quite small). Nonrenal retroperitoneal tumors may be elucidated by CT. In every patient, it is significant for diagnosis that there be the utmost correlation of clinical, laboratory, and imaging results in a tailored, stepwise fashion.

References

1. Kirkpatrick JA (1983) Advantages and disadvantages of nuclear medicine, ultrasound and CT in pediatric radiology. In: Marqulis AR, Burhenne HJ (eds) Alimentary tract radiology, chapter 83. Mosby, St. Louis
2. Kirks DR, Merten DF, Grossman H, Bowie JD (1981) Diagnostic imaging of pediatric abdominal masses: an overview. Radiol Clin North Am 19: 527–545
3. Kuhn JP, Berger PE (1981) Computed tomography of the kidney in infancy and childhood. Radiol Clin North Am 19:445–461
4. Kuhns LR (1981) Computed tomography of the retroperitoneum in children. Radiol Clin North Am 19:495–501
5. Sweet EM (1983) The impact of new imaging systems on paediatric radiology. Clin Radiol 34: 361–365

Consensus on Imaging Pathways: Liver, Gallbladder, and Pancreas

J. T. Ferrucci, A. L. Baert, W. Reichardt, A. R. Margulis, W. Frommhold, and J. A. Kirkpatrick, Jr.

Introduction: Dr. J. Ferrucci

I would like to introduce our discussion by acknowledging the very timely overall theme of this congress, that of critical diagnostic pathways. Certainly, whether in Europe or the USA, we all hear continuously about the inability or unwillingness of government, private industry, or the trade unions to pay the ever-increasing costs of health care. In the USA we have now entered a new era of prospective payment by the federal government for Medicare patients using the Diagnosis-Related Groups. This system has the effect of transforming the Radiology Department from a profit-making center into a cost center, and unlike any period in the past, from now on performing radiologic services in a hospital may lose money rather than make money. Therefore, the pressures to select efficiently among our various competing radiologic techniques have increased dramatically.

Put very simply, health care and radiologic services are now being rationed, and the diagnostic radiologist now has the opportunity and the critical responsibility to organize the diagnostic process to get the very most out of the resources available.

Thus, the concept of critical diagnostic pathways selected by our hosts becomes much more than an academic exercise. It really becomes a strategy for survival. Of course, the concept of critical diagnostic pathways is not new. We have all been familiar with algorithms and decision trees for years and this is really the same music. We have heard these songs before, but now we really have to dance.

Unfortunately, algorithms and decision trees are generally regarded as boring. How many times have you heard a colleague show slides of an algorithm or decision tree during a talk with profound apologies, prompting at least half the audience to respond with a sleepy yawn or by excusing themselves to visit the restroom? Why exactly have algorithms been so tedious and generally ineffective?

Most algorithms contain one or more defects. They are often too complicated and all-inclusive, and thus become ill-suited for spedific patients and specific clinical problems. Technologic or operator bias is common, which distorts the approach and reduces its value for others. Susceptibility to obsolescence is, of course, inevitable, and in some areas the pace of change may require yearly revisions. Finally, these formulas and recipes have rarely been exportable from one institution to another.

On the other hand, I believe there are principles or guidelines which can make the construction of algorithms a more useful exercise.

First, they should be *simple.* If they are to be usable and practical, they must be streamlined to be workable in clinical practice, realizing that an occasional exceptional case may be overlooked or require management outside the algorithm.

They must be *technologically neutral.* Institutional or individual bias must be minimized simply to increase their usefulness to the largest number of institutions.

Availability is important. This refers to local geographic availability of a particular technology, such as CT, or some specific, say interventional, therapy, and to the local demand. Obviously, CT scanning is much more widely available then it was a few years ago, but there still may be a long delay before getting on the CT schedule in any given institution and this has a definite cost associated with it. Other examples might be the delay due to unavailability of an ERCP, angiogram, or needle biopsy.

Cost consciousness is certainly critical. It is not just a question of whether one test is more sensitive or more specific than another, nor is it simply whether one costs more than another. In fact, few tests survive clinical scrutiny if they are less than 75% sensitive, while few ever attain greater than 90% sensitivity. Thus, the most advantage that one

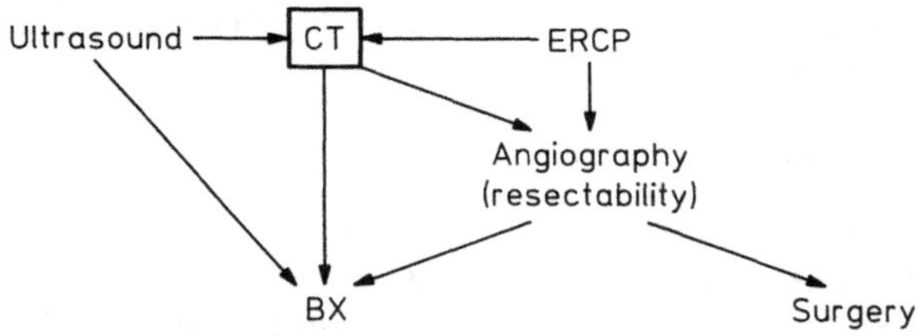

Fig. 1. Algorithm for pancreatic cancer. *BX*, needle biopsy

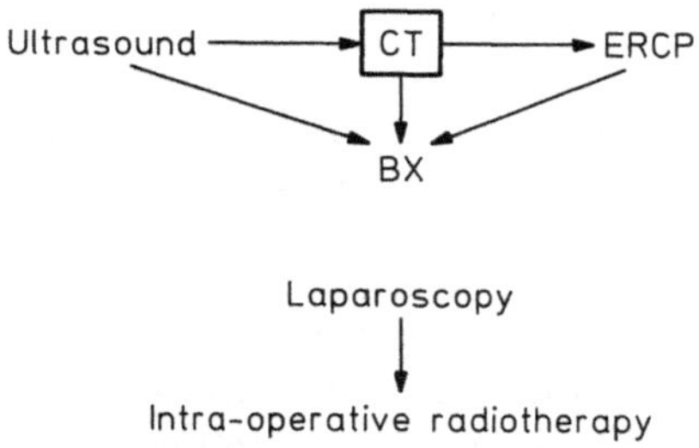

Fig. 2. Modified algorithm for carcinoma of body or tail of pancreas

alternative test usually has over another is perhaps 15%–20%. If the price paid for this marginal benefit is two or three times greater, this may be excessive.

Finally, *relevance to therapeutic choices.* Any diagnostic pathway or algorithm must lead to a therapeutic choice as economically as possible. There is no point in developing radiologic, anatomic, or functional information that will have no impact on the form of therapy. Thus, information has varying degrees of quality as it relates to the ability of the clinicians to make a therapeutic decision. Usually, the type of information provided by a noninvasive vs an invasive test is less specific in this regard. For example, there is no doubt that a CT needle biopsy or an angiogram is much more likely to direct a therapeutic choice than a radionuclide scan or an ultrasound. This is in part true because the information obtained is so much more readily interpretable by the clinicians. So we need to consider the necessary balance between the noninvasive tests which are more available but are sometimes redundant, and the invasive procedures which are more specific although usually more costly and, of course, hazardous.

I believe that if these principles are followed by the pathfinders and algorithm makers among us, they are more apt to win approval from our clinical colleagues.

With that preamble, I would like to start the discussion on what we've heard this morning by showing you one or two of my own algorithm pathways.

First, *pancreatic cancer* (Fig. 1). I have placed CT in the center of the screening tests because when it is available it invariably gives the best combination of anatomic and etiologic information obtainable noninvasively. Ultrasound is occasionally perfectly acceptable and may be followed by CT or by needle biopsy. There is also ERCP, which gastroenterologists seem to do on nearly everybody they can get their hands on, and they occasionally find a pancreatic cancer. With small lesions in the pancreatic head where Whipple resection is being considered, angiography may be a legitimate next step to provide an anatomic road map prior to surgery. However, for the vast majority of pancreatic carcinomas, guided needle biopsy, usually under CT or ultrasound, has become the standard means of establishing the pathologic diagnosis.

In our own institution this general pathway has been modified slightly, especially in the case of cancers of the body and tail (Fig. 2). These are generally considered unresectable and incurable. We follow the biopsy confirmation of the disease with a laparoscopy to detect peritoneal or serosal metastases, and if none are present we then proceed with intraoperative radiotherapy. A number of surprisingly good survivals are now being recorded with this type of aggressive therapy.

If one were to reduce the diagnostic workup to the point where maximum cost-effectiveness might be achieved in pancreatic cancer, it would consist of a CT scan followed by a needle biopsy on an outpatient basis, which, of course, is now a routine procedure yielding considerable cost savings.

In the case of *jaundice* due to obstruction of the bile ducts, the focus shifts to the very critical interrelationship between the diagnostic cholangiogram and the new forms of interventional alternatives using radiologic or endoscopic techniques (Fig. 3). There is fairly broad consensus that ultrasonography is the screening procedure of choice in suspected biliary tract obstruction because of its exquisite sensitivity for delineating both the intra- and extra-hepatic duct systems. CT is occasionally useful as an additive test in problem cases, including cancers of the pancreatic head, where a question of resectability might be answered by showing liver metastases or tumor infiltration of the celiac axis or aorta. However, for the most part, a positive ultrasonogram will be followed either by PTC or ERCP to obtain direct cholangiographic documentation of the level and nature of the obstruction. PTC is best applied for

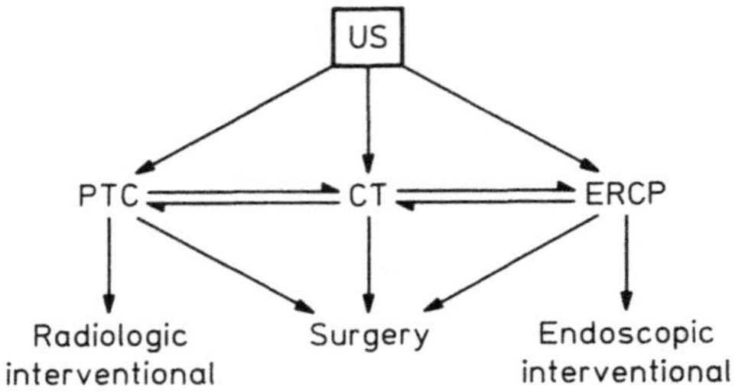

Fig. 3. Algorithm for jaundice due to obstruction of the bile ducts

Table 1. Primary imaging and other diagnostic procedures in the liver

Procedure	Modifications
Radionuclide imaging	ECAT
Ultrasonography	Contrast agents
CT	Dynamic; CTA; EDE-13
Magnetic resonance imaging	Contrast agents
Angiography	Perfusion/embolization
Biopsy	Small vs large needle

high obstructions in the porta hepatis or common hepatic duct, especially if they are malignant, whereas ERCP is most successful in delineating lesions of the distal common bile duct and is especially applicable to common duct stones which may be successfully treated by endoscopic papillotomy and basket extraction. It is now fairly clear that both radiologic and endoscopic interventional stent placement can effectively palliate malignant obstructions and offer a legitimate alternative to surgical palliation. The key in choosing among these alternatives is local expertise and, of course, the underlying biology of the disease process. Pancreatic head cancers have an average survival of 6 months no matter which form of therapy is employed, whereas some metastatic lesions to the periportal area can be effectively managed on a long-term basis with a combination of radiologic catheter drainage, chemotherapy, and irradiation therapy.

With regard to the *gallbladder,* I would only say that in our institution ultrasound is king. We do almost no oral cholecystograms now, and we have found so many problems with technetium HIDA scintigraphy, both false-negatives and false-positives, that we rarely perform it. The patient with acute classic cholecystitis with or without stones does not need a HIDA scintigram, and in a case of acalculous cholecystitis, especially in a postoperative patient who may be fasting, the HIDA study is almost always abnormal because of poor bile flow and will therefore give a very high false-positive rate. In acalculous cholecystitis we still rely mainly on ultrasonography, but recognize the persistent difficulties one may have in establishing the diagnosis.

Finally, with regard to the *liver,* I will basically leave that subject to others but would like to point out that we now have six primary liver imaging or diagnostic tests – radionuclide scanning, ultrasonography, CT, magnetic resonance, angiography, and biopsy – and that each of these has its own specific technical modifications which may extend its accuracy but about which there is still controversy (Table 1). Perhaps nowhere do we have a more outstanding example of the difficulty of applying a uniform algorithm or recipe from institution to institution; there are so many specific modifications that may be applied to increase the accuracy of one of the primary competing techniques.

If, however, one insists on a "bottom line" judgement, as we should, then the standard order of preference for noninvasive liver screening, say for metastatic disease, is first, radionuclide scanning; second, CT scanning; and third, ultrasound.

Radionuclide liver scans rarely overlook a lesion and the question of "rule out lesion" is quickly, easily and accurately answered. False-positive scans occur in 15% of cases but these can be readily evaluated further by CT or ultrasound.

CT is used next because of the highly accurate anatomic detail it provides, especially with various forms of contrast enhancement. Indeed, CT provides the modern benchmark for noninvasive liver imaging.

Ultrasonography, because of its wide application as an inexpensive survey method for upper abdominal complaints, also discloses a significant number of hepatic lesions. However, it has a significant false-negative rate compared to CT and is considerably less specific.

The role of magnetic resonance imaging is undoubtedly going to grow steadily in the near future, but its specific uses, especially vis-à-vis CT, are yet to be ascertained in clinical material.

I should now like to turn to our distinguished panel for their summary remarks on their initial diagnostic pathways.

Dr. A. L. Baert: Because of the generally very negative outcome of *pancreatic carcinoma* the diagnostic workup generally leads to a sentence as much as a diagnosis. Despite major surgery and

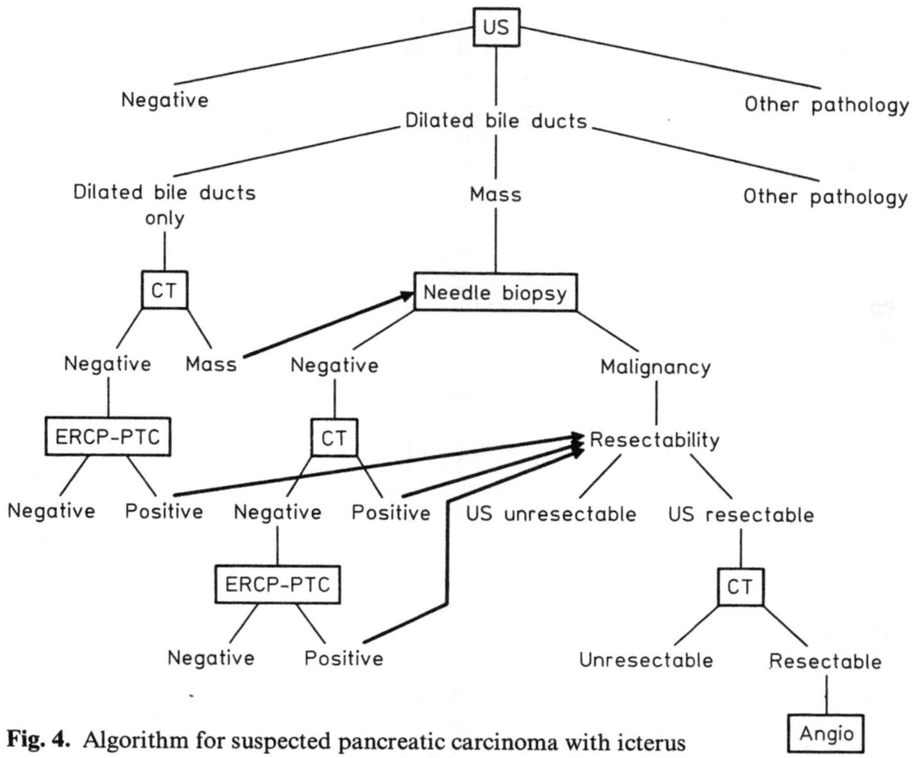

Fig. 4. Algorithm for suspected pancreatic carcinoma with icterus

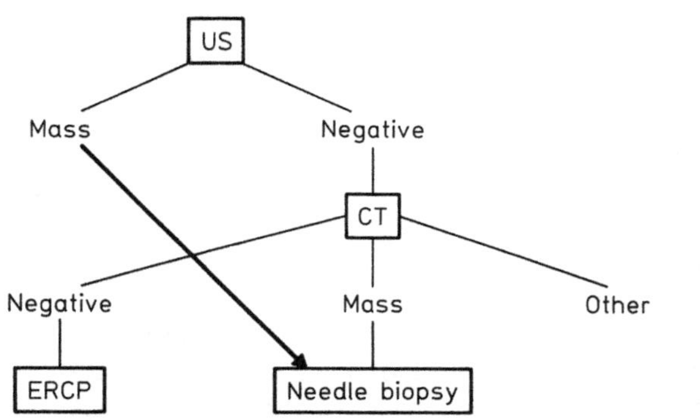

Fig. 5. Algorithm for suspected pancreatic carcinoma without icterus

different types of chemotherapy, survival remains very low. In this context diagnosis should be achieved at the lowest morbidity for the patient and include techniques which can also provide palliation. However, the diagnosis has to be sufficiently specific to avoid overlooking tractable diseases.

From the clinical point of view, two different situations can be recognized: (1) icterus, frequently due to a smaller carcinoma of the pancreatic head (Fig. 4); (2) the non-icteric patient with more diffuse symptomatology (Fig. 5).

In the first category, the diagnostic sequence should be started with ultrasound. If dilated bile ducts are demonstrated, the further sequence will depend upon the presence or not of an obstructive mass. In the presence of a mass the diagnosis has to be specified with cytology and further evaluated for resectability or palliation. If only dilatation is shown CT and possibly ERCP have to be added.

In the nonjaundiced patient the best sequence is to start with CT and continue with needle biopsy and assessment of resectability in the presence of a mass lesion. If CT is negative for a mass, ERCP should be done to rule out pancreatitis.

Dr. W. Reichardt: Four methods are used for localization of *endocrine tumors of the pancreas:*

1. Angiography: Well-documented results since 1963. The reported success rate differs, but even in small tumors is about 60%.
2. CT: The results with older CT machines were poor (about 30%). Using state-of-the-art techniques CT results are improved, especially in larger tumors (> 2 cm). The sensitivity is probably 70%–80%.
3. Ultrasound: Localization of endocrine tumors is possible, but the reliability of the method is not sufficiently documented.

4. Pancreatic venous sampling: This method is the most reliable for localization of insulin-, gastrin-, and glucagon-producing tumors, but has the disadvantage of being the most invasive and time-consuming. The catheterization should be as selective as possible and the individual anatomy should be documented.

I suggest the following procedure. In all patients with clinical evidence of functioning pancreatic endocrine tumors, CT, angiography and ultrasound should be performed. If two of the methods identically localize a tumor larger than 2–3 cm the procedure should be halted. If the tumor is less than 2 cm in size and CT and angiography do not demonstrate identical location(s), venous sampling should be performed. Pancreatic venous sampling is always indicated in patients with Zollinger-Ellison syndrome if radical surgery is anticipated.

Dr. A. R. Margulis: The present applications of *magnetic resonance imaging* (MRI) to the examination of the liver are: (1) diagnosis of hepatoma; (2) metastatic lesions, either bloodborne or by invasion from tumors of surrounding organs; (3) diagnosis of cholangiocarcinoma, particularly of the sclerosing type; (4) diagnosis of diseases of the gallbladder, including tumors and cholelithiasis; (5) diagnosis of portal hypertension, hepatitis, and hemosiderosis. The changes of fatty liver infiltration have so far not been detected by MRI, most likely because the proper technical sequences have not been applied.

Pancreatic pseudocysts and changes of acute pancreatitis, have been demonstrated by MRI. Tumors can apparently be seen better than with X-ray CT. Whether small tumors can be detected has not yet been reliably ascertained because of the lack of a large series of cases.

With proper sequences and the right projections, MRI promises to be the procedure of choice in examining the liver, gallbladder, and pancreas. Even without respiratory gating, one can obtain images with excellent spatial and contrast resolution. As long as the hydrogen density and the T1 and T2 relaxation times of the diseased tissue are different from those of the normal tissue, the proper technique can be designed to enhance the ability of the method to discover and depict lesions.

Dr. W. Frommhold: Any discussion of the rational sequence of radiologic examinations should also take into account the cost-benefit ratio, i.e., clear indications should be established based on the respective clinical symptoms, particularly for high-cost diagnostic procedures.

Three important groups of *biliary diseases* were discussed in this connection: (1) cholelithiasis and cholangiolithiasis, (2) acute and chronic cholecystitis, and (3) differential diagnosis of jaundice.

The possibilities and limitations of ultrasound, which is the method of choice today for all diseases of the biliary tract, were defined. Plain films and oral cholecystangiography are still useful in selecting patients suffering from gallstones for litholytic treatment, whereas the indication for intravenous cholegraphy is rarely established.

Nuclear medical bile flow studies with ^{99m}Tc-labeled test substances provide important clinical information necessary to diagnose initial cystic duct obstruction in patients with cholecystitis.

In the differential diagnosis of mechanical jaundice, sonography helps clarify the etiology of the obstruction in only approximately 60% of the cases. Since the possibility of a tumor should always be considered, CT provides further helpful information in all unclarified cases.

The invasive methods ERC and PTC, the final link in the diagnostic chain, not only demonstrate the exact localization of a stenosis, but also, with their possibility of external or internal biliary drainage, cross the boundary between diagnostic and therapeutic radiology.

There is a close pathophysiologic connection between the biliary tract and the other organs of the right upper abdomen, so these organs should also be included in any diagnostic procedures for unclarified abdominal disorders.

Dr. J. Kirkpatrick: This short discussion is concerned with three benign abdominal masses in children which may have serious consequences if diagnosis is delayed or incorrect.

Choledochal Cyst. This entity is most commonly encountered in children and particularly under 10 years of age. Clinically, the characteristic presentation is of jaundice, abdominal pain, and a right upper quadrant abdominal mass. However, the majority of patients do not present with all three findings. My personal preference is to start the examinations with a plain film of the abdomen to rule out other obvious causes of, or associations with, an abdominal mass, e.g., calcification or an osseous abnormality. This is followed by ultrasonography which demonstrates the dilated common duct and the presence or absence of dilated intrahepatic ducts. A BIDA or HIDA scan then confirms the diagnosis. It is seldom necessary to go further.

Pancreatic Pseudocyst. These pseudocysts are made up of necrotic tissue secondary to escape of secretions from the pancreas as a result of trauma, infection, cystic fibrosis, etc. Characteristically there is abdominal pain, and often a palpable abdominal mass. Again, the plain film examination of the abdomen is of value, followed by ultrasonography; if there is any reason to further document the abnormality of the pancreas and the echolucent pseudocyst, CT may be utilized.

Hemangioendothelioma (Cavernous Hemangioma) of the Liver. This vascular tumor is usually detected prior to 6 months of age and is manifested by an enlarged liver and at times by cardiac failure. The plain film examination of the chest may, of course, document pulmonary edema and cardiac enlargement. Occasionally, the plain film of the abdomen will reveal a calcified mass in the liver. Ultrasonography will demonstrate sonolucent areas of central echogenicity throughout the liver in most instances, but localized in others. Flow studies utilizing technetium sulfur colloid is very helpful in demonstrating the increased blood flow to the area. To separate this lesion more certainly from a vascular hepatic tumor, a scintigraphic examination utilizing technetium-tagged red cells may be of value. Angiography and CT are helpful if a therapeutic procedure, particularly surgical resection, is being considered.

Septic Lesions of the Abdomen

H. Pokieser, H. Czembirek, W. Frank, P. Hajek, H. Imhof, W. Kumpan, G. Lechner, and E. Salomonowitz

Introduction

Within the last five decades, the epidemiology and appearance of septic abdominal processes have changed. Peptid perforations gangrene of the appendix have become infrequent causes for abscesses. Today, the majority of abdominal abscesses develop after surgery [2, 4, 5, 9, 11, 16]. Within the last decade, sonography and CT have markedly increased diagnostic possibilities [6, 8, 10, 12] and allowed the creation of new therapeutic concepts [1, 3, 4, 13, 14, 15]. On the basis of the well-known publications by Meyers [7] and Whalen [17], who investigated extensively the mechanisms of intra-abdominal spread of disease leading to specific abscess formation, this paper will focus on the consequences of modern surgery pertinent to radiologists. It is our intention to demonstrate that postoperative changes of normal anatomical barriers may cause subsequent development of abscesses in unusual or unexpected locations.

Patients and Methods

During 1983 and 1984, 58 patients were investigated by real-time sonography and/or CT for abdominal abscesses (Table 1). 39 patients (67%) developed abscesses following surgery. Septic lesions were verified and treated operatively and by percutaneous drainage procedures. Bacteriological examinations were obtained in all cases. Sterile fluid collections are not included in this report.

Results

Primary abscesses were found to be solitary and predominantly (12 patients) located in the liver, usually in the right lobe. One liver abscess was caused by amebic infestation and another was due to a fish bone which had perforated the stomach and penetrated the liver. Also in this category were four gastrointestinal perforations and three retroperitoneal abscesses.

Postoperative abscesses were mostly located in the subphrenic and subhepatic spaces (Table 2). The largest group (19 patients; 49%) had undergone gastric and colonic surgery. Ten patients developed septic abdominal lesions after hemihepatectomy (8) and liver transplantation (2). The remainder had undergone surgery of the pancreas, biliary system, spleen, or bladder (Table 3).

Changing Intra-abdominal Barriers with Surgical Intervention

Abdominal surgery alters intra-abdominal anatomy in a characteristic way, dissecting natural barriers, connecting normally separated abdominal spaces, and changing the flow of intraperitoneal contents and thus the spread of infection. As a consequence of abnormal communication between intra-abdominal spaces, atypical forms and locations of abscesses may be found (Fig. 1).

Radiologists are faced not only with postoperative changes of cross-sectional anatomy, but also with different logistics of abscess localization. The most important barrier changes are the following:

The coronary ligament is cut in the course of liver mobilization, hemihepatectomy, and liver transplantation. As a consequence, an abnormal communication exists between the right supra- and infrahepatic spaces.

The hepatogastric ligament is divided in selective proximal vagotomy, most types of gastric resection and fundoplication, and exploration of the pancreas. As a consequence, the lesser sac, specifically its superior recess, communicates with the peritoneal cavity and left subphrenic space.

Table 1. Classification of abdominal abscesses

		Solitary	Multiple
Primary	19	19	0
Postoperative	39	31	8

Table 2. Locations of primary and postoperative abscesses ($n = 71$)

Location	No. (%)
Subphrenic R/L	18 (25)
Hepatic	15 (21)
Subhepatic	9 (13)
Pelvic	7 (10)
Inframesocolic R/L	6 (8.5)
Pancreatitic	6 (8.5)
Paracolic R/L	5 (7)
Lesser Sac	3 (4)
Retroperitoneal	2 (3)

Table 3. Operations preceding abscess formation ($n = 39$)

Site	No. (%)
GI tract	19 (49)
Liver	10 (26)
Pancreas	6 (15)
Biliary system	2 (5)
Spleen	1 (2.5)
Urinary bladder	1 (2.5)

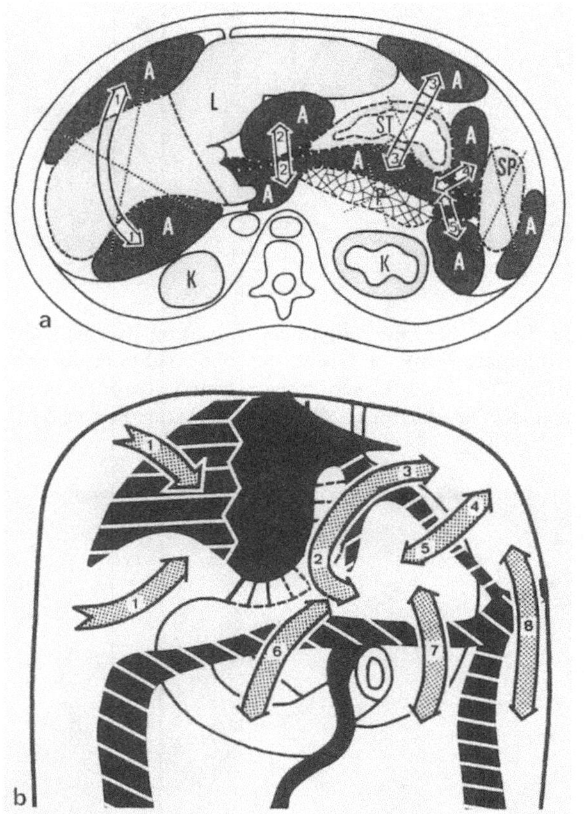

Fig. 1a, b. Cross-sectional (**a**) and supine (**b**) adapted from [7] views of most important upper abdominal peritoneal reflections and recesses, and their alteration by surgical intervention. *A*, abscess; *L*, liver; *K*, kidney; *P*, pancreas; *SP*, spleen; *ST*, stomach. Abnormal communications: *1*, right subphrenic–subhepatic space; *2*, hepatogastric recess – lesser sac; *3–5*, left subphrenic space–lesser sac; *6, 7*, right/left supracolic–inframesocolic space; *8*, left subphrenic–paracolic (rectovesical) space

The gastrosplenic ligament is cut in splenectomy, gastric resections, and fundoplication, and *the splenorenal ligament* in splenectomy. As a consequence, the lower compartment of the lesser sac communicates with the left subphrenic space.

The phrenicocolic ligament is incised in mobilization of the left colonic flexure, resection of the left or sigmoid colon or the rectum, and usually in splenectomy. As a consequence, the left subphrenic space and the paracolic gutter become continuous.

The gastrocolic ligament is split in pancreatic, colonic, rectal, and retroperitoneal surgery. As a consequence, the lesser sac communicates widely with the rest of the peritoneal cavity.

The transverse mesocolon is separated in colonic resections gastric or biliary surgery. As a consequence, the lesser sac and the right subhepatic and left subphrenic spaces become continuous with the inframesocolic spaces.

Representative Cases

Mobilization of the liver is part of some resection procedures, e.g., in tumor or transplant surgery. It is also necessary for mere inspection of the liver, for example after trauma or when the feasibility of resection is being assessed. With mobilization of a liver lobe, the corresponding attachment of the coronary ligament is lacking (Fig. 2). It is im-

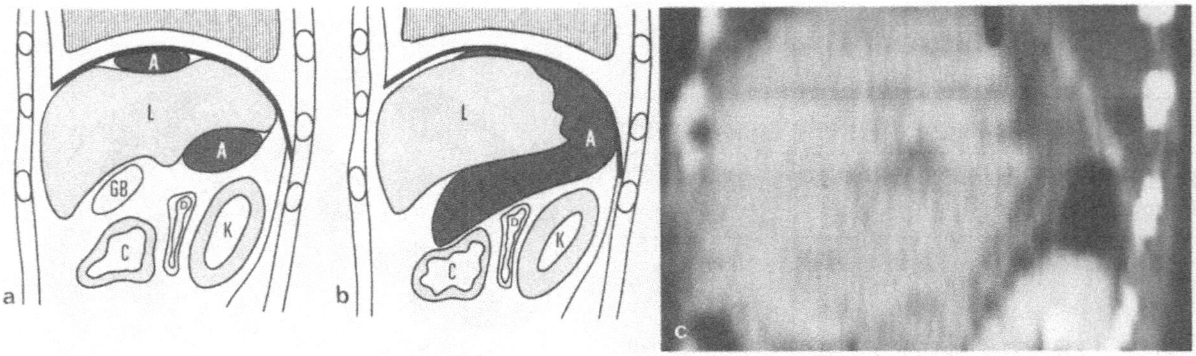

Fig. 2 a – c. Coronary ligament alteration due to right hemihepatectomy. **a** Right posterior subphrenic and subhepatic abscesses separated by intact coronary ligament. **b** With dissection of coronary ligament, an atypical abscess may develop. **c** Reformatted sagittal CT demonstrating large retrohepatic abscess, as indicated in b. *A*, abscess; *C*, colon; *D*, duodenum; *GB*, gallbladder; *K*, kidney; *L*, liver

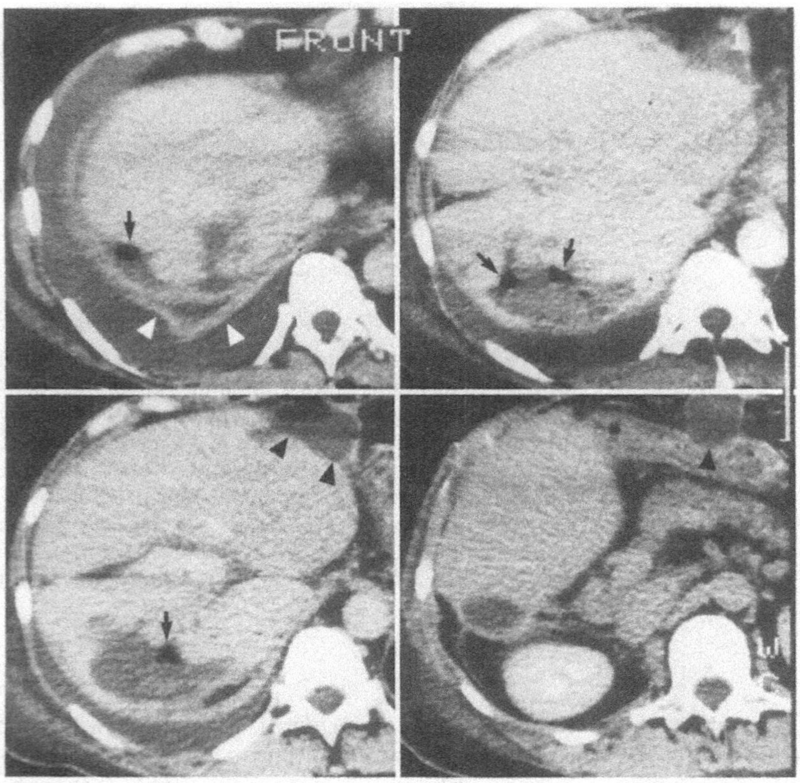

Fig. 3. Same patient as in Fig. 2. CT multi-image of right upper quadrant demonstrating posterior subphrenic – subhepatic abscess with gas bubbles (*black arrows*). There is a concomitant pleural effusion. Note small atelectasis at right posterior lung base (*white arrowheads*) and additional midline abscess in the anterior subphrenic space with gas-fluid level (*black arrowheads*)

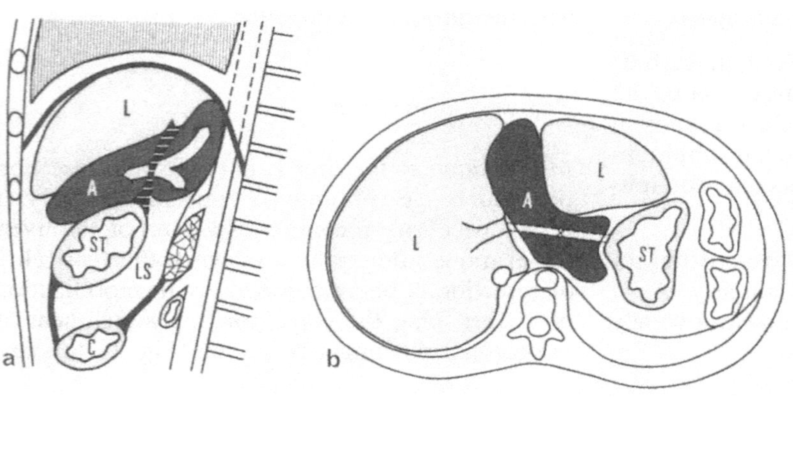

Fig. 4 a, b. Hepatogastric ligament transection, formation of large abscess from hepatogastric space into superior recess of lesser sac. **a** Sagittal view; **b** cross-sectional view. *A*, abscess; *C*, colon; *L*, liver; *LS*, lesser sac; *ST*, stomach

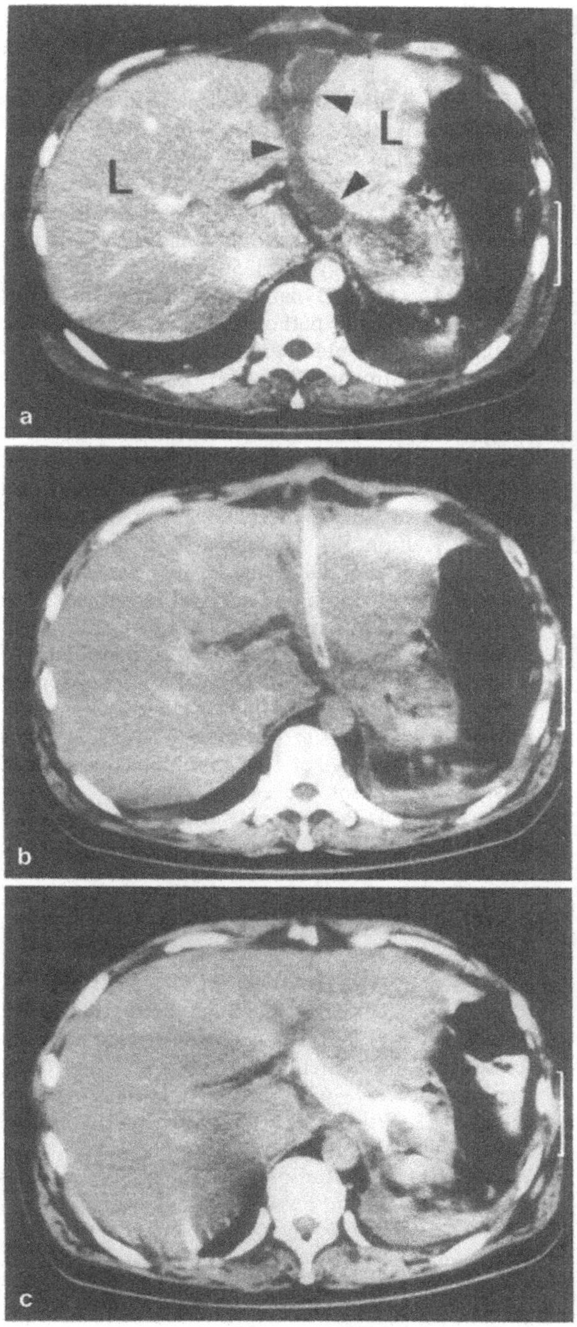

Fig. 5a–c. Percutaneous drainage of abscess as demonstrated in Fig. 4. **a** CT showing ventrodorsal extent of abscess (*arrowheads*) adjacent to liver (*L*). **b** The drainage tube lies with its tip in the superior recess of the lesser sac. **c** Abscessogram showing left posterolateral extent of abscess

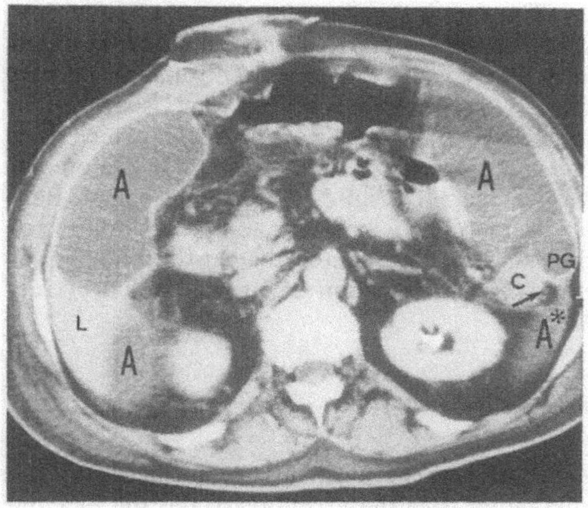

Fig. 6. CT demonstrating four abscesses after right hemicolectomy for carcinoma. Note the intact phrenicocolic ligament (*arrow*) separating abscesses in the inferior left subphrenic space (splenorenal recess) and the left paracolic gutter (*PG*), with the peritoneal cavity adjacent. Due to CT's cross-sectional display, only a small portion of the ligament is seen. *A*, abscess; *C*, colon

portant to know that after abdominal and transplant surgery the ligament is usually not reconstructed. A wide communication of right posterior subphrenic and subhepatic spaces and a potential opening into the ventrally located lesser sac are consequences of coronary ligament alteration. Figures 2 and 3 illustrate the case of a 60-year-old patient who underwent hemihepatectomy for metastatic lesions from a colon carcinoma. She became "septic" on the 12th postoperative day. CT disclosed a large, unusually located *E. coli* abscess which was subsequently drained percutaneously.

Transection of the hepatogastric ligament opens the superior recess of the lesser sac to the ventrally located hepatogastric recess. The 37-year-old patient whose case is illustrated in Figs. 4 and 5 had a selective proximal vagotomy and splenectomy. Septic fever on the 13th postoperative day prompted the radiologic workup, and a large hypodense mass was found beneath the left lobe of the liver, reaching from the hepatogastric recess well into the superior recess of the lesser sac. CT-guided drainage was performed.

Alterations of the phrenicocolic ligament produce a communication between the left subphrenic space and the lowest portion of the peritoneal cavity, the rectovesical space, via the left paracolic gutter. The intact ligament follows an oblique dorsoventral course and is usually not demonstrated in its entirety on CT (Fig. 6). The anatomical barrier of the phrenicocolic ligament is broken in mobilization of the splenic flexure, which is a common procedure in a variety of abdominal surgical techniques. For instance, the splenic flexure is mobilized in splenectomy, exploration of the pancreas, as in acute pancreatitis, follow-up of necroses, and resection of sigmoid colon or rectum.

Conclusion

After surgery, atypical abscess formation is the rule rather than the exception. CT is the imaging technique of choice for adequate search and therapy. Sonography has its merits as primary and bedside technique, and in cases of parenchymal or localized lesions. For the sake of complete examinations and for accurate analysis radiologists should be familiar with the classic surgical steps and with the variations of intraperitoneal anatomy one might expect in a given case. With these prerequisites, both diagnosis and therapy of septic lesions in the abdomen will be adequate.

References

1. Clark RA, Towbin R (1983) Abscess drainage with CT and ultrasound guidance. Radiol Clin North Am 21:445–459
2. Connell TR, Stephens DH, Carlson HC, Brown ML (1980) Upper abdominal abscess: a continuing and deadly problem. AJR 134:759–765
3. Gerzof SG, Robbins AH, Johnson WC, Birkett DH, Nabseth DC (1981) Percutaneous catheter drainage of abdominal abscesses. A five-year experience. N Engl J Med 305:653–657
4. Glick PL, Pellegrini CA, Stein S, Way LW (1983) Abdominal abscess. A surgical strategy. Arch Surg 118:646–649
5. Hiatt JR, Williams RA, Wilson SE (1983) Intraabdominal abscess: etiology and pathogenesis. Sem Ultrasound 4:71–79
6. Knochel JO, Koehler Pr, Lee TG, Welch DM (1980) Diagnosis of abdominal abscess with computed tomography, ultrasound, and 111-In leukocyte scans. Radiology 137:425–432
7. Meyers MA (1982) Dynamic radiology of the abdomen. Normal and pathologic anatomy 2nd edn. Springer, Berlin Heidelberg New York
8. Mueller PR, Simeone JF (1983) Intraabdominal abscess. Diagnosis by sonography and computed tomography. Radiol Clin North Am 21:425–443
9. Ochsner A, DeBakey M (1938) Subphrenic abscess. Collective review and analysis of 3608 collected and personal cases. Surg Gynecol Obstet 66:426–438
10. Saini S, Kellum JM, O'Leary MP, O'Donnell TF, Tally FP, Carter B, Deterling RA, Curtis LE (1983) Improved localization and survival in patients with intraabdominal abscesses. Am J Surg 145:136–141
11. Sanders RC (1970) The changing epidemiology of subphrenic abscess and its clinical and radiological consequences. Br J Surg 57:449–455
12. Schneekloth G, Terrier F, Fuchs WA (1982) Computed tomography of intraperitoneal abscesses. Gastrointest Radiol 7:35–41
13. Sones PJ (1984) Percutaneous drainage of abdominal abscesses. AJR 142:35–39
14. van Sonnenberg E, Mueller PR, Ferrucci JT Jr (1984) Percutaneous drainage of 250 abdominal abscesses and fluid collections. Radiology 151:337–341
15. van Waes PFGM, Feldberg MAM, Mali WPTM, Rujs SHJ, Eenhoorn PC, Buijs PHO, Kruis FJ, Ramos LRM (1983) Management of loculated abscesses that are difficult to drain: a new approach. Radiology 147:57–63
16. Wand SMS, Wilson SE (1977) Subphrenic abscess. The new epidemiology. Arch Surg 112:934–936
17. Whalen JP (1976) Radiology of the abdomen. Anatomic basis. Lea and Febiger, Philadelphia

Percutaneous Drainage of Abdominal Abscesses and Fluid Collections

J. T. Ferrucci, Jr.

Percutaneous drainage of abdominal abscesses and fluid collections has been described as "one of the great advances in modern surgery" [1] and is now a widely performed interventional radiologic procedure. This discussion will review certain current technical concepts [2–12].

Fluid Aspiration

Guidance. Many fluid aspirations can be performed under real-time ultrasound guidance if they are large enough or superficial. The key concern is to be certain that there are no intervening bowel loops. If there is any doubt, CT should be performed. The worst sin is to traverse a loop of bowel and contaminate a sterile fluid collection, converting it into an abscess. However, because a diagnostic tap is so quickly performed and so definitive if fluid is retrieved, all needle procedures should be first considered for ultrasound guidance, and only then triaged to CT.

Localizing Techniques. Using real-time sonography the tip of the needle is relatively easily visible in fluid collections as opposed to solid lesions. Similarly, once a needle tip has entered the fluid collection confirmation is immediately evident because fluid is easily aspirated. Jiggling the needle shaft will cause simultaneous movement of the tip with the transducer probe held off-angle or at right angles. Specialized snap-on needle-holder adaptor assemblies advertised by commercial firms have not proven especially necessary or helpful.

Diagnostic Specificity of Ultrasound and CT. The imaging appearance of fluid collections is often not sufficiently precise to determine whether the fluid is blood, pus, phlegmon, etc. Therefore in the vast majority of cases where a fluid collection is seen in the presence of a fever, needle aspiration will be required. Analysis of the sample should include at least a Gram's stain for white cells and organisms. Pyogenic abscesses will contain both, sterile abscesses will contain white cells but no organisms, and bowel contents will contain organisms but no white cells.

Drainability of Cavity Contents. Usually it is impossible to tell from the ultrasound/CT appearance whether a fluid collection is liquid enough to be drained by a catheter. A therapeutic trial of catheter insertion is often required. The thicker the fluid, the larger the catheter caliber required. Nevertheless, gelatinous nonliquid clot and phlegmonous pancreatic necrosis can rarely be drained successfully.

Abscess and Fluid Drainage

The following comments are based on the author's experience with over 300 cases [2–4].

Indications. These have broadened since the introduction of the technique several years ago. At present, any fluid collection with a safe access route is a candidate for percutaneous catheter drainage. This includes collections in unusual locations such as the presacral space, the lesser peritoneal sac, and the iliopsoas muscle. In most instances a therapeutic trial of drainage will be necessary to determine whether the fluid collection is in fact liquid enough to be drainable. Many abscesses will be shown to have an underlying fistula as the etiology, and this is generally not discovered until several days after the abscess itself has been drained. Acutely ill and/or moribund patients are also candidates for drainage as a temporizing maneuver, even if the percutaneous approach is not considered likely to be curative. Definitive elective surgical drainage can then be carried out after resuscitative measures have been administered.

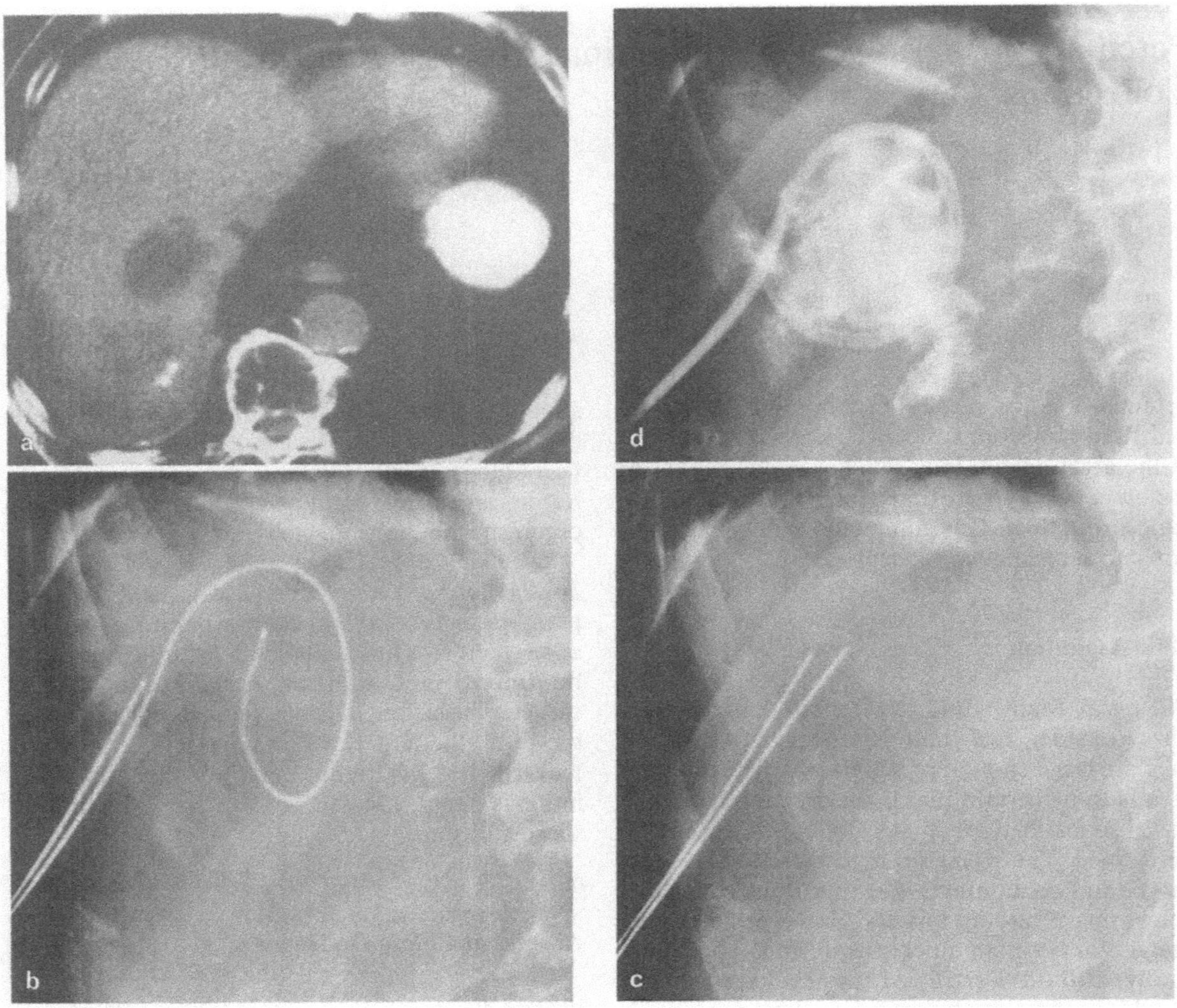

Fig. 1 a – d. Drainage of a liver abscess using combined CT and fluoroscopic guidance and a Seldinger two-step technique. **a** Initial CT scan showing a low-attenuation lesion in the posterior right hepatic lobe. A focus of parenchymal liver calcification is seen immediately behind the lesion. **b** Diagnostic needle aspiration performed under fluoroscopic guidance based on the approximate localization provided by CT. A dual tandem 20-gauge needle and 18-gauge sheath technique has been employed. **c** Following successful aspiration of pus, a guide wire has been inserted through the cannula sheath and coiled within the abscess cavity. **d** An abscess drainage catheter has been inserted and contrast medium injected outlining the extent of the cavity

Access Route Planning. This is the critical issue from a technical standpoint. Originally, retroperitoneal and dependent access routes were the primary approaches employed. At present any access route, including transperitoneal and nondependent routes, is acceptable providing there is no intervening bowel or contamination of sterile spaces (pleura). In addition, transorgan (transhepatic, transgastric) approachės to lesser sac pancreatic collections have also been used successfully.

Image Guidance. CT is particularly valuable for access route planning to establish regional topographic relationships and locate intervening contrast opacified loops of bowel. However, other imaging modalities are often useful, including ultrasonography and fluoroscopy, especially when angled needle approaches are made. Ultrasound and fluoroscopy add tremendous speed and flexibility to the procedure and it is increasingly common to combine CT guidance with real-time ultrasound or fluoroscopy (Fig. 1).

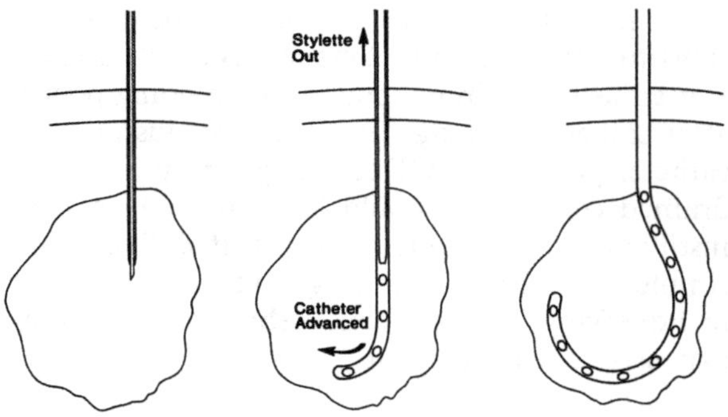

Fig. 2. The single-step trocar technique for draining an abscess or fluid collection

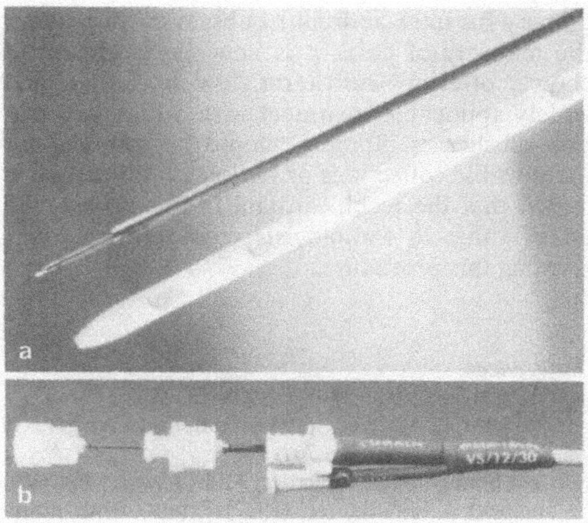

Fig. 3 a, b. The van Sonnenberg double-lumen sump catheter for abscess drainage. **a** Catheter tip, showing the inner stylet and metallic introducer in the large side-holes. **b** Catheter hub, showing the separate side-port for sump effect

Catheter Insertion Technique. Both Seldinger (two-step) and trocar (single-step) techniques are employed. The latter are most widely used for large or superficial collections (Figs. 1, 2).

Catheter Systems. Almost any catheter can be used to drain an abscess/fluid collection, although specially designed double-lumen sump catheters (van Sonnenberg) have been most widely popularized [5]. These are soft-walled catheters, fitted with an inner metal introducer and stylet, and are available in 12–14 F sizes with large side-holes (Fig. 3). The van Sonnenberg catheter can be introduced using either a trocar or Seldinger technique. Pigtails and tip-retention devices are less important in abscess drainage than in biliary or in urinary drainage, because the duration of catheter drainage is seldom more than 10–14 days and catheter dislodgement is less of a problem.

Mechanism of Success: Radiology vs Surgery. The early skepticism of experienced surgeons that small-caliber radiologic catheters could be effective in draining abscesses has given way to a general desire to understand the mechanisms of success [4]. They are as follows:

1. Both surgical and radiologic drainage have their major beneficial effect almost immediately at the time of initial catheter placement. Evacuation of pus can result in recovery of a critically ill unstable patient in a matter of hours with either method. Use of sumps, drains and tubes undoubtedly adds to the long-term therapeutic effect, but the major benefit occurs immediately.
2. The thoroughness of cavity emptying by visual inspection (surgery) vs imaging may favor the radiologic approach, as it is more precise, especially for complex or multiloculated collections. More accurate, tailored placement of side-holes is certainly an advantage of the radiologic approach.
3. Although surgeons have traditionally used large bore catheter drains and sumps, since the major therapeutic effect occurs nearly instantaneously, the smaller bore radiologic catheters are quite adequate to drain residual fluid or convey irrigant solutions. This is especially true since irrigation at the time of initial catheter placement is routinely performed to remove the thickest material.

Pitfalls

Avoiding the Pleura. Localization of the posterior costophrenic sulcus on CT scans is often confusing, especially when there is a combined subphrenic and pleural fluid collection. Use of fluoroscopy – guided needle insertion in combination with initial ultrasound/CT imaging expedites catheter insertion. Transgression of the pleura is probably more frequent in biliary drainage work than in abscess or biopsy work, however.

Special Considerations

Pancreatic Abscess. Catheter drainage of pancreatic abscess can be curative, but patient selection is important. Obviously, with diffuse phlegmonous pancreatic inflammatory disease, especially with thick necrotic pancreatic tissue, complete cure with one or more percutaneous catheters can not be guaranteed. Such patients are obviously moribund, and although complete cure is not possible, a temporizing effect may be achieved with restoration of metabolic, fluid, and respiratory status so that subsequent elective surgery can be carried out [10]. Wherever possible a retroperitoneal route should be chosen.

Pancreatic Pseudocysts. These are a continuing dilemma. The critical issue is to avoid contaminating the cyst, principally by scrupulous attention to access route planning. Recently, transorgan access via transhepatic and transgastric approaches have been used successfully. An issue of secondary importance is the presence of communication with the pancreatic duct and the presence of pancreatic duct obstruction as demonstrated by ductography. If there is open communication with the pseudocyst and the underlying duct anatomy is abnormal, catheter drainage is unlikely to succeed. Few institutions attempt percutaneous drainage of pseudocysts with great enthusiasm.

Abscess-Fistula Relation. Many postoperative abscesses subjected to percutaneous catheter drainage will be found to arise from underlying fistulae from bowel, biliary, or urinary sources. Diagnosis is made by observing a sudden increase in flow via the abscess drainage catheter, usually on the 7th – 10th day after successful abscess drainage [6]. Confirmation is obtained by contrast sinography of the catheter. Complete nonoperative treatment can be accomplished by adjusting the abscess catheter to completely drain the leaking fluid by means of tailored side-hole positioning. Use of a second or third catheter or diversion of the bile, bowel content, or urine flow by another catheter or tube may assist healing. Usually a more prolonged period of catheter drainage of a fistula (2 – 3 weeks) is required, but complete healing can be expected in most cases provided there is no obstruction distally.

Mucomyst. This protein-cleaving agent (acetylcysteine) has been advocated as an aid to liquefying thick tenacious debris [8]. However, there is no convincing experimental or clinical evidence to confirm its efficacy, and it should not be used as a substitute for more direct maneuvers such as catheter adjustments in patients who are doing poorly after catheter drainage [9]. Thus, readjustment of catheter position or CT scanning for multiple undrained collections should be instituted prior to instillation of Mucomyst. In fact, it is likely that simple saline irrigations may have as much effect in liquefying proteinaceous debris as this rather expensive chemical agent.

Conclusion

Percutaneous drainage effectively supplements antibiotics and surgery as an additional mode of therapy for intra-abdominal abscesses. In perhaps the majority of cases it is now the treatment of choice, offering short-term, low-morbidity, and widely applicable treatment with a high expectation of success. Surgery should be reserved for inaccessible collections or radiologic failures. It is hoped that the technical data in this review will be of value to radiologists considering or performing this procedure.

References

1. Welch CE, Malt RA (1983) Abdominal surgery. N Engl J Med 308:753 – 760
2. van Sonnenberg E, Ferrucci JT Jr, Mueller PR, Wittenberg J, Simeone JF (1982) Percutaneous drainage of abscesses and fluid collections: technique, results, and applications. Radiology 142:1 – 10
3. van Sonnenberg E, Mueller PR, Ferrucci JT Jr (1984) Percutaneous drainage of abdominal fluid collections in 250 cases. Part I. Results, failures and complications. Radiology 151:337 – 348
4. Mueller PR, van Sonnenberg E, Ferrucci JT Jr (1984) Percutaneous drainage of abdominal abscesses and fluid collections in 250 cases. Part II. Current procedural concepts. Radiology 151:343 – 348
5. van Sonnenberg E, Mueller PR, Ferrucci JT Jr et al. (1982) Sump catheter for percutaneous abscess drainage by trocar or Seldinger technique. AJR 139:613 – 614
6. Mueller PR, Ferrucci JT Jr, Simeone JF, Wittenberg J, Neff CC, van Sonnenberg E (1983) Detection and drainage of bilomas: special considerations. AJR 140:715 – 720
7. Mueller PR, Ferrucci JT Jr, Wittenberg J et al. (1984) Iliopsoas abscess: treatment by CT guided percutaneous catheter drainage. AJR 142:359 – 362
8. van Waes PM, Feldberg MM, Mali WP et al. (1983) Management of loculated abscesses that are dif-

ficult to drain: a new approach. Radiology 147: 57–63
9. Dawson S, Mueller PR, Ferrucci JT Jr (1984) Mucomyst for abscesses: a clinical comment. Radiology 151:342
10. van Sonnenberg E, Wing VA, Ferrucci JT Jr et al. (1984) Temporizing percutaneous drainage of complicated abscesses in critically ill patients. AJR 142:821–826
11. Nichols DM, Cooperberg PL, Golding RH, Burhenne HJ (1984) The safe intercostal approach? Pleural complications in abdominal interventional radiology. AJR 142:1013–1018
12. Neff CC, Mueller PR, Ferrucci JT Jr et al. (to be published) The pleural space: serious complications following pleural transgression in drainage procedures. Radiology

Radiologic Investigation of the Postoperative Patient

P. E. Peters

In the field of *gastrointestinal radiology,* most centers report decreasing numbers of examinations owing to the performance of endoscopic investigations by gastroenterologists. However, in the postoperative phase, the role of the GI radiologist remains unchallenged – or has even expanded because of improved possibilities for the diagnosis and treatment of postoperative complications. Before *critical diagnostic pathways* can be discussed a few definitions are needed: there are two periods to be considered:

a) The *immediate postoperative phase,* while the patient is still in hospital recovering from the operation.
b) The *followup phase,* which could be defined as the time period following discharge from the hospital.

The first period is mainly the concern of radiologists in hospital departments, while the second is also of interest to those in private practice.

The immediate postoperative phase, at least in our institution, is indubitably the province of the radiologist, while followup studies in postoperative patients often take the form of endoscopic examinations performed by either the surgeon or the gastroenterologist. Thus, the discussion is focused mainly on the immediate postoperative phase.

From the radiologist's point of view, it is necessary to differentiate between

Regular or routine studies performed as a control for the surgeon, and

Irregular or emergency studies performed mainly for the diagnosis of postoperative complications.

Radiologists should know as much as possible about surgical procedures, as otherwise their examinations will be incomplete and inadequate or wrong. As a rule, advanced surgeons have a tendency to be creative. They create their own modifications of standard procedures, either as new *inhouse standard procedures* (e.g. the so-called Billroth 3 operation at the University of Muenster) or as individual solutions to difficult anatomic conditions in particular patients. We therefore ask for the surgical report and, if necessary, for a schematic before starting the postoperative study. Radiologists and surgeons will best understand each other's problems if regular conferences are held between them (Table 1).

It is probably not possible to give general rules as to *when, how,* and *whether* routine postoperative studies should be performed, since this depends mainly on the surgeon. Thus, I will simply discuss the way it is done at our institution, which might be fairly representative for most German surgical hospitals (see Table 2).

Esophageal and gastric anastomoses are studied by means of orally administered water-soluble contrast medium (*Gastrografin*) on the 4th postoperative day. Statistically, most leakages at the anastomotic site will appear between the 3rd and 4th postoperative days, yet they can remain undetected for weeks [1]. The patients do not receive regular meals until the radiographic test has confirmed a tight suture (Fig. 1).

The Gastrografin study also reveals other complications of the immediate postoperative phase, such as stomal edema with concomitant failure of gastric emptying and gastric atony as a result of vagal denervation.

Routine Gastrografin studies of small-bowel anastomoses are carried out between the 4th and 7th postoperative days, depending on the site of anastomosis.

Colonic anastomoses are not studied routinely in the immediate postoperative phase. In patients

Table 1. Prerequisites for performance of routine studies in the immediate postoperative phase

1. Precise knowledge of operative procedure performed; report of operation and schematic
2. Standardized radiologic study
3. Regular conferences

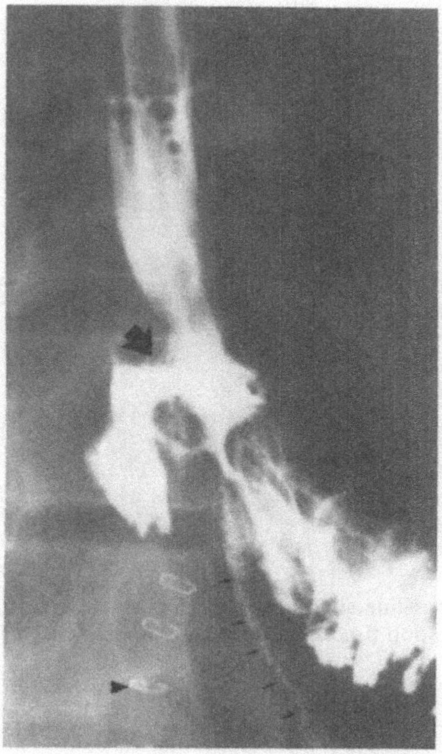

Fig. 1. Anastomotic leakage following total gastrectomy for gastric cancer. ➡, extravasation of contrast medium; →, surgical staples in the small bowel; ▸, surgical clips in the skin wound

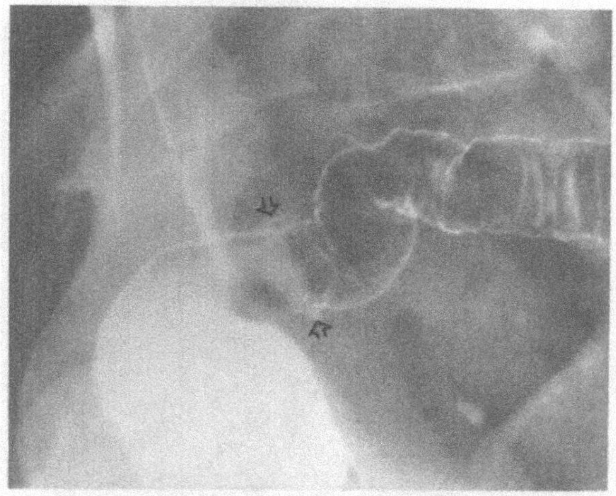

Fig. 2. Ring anastomosis following resection of sigmoid colon for cancer. Air contrast enema. Normal postoperative findings prior to closure of the temporary stoma

Table 2. Standardized procedures for radiologic investigation of the postoperative patient

Esophagus	Gastrografin	Day 4 after operation
Stomach	Gastrografin	Day 4 after operation
Small bowel		
Anastomoses	Gastrografin	Day 4–7 after
Colon, gall-bladder, etc.	No standardized procedure	operation

with a temporary cecal or transverse stoma, the unused colon will be investigated by means of a contrast enema prior to closure of the stoma (Fig. 2).

According to most investigators, the contrast medium of choice in the immediate postoperative phase is a water-soluble iodinated solution, although there are reports in the literature emphasizing that small leaks are relatively easy to overlook due to the poor contrast Gastrografin gives. These authors recommend the use of *barium sulfate* for the following reasons:

If there is no leak, it will not be harmful.

If the leak is partly sealed, it will still not be harmful.

If there is free communication with the peritoneal cavity the patient will need surgery. At that time, the barium sulfate can be removed [3].

We normally do not use barium sulfate in the early postoperative phase, but we use it occasionally at a later time in patients with fistulas, with the purpose of creating a strong foreign body reaction which may help to close the fistula.

Before entering the field of acute postoperative complications, I would like to stress the importance of postoperative *baseline studies.* If the patient, particularly the patient with malignant disease, is to be followed up radiographically, a double-contrast baseline study should be performed when the postoperative edematous changes have disappeared and while there is still no recurrent disease. Partial gastrectomy involving wedge or sleeve resection usually results in a radiographic deformity where the gastric wall is inverted and sutured. Without a baseline study, these defects may easily be mistaken for recurrent disease (Figs. 3 and 4). The radiologist should bear in mind that postoperative changes are also very difficult to analyze endoscopically. The new surgical suture machines using radiopaque staples facilitate radiographic recognition of the anastomosis. Even the plain film can suggest an anastomotic leakage or local tumor recurrence in patients with broken anastomotic rings [9, 11].

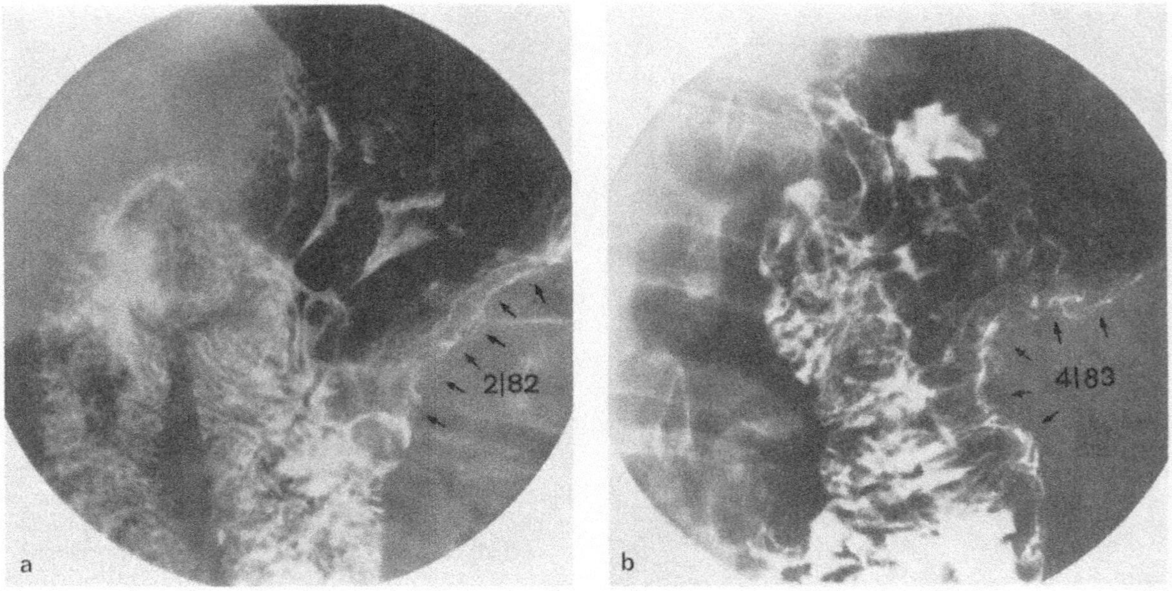

Fig. 3. a Partial gastrectomy (Billroth II) for cancer. Double contrast baseline study. Pseudolesion at the greater curvature following gastric surgery; **b** no change with 14 months observation time. Endoscopically no evidence of recurrent disease

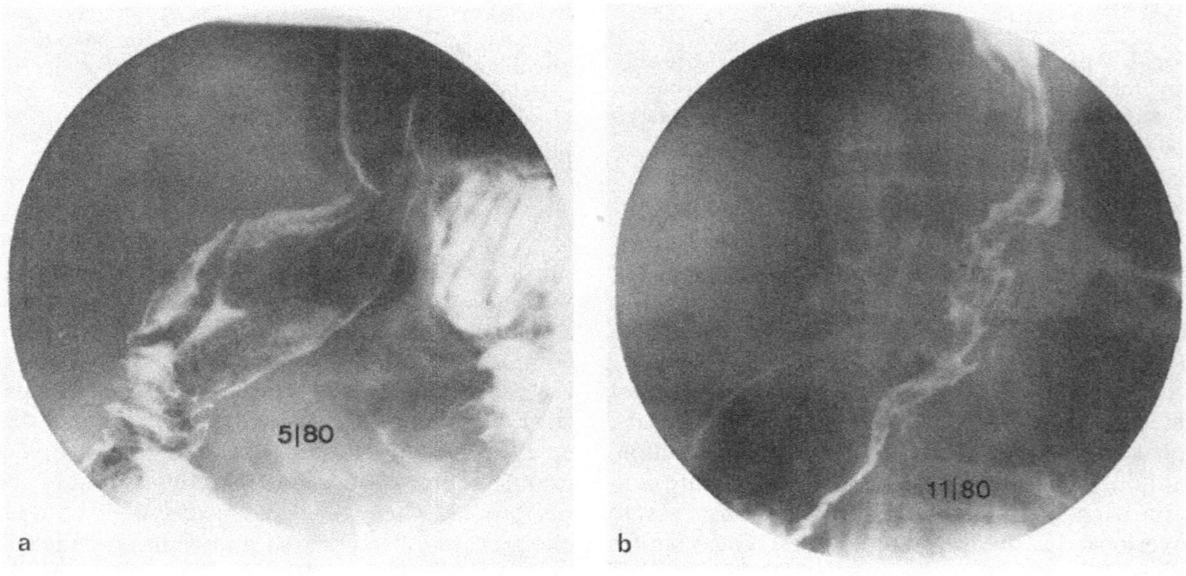

Fig. 4. a Subtotal gastrectomy for gastric cancer (5/80). Double contrast baseline study. Normal findings; **b** recurrent cancer in the gastric remnant 6 month later

Imaging modalities for the detection of *postoperative complications* include conventional radiography (CR), ultrasonography (US), computed tomography (CT), radionuclide studies (NUC) and conventional or digital subtraction arteriography (see Table 3). The most common postoperative complications requiring radiographic examinations are infected or uninfected fluid collections, ileus, bleeding, and thromboembolic complications [14].

Postoperative Fluid Collections

Fluid collections are very common following abdominal surgery. In a prospective sonographic

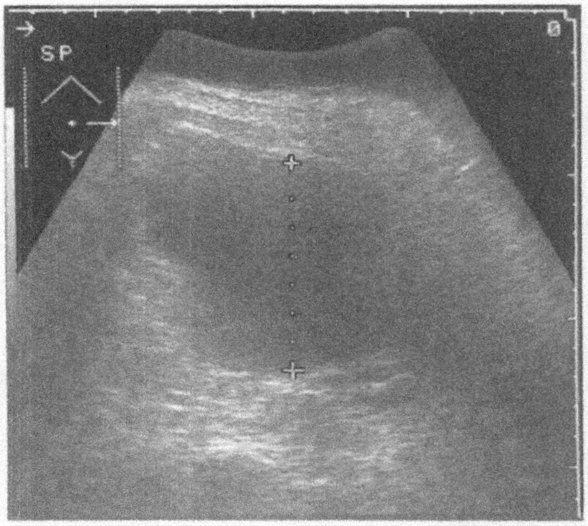

Fig. 5. Large postsurgical hematoma in the left lower abdomen. Lesion gave poor echo on sonography

Table 3. Imaging modalities for radiologic investigation of emergencies/complications in the postoperative patient

Conventional radiography
Ultrasonography
Computed tomography
Radionuclide studies
Arteriography/DSA

Table 4. Value of different imaging modalities for investigation of postoperative fluid collections

	Conventional radiography	Ultrasonography	Computed tomography
Right upper quadrant	(+)	+++	+++
Left upper quadrant	(+)	++	+++
Mid-abdomen	+	(+)	+++
Pelvis	+	++	+++

survey, Neff et al. observed fluid collections in 19% of asymptomatic patients recovering from various abdominal surgical procedures on the 4th postoperative day [8]. In most cases, the fluid collections were reabsorbed by the 8th postoperative day. Only 1 of 80 patients under investigation developed an abscess, which was sonographically characterized by an increasing amount of fluid over the observation period [8]. Pathologically, postoperative fluid collections can be seromas, hematomas, and bilomas. They can be infected, like pyogenic abscesses, or uninfected, sterile abscesses. Both pancreatic pseudocysts and cystic lesions can be mistaken for encapsulated fluid collections. Less common complications following gastrointestinal surgery are lymphoceles and urinomas. A necrotic tumor may appear as a postoperative fluid collection. Anatomically, postoperative fluid collections are located within the peritoneal cavity, in the extraperitoneal spaces, or within parenchymatous organs. The typical spreading of abdominal fluid collections has been extensively studied by Meyer [5, 6] and Whalen [15].

In the postoperative phase, however, the normal anatomic pathways are often interrupted surgically or obstructed by adhesions and scar formation. Thus, for practical purposes, it seems to be more appropriate to divide the abdomen into four regions:

Right upper quadrant
Left upper quadrant
Mid-abdomen
Pelvis

and to discuss the different imaging modalities applicable to suspected abscess formation within these regions (see Table 4).

Conventional radiography is of very limited value for the detection of abdominal fluid collections. They must be rather large to be recognized, unless they are infected and contain gas bubbles. Ultrasonography, in contrast, is an extremely sensitive tool for detecting fluid collections in the abdomen and pelvis. Its performance is only hindered by bowel gas and bone. Therefore, anatomic regions providing gas-free acoustic windows, such as the liver, the spleen, and the fluid-filled bladder, are best suited to sonographic examinations [7] (Fig. 5).

Computed tomography is even more accurate. It gives detailed and reproducible information on the cross-sectional anatomy, which can be easily understood by the referring physician and can form the basis of a surgical or interventional treatment plan. It is difficult to determine the nature of a given fluid collection, except in the case of fresh blood, which is characterized by its rather high attenuation values. However, other protein-rich fluids may look fairly similar (Fig. 6).

My suggestion for a critical diagnostic pathway in the case of suspected postoperative abdominal abscess formation is outlined in Fig. 7.

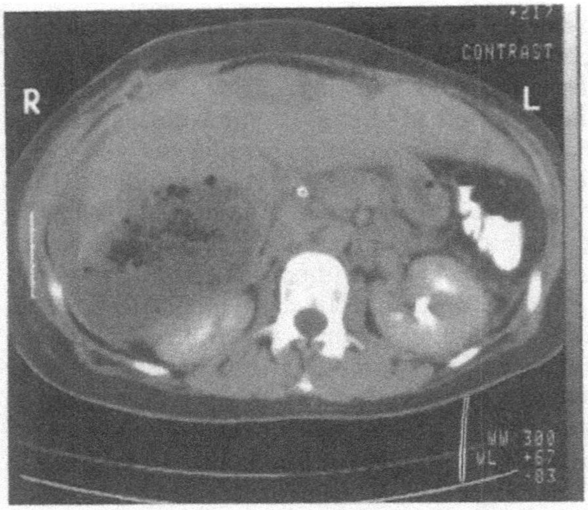

Fig. 6. Subhepatic abscess following cholecystectomy with secondary bleeding complication. Computed tomography following IV administration of contrast medium reveals subhepatic fluid collection with air bubbles

Plain film supine + left lateral decubitus
↓
Ultrasonography *and* computed tomography
↓ (two branches)

- Both normal → Stop
- Definite fluid collection shown by either or both → Percutaneous needle aspiration US/CT-guided
  - Removal of fluid collection by repeated FNP
  - Percutaneous catheter drainage
  - Surgical drainage

Fig. 7. Critical diagnostic pathway suggested for application when abdominal abscess is suspected

In spite of its well-known limitations, I still recommend the use of conventional radiography (i.e., plain film of the abdomen and left lateral decubitus), since it is a very quick procedure which can be performed everywhere, even in the intensive care unit. Conventional radiology gives an anatomic overview that is familiar not only to the radiologist but also to the surgeon. The plain film of the abdomen gives the best detection of foreign bodies and it outlines bowel changes secondary to abscess formation. In addition, it may direct the attention of the sonographer or CT expert to a certain suggestive region.

If the patient is in really poor condition, the next step should be ultrasonography followed by CT. This is admittedly not a suggestion designed to save time or costs in the short term, but in the end it may well save time and costs, and even the patient's life. US and CT are truly complementary studies. US is better for detecting internal structures and morphology, e.g., septations and cavitations within abscesses. Due to its ability to "fluoroscope" the moving diaphragm, US gives much better delineation of subphrenic and subpulmonic fluid collections. CT, on the other hand, is not impeded by air, bone, or wound dressings and is superior in the recognition of retroperitoneal disorders. If both tests are negative no further test is necessary. A definite fluid collection can be approached by surgical or radiologic means [2].

Ileus

The diagnosis of postoperative ileus is much less complicated. The old-fashioned standard procedure consisting in a plain film of the abdomen and left lateral decubitus view remains the radiologic procedure of choice. The radiographic signs of mechanical and paralytic ileus have been carefully analyzed by Swart and Meyer [13]. Occasionally, it might seem desirable to perform a Gastrografin follow-through study, which often stimulates bowel movements as an intended secondary effect. Even in patients with suspected perforation of the bowel, iodinated water-soluble contrast materials can be given orally as they are readily absorbed from the peritoneal cavity, pleural cavities, and interstitial tissues. In children and infants, Gastrografin must be diluted or it replaced by a nonionic contrast medium to avoid the sequelae of its hypertonicity [6]. Due to its renal excretion, leakage of orally administered Gastrografin into the peritoneal cavity causes opacification of the renal collecting system, the ureters, and the bladder. However, renal excretion of orally ingested Gastrografin has also been observed in patients without any evidence of leakage into the peritoneal cavity. "Heterotopic excretion" of this kind was found in 5% of Janson's series of 110 patients [4] (Fig. 8).

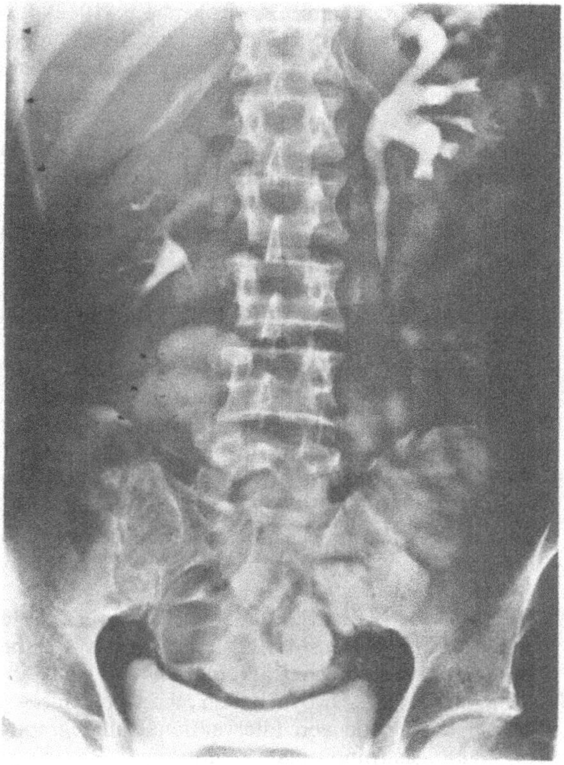

Fig. 8. Renal excretion of orally administered Gastrografin. Anastomotic leakage following gastrectomy for cancer (not shown). Water-soluble iodinated contrast medium within the small bowel and the peritoneal cavity outlining the inner and outer contour of bowel loops. ▸, drain to right of colon; →, bowel wall; ➛, gastrografin between bowel loops

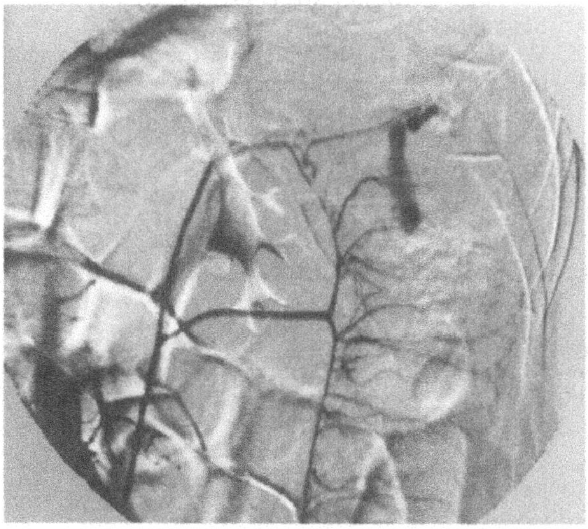

Fig. 9. Necrotizing colitis. IA-DSA discloses bleeding site in the left colonic flexure following injection into the inferior mesenteric artery

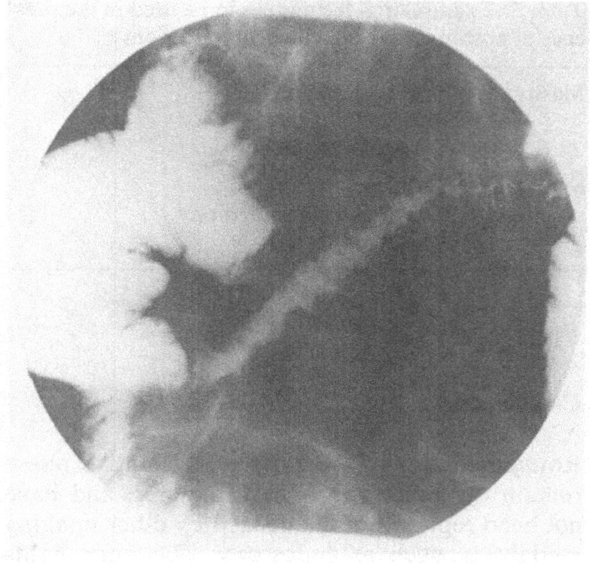

Fig. 10. Postoperative bleeding complication during anticoagulant therapy. Small-bowel examination reveals "stacked coin" appearance

Postoperative Bleeding and Thromboembolic Complications

Massive postoperative bleeding complications require emergency arteriography. The greater the blood loss per time unit, the greater the chance of detecting the bleeding site. The lower threshold of arteriographic recognition is a blood loss of 1 – 2 ml/min. Selective or superselective arteriography is performed with the object of achieving the best diagnostic results. If the patient is able to cooperate, intra-arterial digital subtraction arteriography may provide superb images with a very low dosage of contrast medium, and this is the quickest possible means of diagnosis (Fig. 9). However, under normal postoperative conditions there will be too much bowel gas and too little patient cooperation to achieve images of diagnostic quality. Thus, conventional arteriography remains the procedure of choice. Therapeutic possibilities include intra-arterial drug infusion and transcatheter embolization [10] (Table 5).

In moderate postoperative bleeding complications, endoscopic means are used in diagnosis and treatment. Small-bowel hemorrhage as a complication of treatment with anticoagulants can best be seen by a barium study revealing edematous mucosal folds and thickened bowel wall [12] (Fig. 10). Quite similar observations can be made in thromboembolic complications.

Table 5. Examination techniques to be used in the presence of postoperative bleeding complications

Massive	Arteriography/IA DSA IA drug infusion Transcatheter embolization
Moderate	Endoscopy Conventional radiography Arteriography

Conclusion

Routine studies in the early postoperative phase remain the preserve of the radiologist and have not been replaced or challenged by other imaging modalities, such as endoscopy. The same holds true for the diagnosis of postoperative ileus. Fluid collections, including abscesses, are best studied by ultrasonography *and* computed tomography, and if the patient is seriously ill *both* techniques should definitely be applied. Bleeding complications and postoperative thromboembolic complications require selective arteriography, which in suitable cases allows treatment by selective drug infusion and/or embolization.

References

1. Burrell M, Jay BS (1981) Complications of gastric and duodenal surgery. In: Meyers MA, Gharemani GC (eds) Iatrogenic gastrointestinal complications. Springer, Berlin Heidelberg New York
2. Clark RA, Towbin R (1983) Abscess drainage with CT and ultrasound guidance. Radiol Clin North Am 21:445–459
3. Foley MJ, Gharemani GC, Rogers LF (1982) Reappraisal of contrast media used to detect upper gastrointestinal perforations: comparison of ionic water-soluble media with barium sulfate. Radiology 144:231–237
4. Janson R, Christ F, Schneider B, Engel C (1982) Wertigkeit der oralen Gastrografin-Passage in der Ileus-Diagnostik. Fortschr Rontgenstr 136:641–648
5. Meyers MA (1982) Dynamic radiology of the abdomen, 2nd edn. Springer, Berlin Heidelberg New York
6. Meyers MA, Gharemani GG (1981) Iatrogenic gastrointestinal complications. Springer, Berlin Heidelberg New York
7. Mueller PR, Simeone JF (1983) Intraabdominal abscesses. Diagnosis by sonography and computed tomography. Radiol Clin North Am 21:425–443
8. Neff CC, Simeone JF, Ferrucci JT et al. (1983) The occurrence of fluid collections following routine abdominal surgical procedures: sonographic survey in asymptomatic postoperative patients. Radiology 146:463–469
9. Ott DJ, Munitz HA, Gelfand DW, Lane TG, Wu WC (1982) The sensitivity of radiography of the postoperative stomach. Radiology 144:741–743
10. Rahn NH, Tishler JMA, Han SY, Russinovich NAE (1982) Diagnostic and interventional angiography in acute gastrointestinal hemorrhage. Radiology 143:361–366
11. Sapounov S (1982) Doppelkontrastuntersuchung der zuführenden Schlinge des Billroth-II-Magens. Fortschr Rontgenstr 136:543–545
12. Sellink JL, Miller RE (1982) Radiology of the small bowel. Nijhoff, The Hague
13. Swart B, Meyer G (1974) Die Diagnostik des akuten Abdomens beim Erwachsenen – ein neues klinisch-röntgenologisches Konzept. Radiologe 14:1–57
14. Teplick JG, Haskin ME (1981) Surgical radiology. Saunders, Philadelphia
15. Whalen JP (1976) Radiology of the abdomen: anatomic basis. Lea and Febiger, Philadelphia

Diagnostic Pitfalls of Double-Contrast Gastrointestinal Studies and How to Avoid Them

I. Laufer

Introduction

The double-contrast approach to radiologic investigation of the gastrointestinal tract differs substantially from the single-contrast approach. These differences extend to both the performance and interpretation of these studies [1]. Many potential diagnostic pitfalls may confuse or deceive the unwary radiologist. However, with an awareness and understanding of these pitfalls, they are easily avoided.

Performance

The major pitfalls in the performance of double-contrast studies relate either to a poor choice of materials or to inadequate technique.

Materials

In double-contrast studies, the diagnostic content is in the mucosal coating. Therefore, it is crucial to choose a barium suspension that results in good mucosal coating in the organ under investigation. Inappropriate barium suspensions produce very faint coating and may produce artifacts such as precipitation or cracking which interfere with the diagnosis of mucosal lesions [2]. Thus, the radiologist must be familiar with the properties and qualities of a variety of barium suspensions and must also be familiar with their preparation. Improper preparation of a good barium suspension will also give poor results.

Effervescent Agents

An effervescent agent is used to produce gas in the stomach for upper gastrointestinal studies. These agents should contain an antifoaming agent such as simethicone in order to reduce bubble formation. In addition, the effervescent agent should release CO_2 quickly so that undissolved granules do not remain and produce artifacts.

Technique

A good technique ensures uniform coating on the entire mucosal surface and adequate distention to efface normal mucosal folds, and demonstrates each area of the organ being examined free of overlapping loops. Failure to achieve any of these goals may result in diagnostic error.

Mucosal Coating

Poor mucosal coating may be due to the choice of an inappropriate barium suspension which coats poorly or produces artifacts (see above). It may also be due to a failure to wash the entire mucosal surface with the barium suspension. This is a frequent problem when an inadequate volume of barium is given. Poor coating may not only result in artifacts, but in the presence of poor or patchy coating, many subtle or even large lesions may be missed.

Distention

It is easy to understand that inadequate distention can hide substantial lesions. However, it should also be appreciated that overdistention may also obscure lesions. Therefore, a routine study should utilize an intermediate degree of distention, and if a lesion is suspected but not well demonstrated, the degree of distention may then be varied (Fig. 1). With overdistention, areas of rigidity or nondistensibility are emphasized, while with partial collapse, mucosal detail may be easier to appreciate.

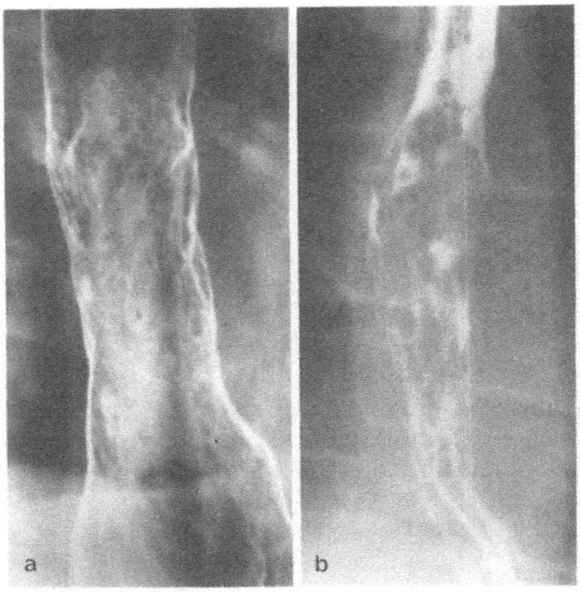

Fig. 1 a, b. Esophageal carcinoma: the influence of varying distention. **a** With complete distention, the diffuse surface abnormality is seen *en face* and in profile, and the extent of the lesion is easily appreciated. **b** With collapse, the nodularity of the mucosal surface becomes more evident

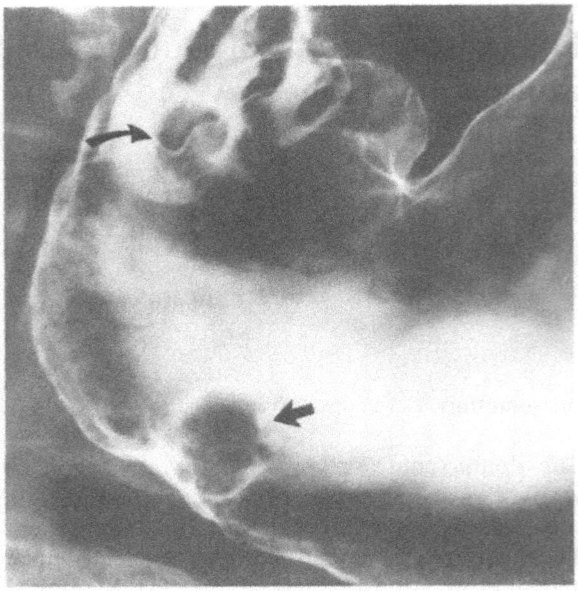

Fig. 2. Polyps on the posterior and anterior wall of the stomach. A supine film shows a filling defect due to a polyp on the posterior wall (*curved arrow*). The proximal polyp (*straight arrow*) is etched in white and is therefore on the anterior wall. Reproduced with permission from [1]

Projection

Lesions anywhere in the gastrointestinal tract can be obscured by overlapping, barium-filled loops of bowel. Therefore, a sufficient number of views must always be obtained in order to show each area free of overlapping loops.

Radiographic Factors

Whereas single-contrast films require high penetration, double-contrast films should be somewhat lighter so that surface detail in the air-filled segments is not lost. Low kilovoltage has the advantage of producing superior contrast in the center of a film which is perfectly exposed. However, this technique has several disadvantages. The exposure time is longer, and the peripheral parts of the film may be too dark or too light, with loss of useful information. As a result, we prefer to use a higher kilovoltage, in the range of 105 to 110 kVp, with as high a milliamperage as possible. We also recommend the use of a 400-speed film screen combination to minimize blurring due to motion.

Interpretation

The interpretation of double-contrast studies differs substantially from the interpretation of conventional single-contrast examinations. A failure to appreciate this difference may result in serious error.

Dependent Versus Nondependent Surface

There are two basic types of pathology in the gastrointestinal tract. Lesions may either be protruded, as with polyps or tumors, or they may be depressed, as with ulcers or diverticula. On the dependent surface, protruded lesions appear as radiolucent, filling defects, whereas depressed lesions collect barium. On the nondependent surface, the edges of a protrusion or the edges of a depressed lesion will be seen in profile, and the lesion itself will be etched in white. This etched-in-white appearance of a lesion on the nondependent surface is characteristic of double-contrast studies. The location and nature of the lesion should be confirmed by obtaining supine and prone films and by compression (Figs. 2, 3).

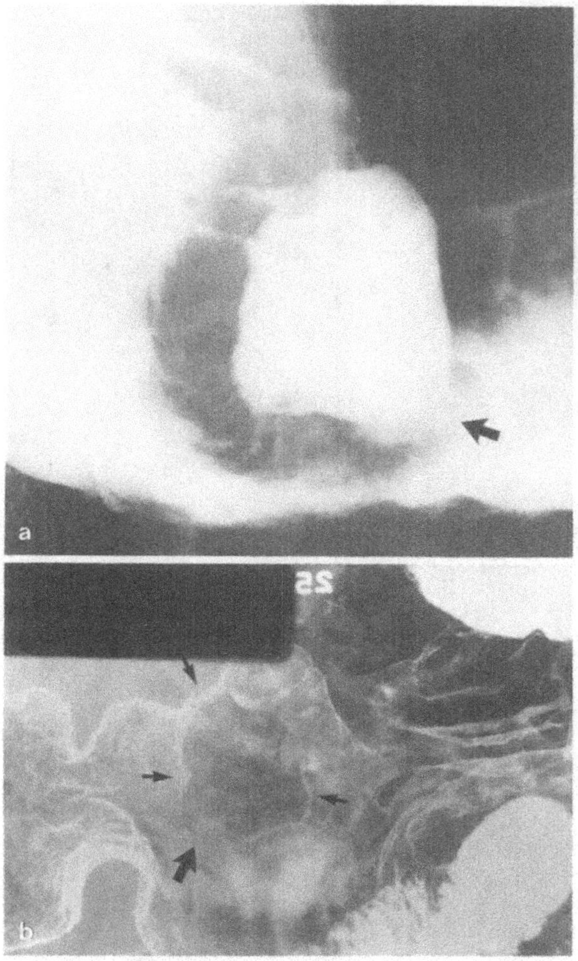

Fig. 3 a, b. Ulcerated gastric carcinoma visualized on the dependent and nondependent surfaces. **a** With the patient prone, a large, ulcerated mass is seen on the dependent or anterior surface. **b** With the patient supine, the ulceration is now on the nondependent or anterior wall and is etched in white (*arrows*)

Morphology

The radiologic appearance of a depressed lesion is also determined by the shape of its margins. In particular, lesions with gradually sloping margins may not be seen when they are located on the nondependent surface. The presence of a "stalactite" or hanging droplet of barium may be the only clue to the presence of such a lesion (Fig. 4) [3]. Such lesions are best demonstrated when placed in a dependent position or when compression is used.

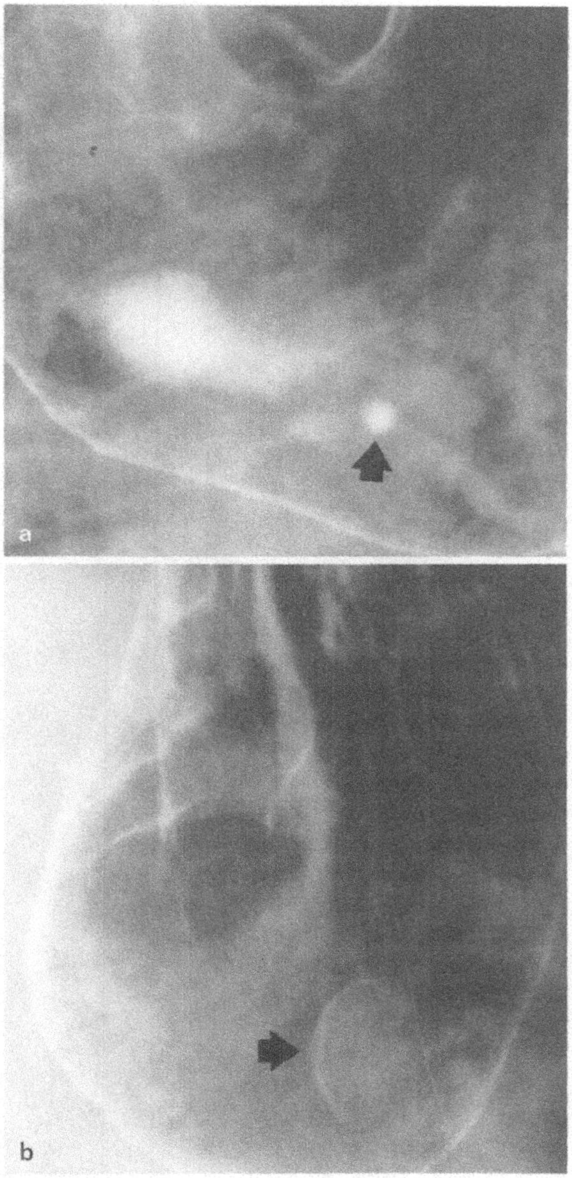

Fig. 4 a, b. A polypoid lesion with tapered margins on the anterior wall. **a** A supine film shows a stalactite (*arrow*) as the only clue to the presence of a leiomyoma on the anterior wall. **b** A subsequent, steep, oblique projection shows the etched-in-white appearance of the leiomyoma. Reproduced by courtesy of Dr. R. Siren, Columbus, Ohio, from [3]

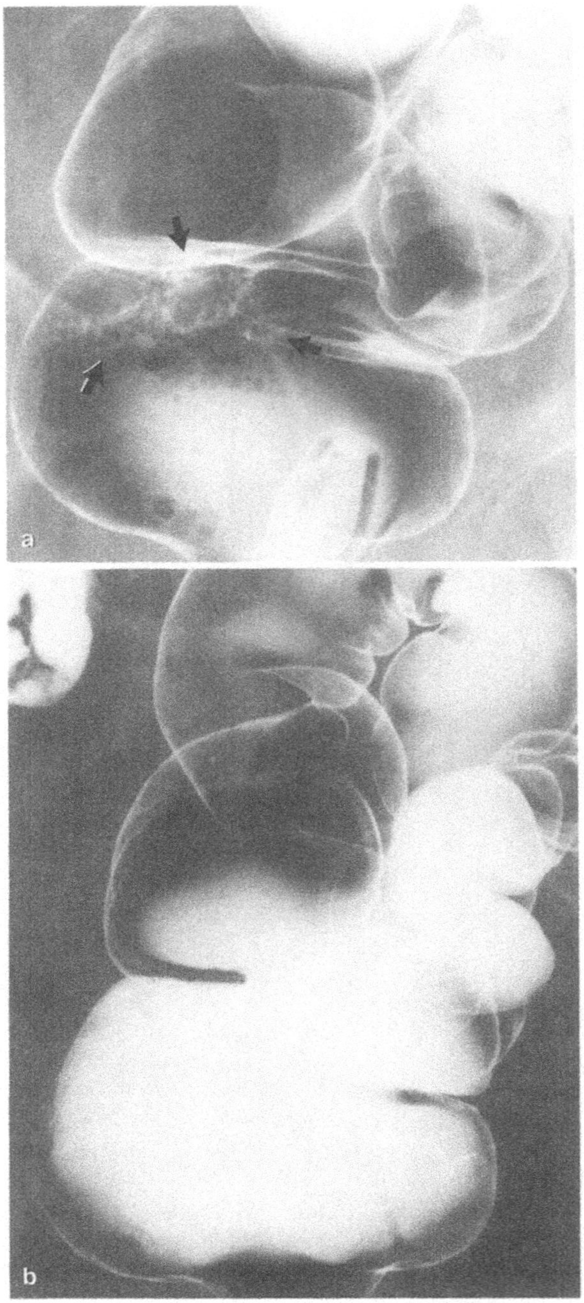

Fig. 5a, b. Rectal carcinoma obscured by the barium pool. **a** A villous carcinoma (*arrows*) clearly seen in the rectum. **b** The lesion is entirely obscured by the barium pool. Reproduced with permission from [5]

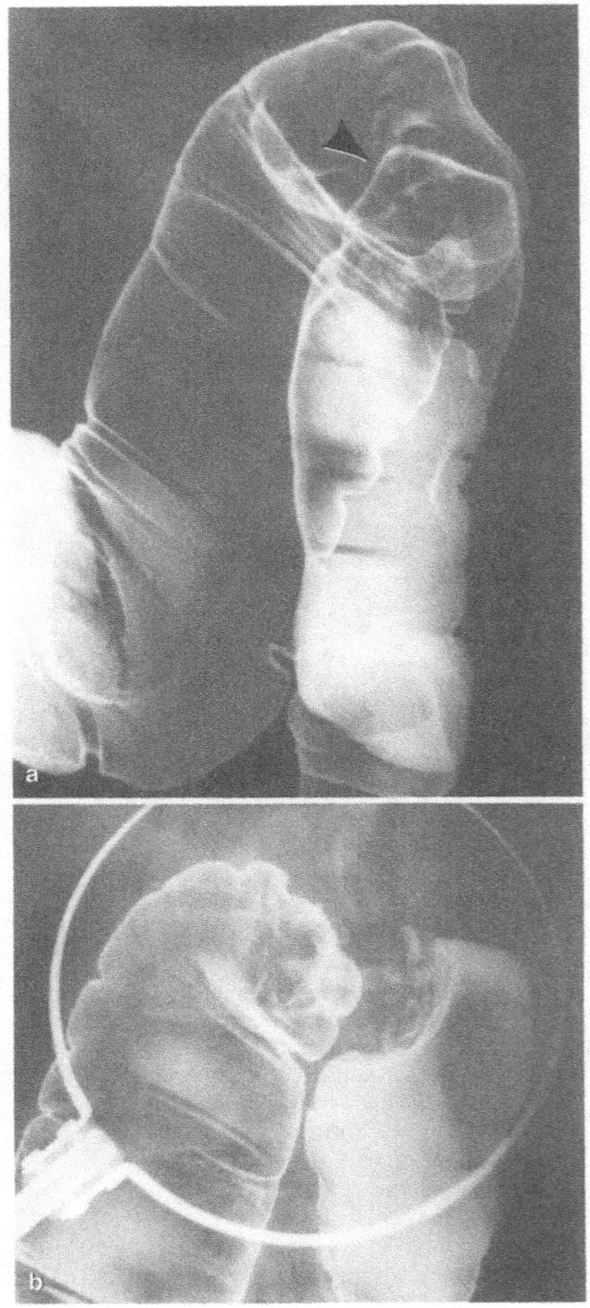

Fig. 6a, b. *En face* appearance of an annular carcinoma. **a** In the frontal projection, the lumen of the annular carcinoma is seen *en face* (*arrow*). The abnormal lines and nodularity of the surface should be recognized as a carcinoma. This is confirmed when the lesion is seen in profile in **b.** Reproduced with permission from [5]

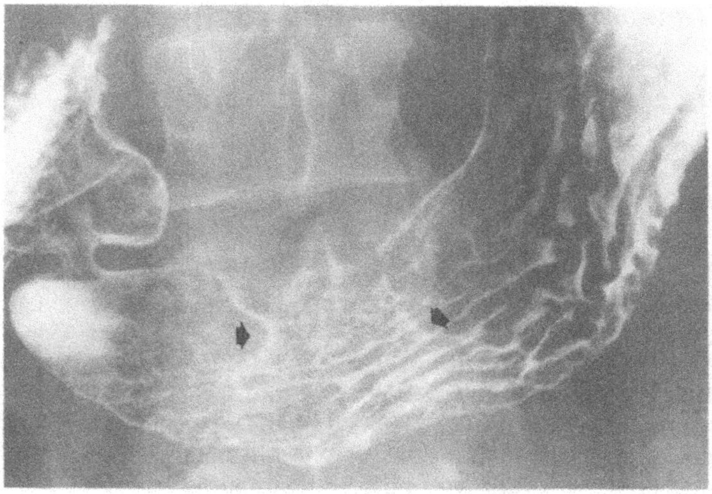

Fig. 7. Kissing artifact. A prominent aorta impresses the posterior wall of the stomach and brings it in opposition to the anterior wall, causing the kissing artifact (*arrows*). Reproduced with permission from [5]

Barium Pool

The barium pool is used to achieve uniform mucosal coating and to demonstrate lesions on the dependent surface. A shallow barium pool is particularly useful for demonstrating flat lesions on the dependent surface. However, a deep barium pool may cover lesions on the dependent surface and may obscure the "etched-in-white" appearance of a lesion on the nondependent surface (Fig. 5). Therefore, it is essential that each area be viewed without a deep barium pool. In general, supine and prone films suffice to redistribute these pools.

En Face Appearance of Annular Lesions

Profile views of annular lesions are identical for both double contrast and single contrast. However, with double contrast, an annular lesion can also be seen *en face* and recognized by the nodular contour of the lumen as seen down the barrel (Fig. 6). It is important that this be borne in mind so as not to miss short annular lesions which are not demonstrated in profile.

Double-Contrast Artifacts

Double-contrast artifacts [2] can be divided into three different categories.

Barium-Related Artifacts

The unique properties of the barium suspensions used in double-contrast studies give rise to characteristic artifacts. These include:

The Stalactite Phenomenon. This refers to a droplet of barium hanging down from a protrusion on the nondependent surface [4]. When viewed end on, these droplets are seen as rounded, dense barium collections which disappear after a few moments (Fig. 4). They are usually associated with a protrusion (fold or polyp) on the nondependent surface and, indeed, in some cases, the stalactite may be the only clue to the presence of a protruded lesion on the nondependent surface. Stalactites should not be mistaken for ulcers.

Kissing Artifact. When there is insufficient distention of the viscus, the anterior and posterior walls may adhere, and the margin of adherence may simulate a polypoid or ulcerated lesion (Fig. 7). With further distention, the artifact disappears.

See-Through Artifacts

Because of the transradiant nature of air-filled bowel, portions of the skeleton, calcifications, or contrast-filled structures may resemble intraluminal lesions. The structures which may cause confusion include portions of the lumbar spine, the greater trochanter of the femur, calcified lymph nodes, fibroids, phleboliths, calculi, and barium-filled diverticula.

Extraneous Material

A variety of extraneous materials within the bowel can produce confusing images. These include air bubbles (particularly in the esophagus), undissolved effervescent agents in the stomach, and mineral oil droplets in the colon.

Summary

The use of double-contrast techniques in the gastrointestinal tract offers the potential for improved diagnosis of a variety of benign and malignant conditions. However, these techniques also produce a variety of misleading appearances which must be recognized and should not be mistaken for disease. Furthermore, the language of double contrast is quite different from the language of single contrast. An appreciation of these differences allows the radiologist to extract all the diagnostic information which is on the films. It will also help to avoid many potential pitfalls in the interpretation of these studies.

References

1. Kressel HY, Laufer I (1979) Principles of double contrast diagnosis. In: Laufer I (ed) Double-contrast gastrointestinal radiology with endoscopic correlation. Saunders, Philadelphia, pp 11–58
2. Gohel VK, Kressel HY, Laufer I (1978) Double-contrast artifacts. Gastrointest Radiol 3:139–146
3. Aronchick J, Laufer I, Glick S (1983) Barium stalactites: observations on their nature and significance. Radiology 149:588–591
4. Op den Orth JO, Ploem S (1975) The stalactite phenomenon in double-contrast studies of the stomach. Radiology 117:523–525
5. Laufer I (1983) Double-contrast examination of the gastrointestinal tract. In: Margulis AR, Burhenne HJ (eds) Alimentary Tract Radiology, vol 1. Mosby, St. Louis, pp 148–191

GENITOURINARY TRACT

Radiology of Renal Masses

H. Hricak

Introduction

Excretory urography is considered a primary screening examination in the diagnostic workup of a suspected renal mass. When an excretory urogram reveals a mass, another cross-sectional imaging method, either sonography or CT, is employed to define the nature of the lesion. However, when the excretory urogram is considered normal, further studies are usually abundant. The importance of further diagnostic imaging for clinically suspected renal masses undetected by excretory urography should be underlined (Figs. 1–3). Literature reviews of radiology, urology, and pathology experience emphasize the need for vigorous radiologic evaluation in a clinical setting of suspected renal mass [1, 2, 3]. In about two-thirds of 100 patients with renal cell carcinoma, the diagnosis had not been established before death [3]. When and how aggressively to pursue the diagnosis of renal cell carcinoma is difficult to answer. Clinical suspicion of renal cell carcinoma arises from a variety of clinical and laboratory findings. Two-thirds of all renal cell carcinomas diagnosed present with either microscopic or gross hematuria. About half of the patients have abdominal pain. A palpable renal mass is found in about one-third. A smaller, but still significant proportion of renal carcinoma patients have toxic hepatic dysfunction, fever, hypertension, or hyperglycemia. An acute left varicocele strongly suggests the presence of a left renal tumor. However, many patients are asymptomatic [2, 4]. Primary presentation with lung, liver, of bone metastases is seen in about 10% of patients.

When an excretory urogram is performed for a clinically suspected renal mass, nephrotomograms after bolus injection of contrast medium should be included [5]. The small exophytic mass arising from the anterior or posterior aspect of the kidney will not alter the renal outline and will not displace the pelvocaliceal system. Therefore, tomograms obtained in the nephrographic phase will be the most valuable. However, even when nephrotomographs are obtained, the lesions might go undetected. This indicates the need for further investigations [1, 4].

The relative role of sonography or CT as a second step in the diagnosis of occult renal cell carcinoma should be clarified. Diagnostic ultrasound is noninvasive, nonionizing, and often extremely helpful in evaluation of renal masses. However, it should be remembered that sonography is operator-dependent and often limited by the patient's physique or by the amount of mesenteric fat or bowel gas. Furthermore, if the lesion is small and confined to the renal outline, it will be distinguished from the normal parenchyma only by the difference in echogenicity, the yield of which is low. Furthermore, in the case of lesion involving the left kidney, specifically the upper pole, difficulties are even more extensive. In obese or very tall patients, the evaluation of the left upper quadrant by sonography can be very limited. In those cases, CT should be used for further evaluation of the lesion. Contrast-enhanced CT is more sensitive and specific in analyzing a renal mass than sonography [6, 7]. In addition, if a renal cell carcinoma is detected, CT is accurate and sensitive in preoperative staging [8]. If magnetic resonance imaging is available, it can be used for further evaluation of renal masses [9]. Magnetic resonance is a noninvasive, nonionizing, and non-

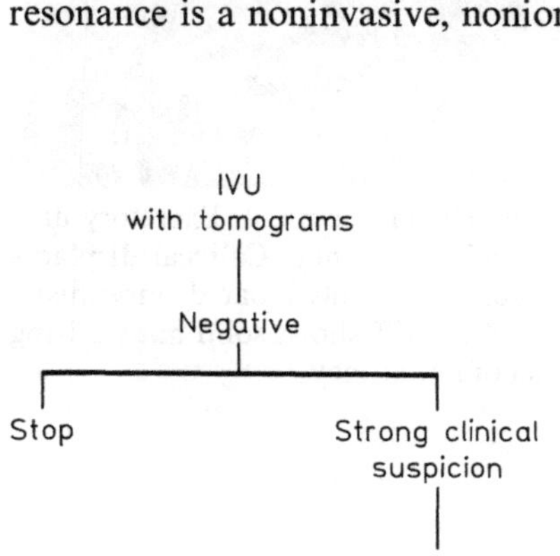

Fig. 1

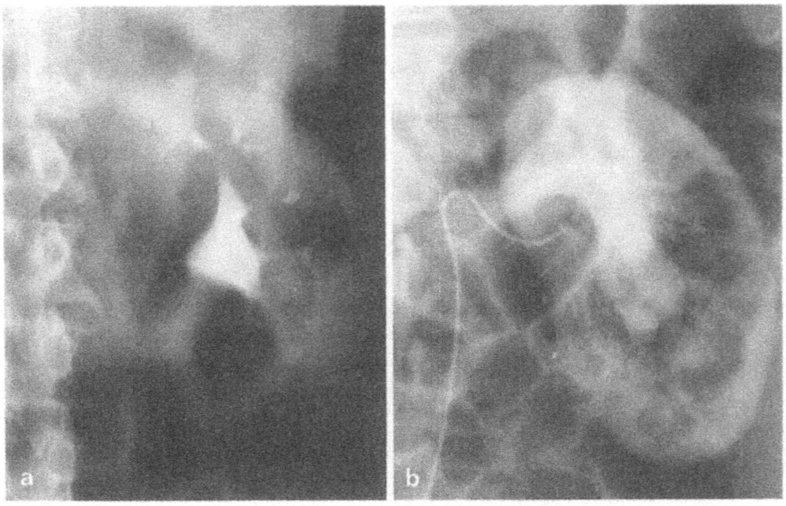

Fig. 2 a, b. Multiple renal metastases. **a** Tomogram obtained during excretory urogram shows normal left kidney. Renal outline smooth, normal. Nocaliceal displacement is seen. **b** Selective left renal angiography obtained next day. Multiple solid lesions in left kidney are demonstrated

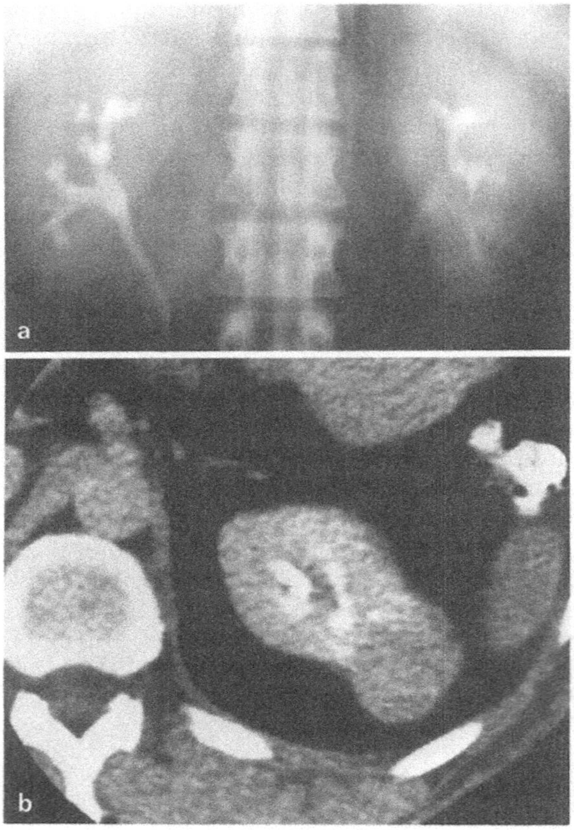

Fig. 3 a, b. Left renal cell carcinoma. **a** Excretory urogram: normal right and left kidney. Caliceal displacement of left upper pole represents lobar dismorphism. **b** Contrast-enhanced X-ray CT shows solid mass arising from posterior aspect of left kidney

operator-dependent, and, most important for diagnostic evaluation of the genitourinary tract, no iodinated contrast media are required. The ability of direct multiplanar imaging further increases the value of magnetic resonance in diagnosis and staging of renal neoplasms.

Is the Renal Tumor Cystic or Solid?

Once a renal mass is displayed on excretory urography, further evaluation is mandatory. The question of whether the mass is a benign simple renal cyst or a solid lesion needs to be resolved. If on excretory urography a lesion raises a suspicion of renal cyst, sonography is utilized for further evaluation (Fig. 4). If all four sonographic features characteristic of renal cyst are present, the lesion is considered a simple cyst and no further evaluation is needed (Table 1, Fig. 5). Cyst puncture is today performed only for symptomatic relief in a patient with a large cyst or in cysts that are indeterminate on sonography and CT. If the sonographic criteria for renal cysts are not fulfilled, CT is the next procedure, and should be performed with bolus injections of iodinated contrast media [10]. If on CT the lesion is considered a simple cyst, no further evaluation is needed (Table 2). However, if the lesion is classified as indeterminate, skinny needle biopsy or surgery should be performed [11, 12]. The role of angiography is nowadays limited to tumor embolization.

If, on excretory urography, a lesion is considered possibly solid, CT is the next step (Fig. 6). In addition to being sensitive in diagnosing a solid lesion, CT offers valuable preoperative staging of renal malignancies (Fig. 7) [7, 8]. Magnetic resonance imaging can be substituted for CT [9]. Magnetic resonance will accurately distinguish whether the lesion is solid or cystic in nature. Simple renal cysts are clearly visualized by magnetic resonance as low intensity masses whose T1 is greater than 1500 ms, T2 greater than 200 ms. Furthermore, fluid characterization on MRI is more precise than with CT, classifying the cyst as simple, hemorrhagic or indeterminate. In staging of renal malignancies, magnetic resonance is superior to CT in evaluating venous extension of the tumor thrombus into the renal vein or inferior vena cava (Fig. 8). Differentiation between direct tumor extension and blood clot is also possible. As the vessels are clearly visualized by magnetic resonance it is more sensitive than CT in distinguishing between vessels and lymph nodes. The depiction of lymph nodes in the renal hila by magnetic resonance is superior to CT. Also, there is no problem in differentiating thickened diaphragmatic crura from lymph nodes. Information regarding renal parenchyma can also be obtained by magnetic resonance without the need for contrast media, whether the kidney is excreting or nonexcreting. Multiplanar imaging offers better evaluation of direct extension of the

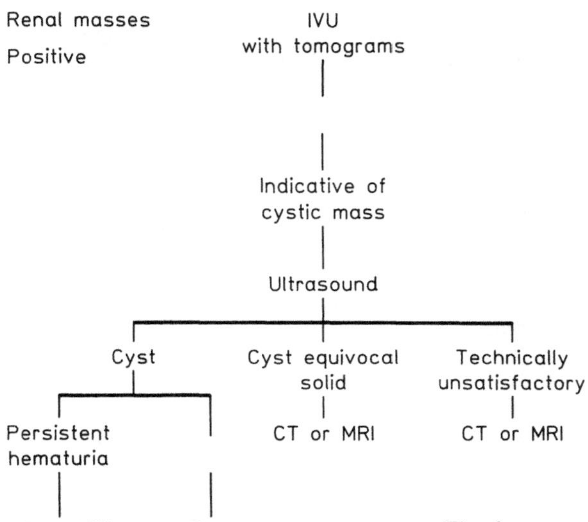

Fig. 4

Table 1. Renal Cyst: Sonographic criteria

No internal echoes present
All walls smooth and sharply defined
Acoustic enhancement beyond the posterior wall proportional to the fluid content
Narrow band of acoustic shadowing beyond the outer margin

Table 2. Renal cyst: CT criteria

Homogeneous attenuation value near water density
No measurable thickness of the cyst wall
Smooth interface with renal parenchyma
No enhancement after intravenous injection of contrast material

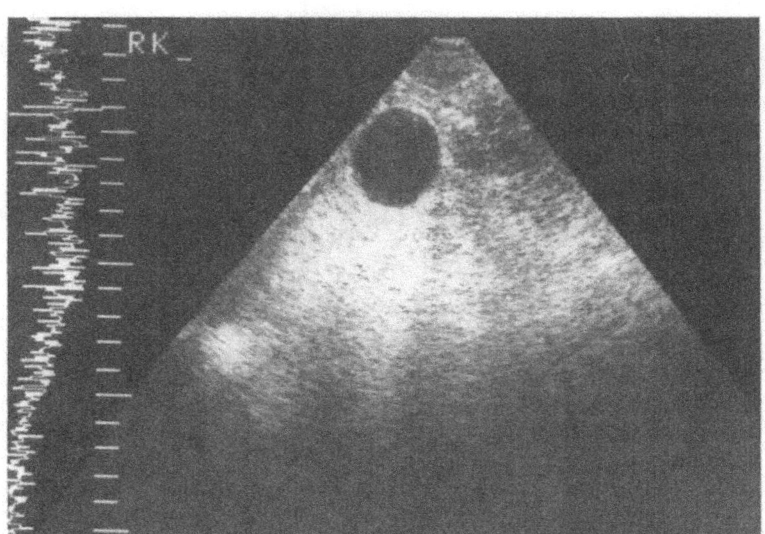

Fig. 5. Diagnostic ultrasound of simple renal cyst

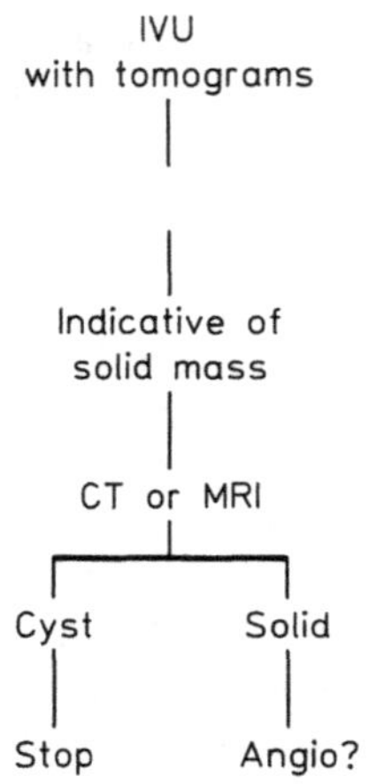

Fig. 6

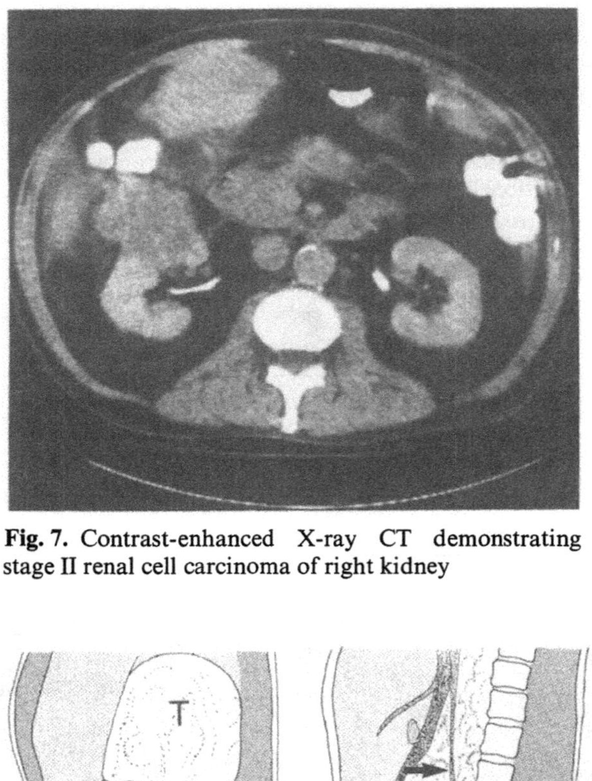

Fig. 7. Contrast-enhanced X-ray CT demonstrating stage II renal cell carcinoma of right kidney

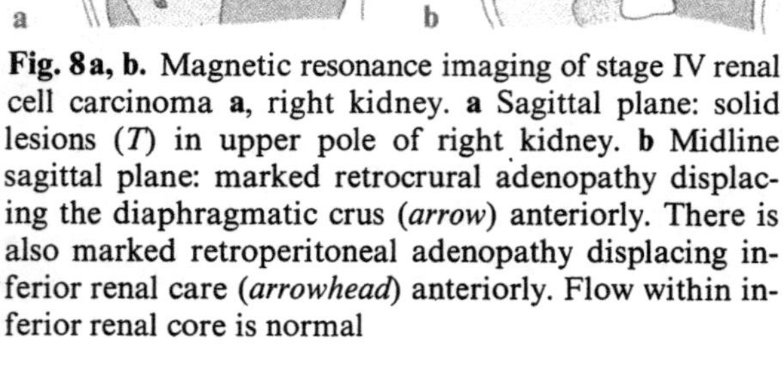

Fig. 8 a, b. Magnetic resonance imaging of stage IV renal cell carcinoma **a**, right kidney. **a** Sagittal plane: solid lesions (*T*) in upper pole of right kidney. **b** Midline sagittal plane: marked retrocrural adenopathy displacing the diaphragmatic crus (*arrow*) anteriorly. There is also marked retroperitoneal adenopathy displacing inferior renal care (*arrowhead*) anteriorly. Flow within inferior renal core is normal

tumor into the perirenal space. Also, the superior tissue contrast enhances the ability of magnetic resonance to differentiate a direct extension of the tumor to the psoas muscle or diaphragmatic crura.

Magnetic resonance imaging has in a short time demonstrated its value in the study of renal disease, especially in distinguishing solid from cystic renal lesions.

The introduction of CT and ultrasound has raised the percentage accuracy of diagnosis of renal lesions to the high 90 s. Magnetic resonance further enhances accuracy in diagnosis and staging.

The advantage of magnetic resonance lies in its superior contrast resolution combined with the ability to obtain direct multiplanar images and to provide a diagnosis without the need to use iodinated contrast media. This is particularly of value in patients who exhibit contrast media sensitivity or present with compromised renal functions.

References

1. Kass D, Hricak H, Davidson A (in press) Normal excretory urogram in the presend of renal cell carcinoma. AJR
2. Clayman RV, Williams RD, Fraley EE (1979) The pursuit of the renal mass. N Engl J Med 300:72
3. Hajdu ST, Thomas AG (1967) Renal cell carcinoma at autopsy. J Urol 97:978
4. Plaine LI, Hinman F Jr (1965) Malignancy in asymptomatic renal masses. J Urol 94:342
5. Ladwig SH et al. (1981) Ultrasonic, angiographic, and pathologic correlation of non-cystic appearing renal masses. Urology 17:204
6. Levine E, Maklad NF, Rosenthal SJ, Lee KR, Weigel J (1980) Comparison of computed tomography and ultrasound in abdominal staging of renal cancer. Urology 16:317
7. Cronan JJ, Zeman RK, Rosenfield AT (1982) Comparison of computerized tomography, ultrasound and angiography in staging renal cell carcinoma. J Urol 127:712
8. Levine E, Lee KR, Weigel J (1978) Preoperative determination of abdominal extent of renal carcinoma by CT. Radiology 122:395
9. Hricak H, Williams RD et al. (1983) NMR imaging in renal mass lesions. Radiology 147:765
10. Englestad B, McClennan BL, Levitt RG (1980) The role of precontrast images in CT of the kidney. Radiology 136:153
11. McLennan BL, Stanley RJ, Melson GL, Levitt RG, Sagel SS (1979) CT of the renal cyst: is cyst aspiration necessary? AJR 133:671
12. Balfe DM et al. (1982) Evaluation of renal masses considered indeterminate on computed tomography. Radiology 142:421

Diagnostic Approach to the Dysplastic Kidney

H. Treugut and M. Zieger

In anomalies, as in normal kidney diagnostics a three-step procedure is followed. This sometimes results in increased diagnostic accuracy, but concomitantly means more invasiveness and higher costs.

We find that anomalies of the kidney present not so much of a diagnostic challenge, but demand a well-founded understanding of the pathologic-physiologic process. Most anomalies are clearly diagnosed by the first step of basic examination, a combination of IVP and ultrasound. Only very few anomalies necessitate a second step, CT or nuclear medicine. Nuclear medicine is suitable mainly for general renal diagnostics, not so well equipped as CT to diagnose renal anomalies, but if questions arise which go beyond diagnosing anomalies, and for example refer to functional values, this would be an indication for a corresponding nuclear medicine and comes within the range of general renal diagnostics.

The third diagnostic step, involving invasive methods, is required in only very few situations. Two examples are vascular anomalies and the very rare cases of agenesia that cannot be diagnosed occurately with the first two steps. From the broad spectrum of renal anomalies we want to focus on five situations that may cause major diagnostic problems.

One Kidney Not Visualized on IVP

When one kidney is not visualized on IVP we have to differentiate between agenesia/hypoplasia and a pathologic process. Differential diagnosis covers a wide range, includes hydronephrosis, arterial and venous occlusion, and tumorous and infectious processes.

It is sometimes difficult to locate a kidney smaller than 3 cm by sonographic methods. In left agenesia the renal fossa is filled by the splenic flexure, and diagnostic mistakes occur easily. Fluid in the flexure mimics a cystic process, feces give the impression of solid tissue or a normal kidney. An examination with negative results in the lumbar area should be extended to the pelvis in order to exclude caudal ectopia. If no kidney can be located, a CT examination has to follow, sometimes with additional invasive methods.

A very small kidney can be clearly recognized on CT, even if located in the pelvis. Contrast media are usually needed in order to distinguish it from other structures, e.g., small bowel loops.

The renal artery may be extremely thin or secondarily occluded and thus escape identification by aortography, or a suprarenal artery may be mistaken for a renal vessel. If a selective search is carried out, the risk of a lesion of the spinal cord has to be taken into consideration.

Venography is of advantage in combination with renin sampling. Sometimes, due to abnormal anatomy, contrasting of the renal vein is only secured via the spermatic or ovarian vein. If the search for the renal vein remains unsuccessful in the usual level, L1/2, a caudal search is required (Fig. 1) [2–4, 10, 13, 14].

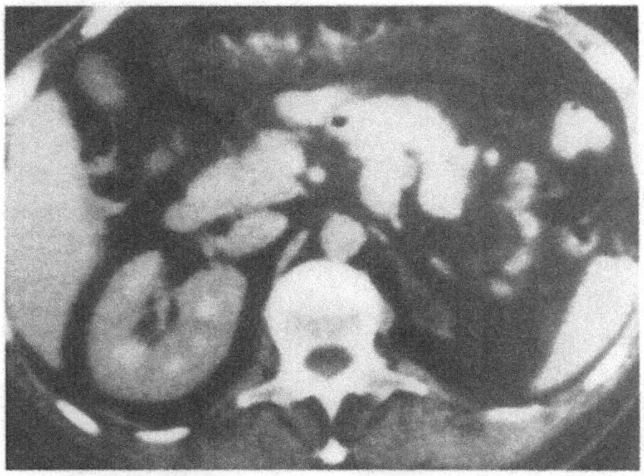

Fig. 1. CT displays this 3-cm-long hypoplastic left kidney that was not identified on ultrasound and not visualized on IVP, leading to the false diagnosis of left agenesia

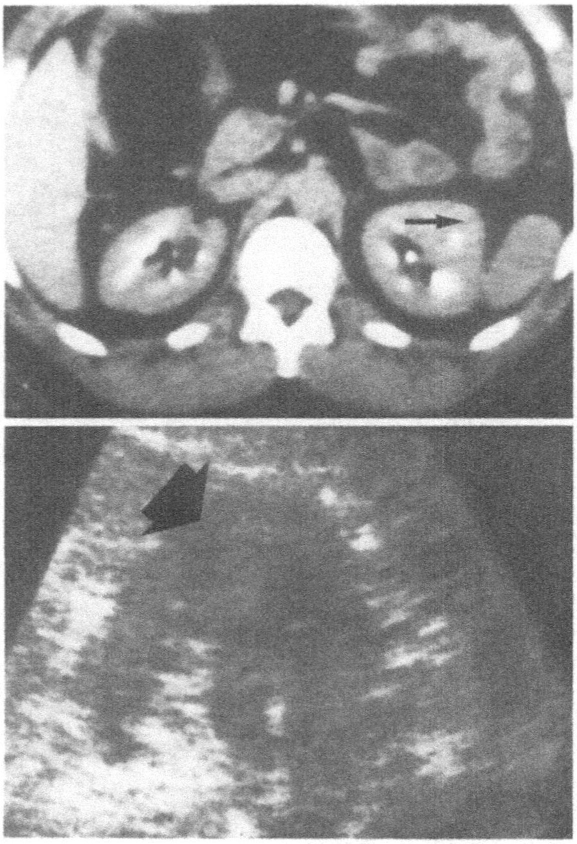

Fig. 2. Renal pseudotumor on ultrasound and CT (*arrows*)

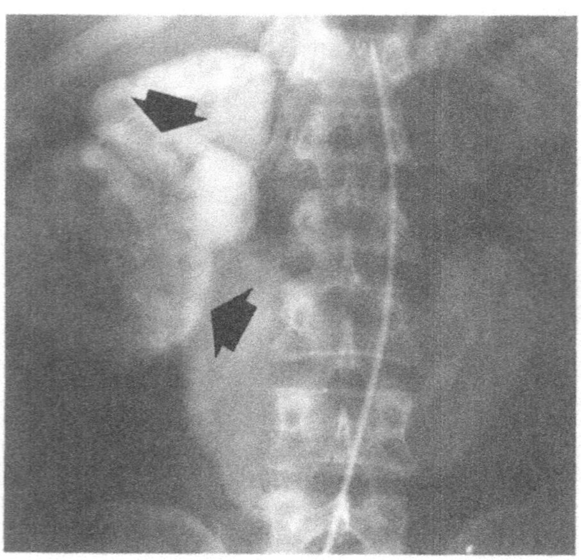

Fig. 3. Hypernephroma in a horseshoe kidney (*arrows*)

Pseudotumors

Pseudotumors are localized concentrations of normal renal cortex tissue within the kidney, also known as aberrant lobules, lobar dysmorphism, benign cortical rest, and focal renal hypertrophy. At first glance they do not fit the three known localizations of cortex tissue: subcapsular, on the hilar lips, and on the renal columns.

On sonography, pseudotumors are recognizable as structures related to parenchyma, bulging towards the center and having the same echogenicity as the cortex. Small central cysts, tumors, or parenchymal bands in renal pelvis duplication have to be distinguished in differential diagnosis.

In CT, pseudotumors show the same enhancement as the normal cortical tissue, sometimes marked clearly by fat. If the renal columns are within the same dynamic CT scan they may cause misinterpretation of pseudotumors as hypervascularized tumors. An identical phase and peak of enhancement in the area of intrarenal and subcortical cortex tissue give clear proof as to where the renal columns belong (Fig. 2) [5, 6, 9, 15, 17, 18].

Horseshoe Kidney

Diagnosis of horseshoe kidney is clear on IVP, but problems arise in sonography, increased by a fibrous bridge or an aortic aneurysm. A parenchymal bridge, on the other hand, may be mistaken for a solid process. Furthermore, judgement is impaired by a caudal position behind air-filled intestinal loops.

The typical picture is a bow-shaped structure ventral of the lower lumbar spine with the same echogenicity as kidney tissue, poor demarcation of the lower kidney poles, and an altered longitudinal axis. Differential diagnosis includes Ormond's disease and retroperitoneal lymphoma, in cranial fusion also pancreatic processes.

In this case, too, CT clears the situation and allows reliable definition of the bridge tissue. A special advantage is the demonstration of additional pathologic processes (Fig. 3) [1, 8].

Renal Pelvis Duplication

In the case of a double renal pelvis, the ureter draining the caudal pelvis ends at the trigonum vesicae and the one draining the cranial pelvis leads caudally, sometimes ectopically outside the urinary bladder. In males, the orifice is proximal of the external sphincter, in females however it lies outside the external sphincter within the urethra, vagina, or uterus, which leads to incontinence of urine. Quite often, this is accompanied by a ureterocele. Impaired flow promotes formation of hydroureter and of hydronephrosis in the upper kidney and carries the danger of infection, which may lead to parenchymal atrophy.

A vesicoureteral reflux may often be noted in the ureter draining the caudal part of the kidney. Infections are the outcome, and the parenchyma may become atrophic. Sonography diagnoses a long kidney, as well as cortical tissue between the two kidney sections. An enlargement of renal pelvis or ureter caused by obstruction or reflux as may parenchymal atrophy may be diagnosed by this method, the existence of a ureterocele can be distinguished, but it has to be differentiated from an ovarian cyst, a vesical diverticulum, and hydrosalpinx.

Due to reduced excretion of contrast media, IVP is diagnostic in only 50% of cases. The marked obstruction of the upper part of the kidney induces an inferior-lateral shift and may cause tortuosity of the other ureter. In marked reflux of the ureter draining the lower pelvis, we see flattening of the lower kidney pole that looks like a partial resection and the so-called "nubbin sign". A clear definition by means of differential diagnosis excludes renal tumors, adrenal tumors, segmental infarction, and Ask-Upmarkkidney.

In exceptional cases it might be necessary to define preoperatively the exact location of the ureter orifice by antegrade pyelography following puncture (Fig. 4) [1, 12].

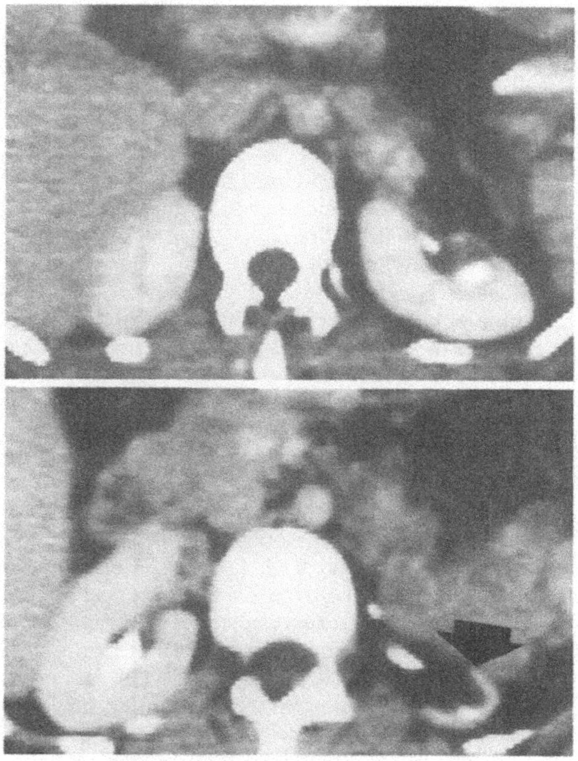

Fig. 4. Left renal pelvis duplication with atrophic caudal part of the malrotated kidney ("nubbin sign"; *arrow*) due to parenchymal atrophy in long-standing vesicoureteral reflux

Cystic Disease

Ultrasound encounters special problems in cystic disease:

- Echoes within the cysts, depending on gray scale equipment, hemorrhage, or infection
- No reliable differentiation between solid and liquid small structures (< 2 cm)
- Occasional smoothness of the opposite wall in tumors
- Occasionally sharp demarcation of tumors
- Echoes like normal sinus echoes caused by septa between cysts.

The special problems of CT are high attenuation values within the cyst, due to hemorrhage or infection, and artifacts caused by partial-volume effect, calcification of the wall, and streaks.

The main diagnostic problem is differentiation of centrally located cysts from hydronephrosis. Ultrasound shows interfaces between cysts, smoothness of the opposite cyst wall, and posterior acoustic enhancement with no visible ureter. In mild hydronephrosis there is a central sonolucent zone replacing the dense central echoes, in advanced hydronephrosis the "ring sign" with hypoechoic nonspherical areas radiating from a central renal pelvis and possibly a dilated ureter [7, 11,16].

On CT cysts display homogeneous low attenuation values (0 – 15 HU) without enhancement and appear round with smooth outer margins, no discernible wall, and sharp delineation from the surrounding parenchyma. Hydronephrosis is characterized by clear demarcation of dilated renal collecting structures and enhancement depending on renal function.

References

1. Anderegg LA (1983) Ultraschalldiagnostik der Nierenfehlbildungen. Ultraschall 4:160–165
2. Arafa NM, Fathi MM, Safnat M et al. (1982) Accuracy of ultrasound in the diagnosis of nonfunctioning kidneys. J Urol 128:1165–1169
3. Boijsen E (1983) Anomalies and malformations of the kidney. In: Abrams HL (ed) Angiography. Little Brown, Boston
4. Braedel HU, Schindler E (1981) Die Phlebographie, eine sichere und einfache Methode in der Diagnostik der Nierenagenesie/-dysgenesie. Röntgenblätter 34:180–184
5. Fiegler W, Friedrich M, Sörensen R (1975) Der Wert der Sonographie in der Diagnostik renaler raumfordernder Prozesse. Fortschr Röntgenstr 122:99–103
6. Fiegler W, Felix R (1981) Der Nierensinus im Sonogramm. Fortschr Röntgenstr 134:540–545
7. Jaschke W, van Kaick G, Palmtag H (1980) Vergleich der Wertigkeit von Echographie und CT bei der Diagnostik raumfordernder Prozesse der Nieren. Fortschr Röntgenstr 132:145–151
8. Jenss H, Schulze K, Klott KJ (1980) Hufeisenniere – ist sonographisch die Diagnose möglich? Fortschr Röntgenstr 133:71–74
9. Kolbenstvedt A, Lien HH (1982) Isolated renal hilar lip on CT. Radiology 143:150
10. Love L, Des Rosiers RJ (1966) Angiography of renal agenesis and dysgenesis. AJR 98:137–142
11. Madewell JE, Hartman DS, Lichtenstein JE (1979) Radiology – pathologic correlations in cystic disease of the kidney. Radiol Clin North Am 17(2): 261–279
12. Mascatello VJ, Smith EH, Carrera GF et al. (1977) Ultrasonic evaluation of the obstructed duplex kidney. AJR 129:113–120
13. Reed M, Friedman A, Nealey P (1982) Anomalies of the left renal vein: analysis of 433 CT scans. J Comput Assist Tomogr 6:1124–1126
14. Rosenfield AT, Hobbins JC, Taylor KJW, Cook JH (1979) Renal ultrasound. In: Rosenfield AT, Blickman MG, Hodson J (eds) Diagnostic imaging in renal disease. Appleton Century Crofts, New York
15. Stephenson T, Paul G (1979) Accessory renal hilus. AJR 132:765–768
16. Stuck KJ, Koff SA, Silver TM (1982) Ultrasonic features of multicystic dysplastic kidney: expanded diagnostic criteria. Radiology 143:217–221
17. Thornbury JR, McCormick TL, Silver TM (1980) Anatomic/radiologic classification of renal cortical nodules. AJR 134:1–7
18. Welter G, Schmidt KR, Rothenberger K et al. (1980) Bedeutung der Sonographie für die Differentialdiagnose von Pseudotumoren der Niere. Fortschr Röntgenstr 133:621–624

Diagnostic Workup of Ureteral Obstruction in the CT Era

M. A. Bosniak

Obstruction to the flow of urine is one of the most common problems affecting the urinary tract. Obstruction can occur anywhere along the system from the renal tubules to the urethral meatus. In this presentation, we will confine our discussion to hydronephrosis due to ureteral obstruction and particularly stress the role of CT in diagnosis and management of these cases.

Obstruction is often first discovered because of symptoms and signs pointing to urinary tract disease, but may also be discovered incidentally in the study of other abdominal conditions. In general, the radiologic workup to determine the site of the obstruction, the cause of the obstruction, and hence the treatment depends primarily on clinical parameters. These include the presenting complaint, the past medical history, and the results of laboratory testing (urinalysis, BUN, and creatinine).

The initial radiologic examination is greatly influenced by the clinical presentation. For example, if a patient has acute flank pain, then an intravenous urogram is the initial study. If the urogram reveals an obvious stone, further radiologic studies are not usually needed. On the other hand, if the patient presents with weakness and weight loss, and has a history of a previous malignancy, then CT probably should be the initial examination. However, if the BUN and creatinine are elevated, then the initial radiologic study might be an ultrasound examination or a CT scan without intravenous contrast. Not uncommonly, hydronephrosis is found incidentally when studying the patient for other abdominal disease with CT or sonography.

Techniques of Study

The radiologic studies that are currently used in the evaluation of the upper urinary tract include: intravenous urography, sonography, CT, pyelography (retrograde and antegrade), needle aspiration biopsy, nuclear medicine (for functional analysis), and magnetic resonance imaging (MRI).

Intravenous urography remains the most important initial radiologic examination of the urinary tract and is usually the examination first used in detecting obstruction and determining the likely cause. Urography will be used unless a specific contraindication to its use is present, such as laboratory evidence of renal failure or a strong history of contrast allergy. Urography would have less value in the staging or detection of abdominal neoplasm, in which case CT would be of more value. A limited urogram might be performed in association with CT by obtaining an abdominal film after the performance of the IV contrast-enhanced scan. Urography is of value because it can sensitively determine whether urinary tract obstruction is present and if so, whether unilateral or bilateral. The nature, degree, site, and in some instances, the etiology of any obstruction present can be determined. Urography also serves as a rough guide to the functional capacity of the obstructed kidney(s).

Sonography has particular use in evaluation of the urinary tract when there is evidence of renal failure and in helping determine whether the renal failure is due to bilateral hydronephrosis or due to other medical renal disease or vascular disease. It also has great value in the study of the nonvisualized kidney on urography to determine the presence of hydronephrosis. It is particularly important in pediatric practice, where radiation and instrumentation should be avoided as much as possible.

Computed tomography is indicated when the urogram is not specific in determining the etiology of obstruction and often as part of the evaluation and staging of a neoplasm. This technique can determine not only the presence of obstruction, but usually also the site and likely etiology. It obviates the need for pyelography (retrograde or antegrade) in many cases and enables accurate percutaneous needle biopsy for histologic confirmation when necessary.

Retrograde pyelography is needed less often in diagnosis, but is still necessary for evaluation of intrinsic collecting system diseases and for relief of obstruction in some instances. The urologist's collection of urine samples and performance of brush biopsy samples for diagnosis of urothelial tumors is facilitated by this approach.

Antegrade pyelography has been used when the retrograde technique has failed to determine the nature of the ureteral obstruction. However, both techniques have decreased application in the age of CT. Antegrade pyelography as part of the Whittaker test to determine urinary tract dilatation vs obstruction has occasional use for functional analysis [22].

Nuclear medicine studies are primarily used for determining the functional capacity of the obstructed kidney, and therefore the technique is important in some therapeutic decisions in hydronephrosis [6]. However, it has little use in determining the etiology of obstruction.

Percutaneous needle (aspiration) biopsy: The ability to detect periureteral disease by CT and then to obtain tissue for histologic diagnosis by percutaneous biopsy has been one of the important advances in medical diagnosis over the past 10 years. An untold number of exploratory abdominal surgeries to obtain tissue for diagnosis have been avoided.

Magnetic resonance imaging: The ability of MRI to image the urinary tract and retroperitoneum has already been shown to be a potentially great advance in radiologic diagnosis. However, the experience accumulated so far is insufficient to determine its role, and the technique is not yet readily available.

The Use of CT in Ureteral Obstruction

The ureter is one of the more common sites of urinary tract obstruction and the use of CT in the diagnosis of ureteral obstruction will be emphasized and demonstrated. As mentioned before, urography is often the initial radiologic study for the evaluation of most patients with hydronephrosis. If the etiology of the obstruction is evident from the urogram, treatment is directed at relieving the obstruction and treating the underlying etiology. If the etiology of the obstruction is not clear, then depending on either the clinical story or the urographic appearance, retrograde pyelography or CT is often performed for further evaluation. If the patient has a history of hematuria or the urographic appearance suggests an intraluminal ureteral abnormality, retrograde pyelography should be performed. On the other hand, if the patient has a history of previous malignancy, CT would be in order.

Table 1. Etiology of ureteral obstruction studied by CT

1. Malignant disease
   a) Metastatic neoplasm of retroperitoneum and/or periureteral tissues (malignant retroperitoneal fibrosis)
   b) Lymphoma
   c) Primary ureteral tumors
2. Benign conditions
   a) Calculus disease
   b) Retroperitoneal fibrosis
      Benign causes
      – Perianeurysmal fibrosis
      – Radiation fibrosis, postsurgical fibrosis, and inflammatory fibrosis
      – Secondary to methysergide use
      – Idiopathic
3. Miscellaneous conditions
   a) Inflammatory bowel disease
   b) Retroperitoneal or pelvic abscess, hematoma, or urinoma
   c) Gynecologic tumors, benign or malignant
   d) Endometriosis
   e) Ovarian vein syndrome

We have found CT to be diagnostic or very helpful in determining the etiology of ureteral obstruction whose nature is unclear on the preliminary urogram in well over 95% of patients studied [7]. The various etiologies of ureteral obstruction seen in our experience are listed in Table 1 and comprise a wide range of disease processes, both malignant and benign. By far the most frequent cause of ureteral obstruction in which CT was used (over three-quarters of the cases) was metastatic carcinoma to the ureter or periureteral tissues.

In the great majority of cases, the patient had a known, previously treated primary malignancy but no evidence of metastatic disease at the time of presentation with ureteral obstruction. In a small percentage of cases, the patient had no history of primary malignancy, and ureteral obstruction was the initial manifestation of what proved to be malignant disease. Patients with malignant disease were eventually diagnosed either by tissue biopsy or by the appearance of widespread metastatic disease and by the clinical course. The remaining cases are a mixture of benign and malignant conditions that could not be diagnosed accurately by routine urography or pyelography but whose etiology could be determined with CT.

CT has been least helpful in patients with a history of malignant disease who do not have a distinct mass seen at the site of ureteral obstruction. CT is able to determine the level of obstruction, but because the usual sharp tissue planes may be obscured in these patients, particularly if they have received radiation therapy, it may not be possible to specify whether the ureteral obstruction is due to recurrent tumor or to fibrosis secondary to radiation or previous surgery. If a defined mass of tissue greater than 2–3 cm is seen, this generally indicates recurrent tumor, which can be confirmed by percutaneous aspiration biopsy. However, failure to obtain malignant cells by biopsy in such a case does not rule out malignancy, and repeat biopsy or surgical exploration might be necessary. Equally important is the realization that not seeing a defined mass on CT does not rule out malignancy. We have seen several patients in whom the point of ureteral obstruction was identified but a specific periureteral mass could not be identified on CT. Two of these patients were surgically explored, and although no periureteral tumor mass was seen at surgery, biopsy of the periureteral tissue at the point of obstruction revealed malignancy [16]. Fortunately, this is not a common presentation of metastatic malignancy.

The use of CT in evaluating ureteral obstruction has become more widespread as CT equipment has become more available. In many cases where retrograde or antegrade pyelography were used in the past, CT is now used, because it is less invasive and in most instances more definitive.

CT performed without IV contrast enhancement has an obvious application (as does sonography) in patients with urinary tract obstruction who have contrast allergy, renal failure, or a nonfunctioning kidney on urography. However, because of its ability to visualize the retroperitoneum more clearly than sonography, CT can be more specific. Likewise, CT has an advantage over retrograde pyelography in periureteral disease in that it can evaluate the ureteral surroundings; pyelography merely visualizes the affect of the disease on the ureteral lumen. Another major advantage of CT is that it outlines the periureteral disease process for percutaneous biopsy.

Ureteral Obstruction Due to Malignant Disease

Metastatic Neoplasm to Retroperitoneum and Periureteral Tissues

Urinary tract obstruction secondary to malignant neoplasm has been the most common use for CT in ureteral obstruction. Metastases reach the periureteral tissues either by hematogenous or lymphatic dissemination or by direct extension [2, 13, 14]. The primary tumors that most commonly metastasize to the retroperitoneum are carcinoma of the breast, stomach, prostate, pancreas, lung, and colon [20, 9]. The tumor obliterates tissue planes and envelops the ureter. Some neoplasms incite an intense desmoplastic response – "malignant retroperitoneal fibrosis" – in the surrounding tissues which obstructs the ureter. These cases can be difficult to prove by percutaneous aspiration biopsy or even surgical biopsy, as the nests of tumor cells may be widely scattered in the mass of fibrous tissue.

The findings on urography in patients with metastatic neoplasm in the retroperitoneum will vary considerably depending on the level and degree of obstruction. Retrograde pyelography can usually differentiate intrinsic from extrinsic ureteral disease, but in many cases the etiology of the narrowing or obstruction of the ureter is unclear (Fig. 1). CT offers the opportunity to visualize the periureteral tissues, determine the existence and extent of a periureteral mass, and localize it specifically for needle biopsy, so that in patients with urinary tract obstruction and a history of previous malignancy, pyelography is usually noncontributory and CT should be performed instead (Fig. 2).

The appearance of metastatic disease of the retroperitoneum on CT is somewhat variable. It appears most commonly as lobulated para-aortic and paracaval masses resembling lymphadenopathy, but also as solitary masses or as infiltrating mantles of tissue surrounding and obliterating tissue planes. In most instances in our experience, the CT appearance was characteristic of neoplasm, but occasionally a nonmalignant fibrotic process can give a very similar picture. For this reason, histologic confirmation is necessary.

In our experience, over 95% of patients with metastatic disease of the retroperitoneum causing ureteral obstruction show a mass of tissue at the point of obstruction which can be percutaneously biopsied, and over 90% of the biopsies are positive for metastatic malignancy. Often, extensive retroperitoneal and/or focal metastatic disease to

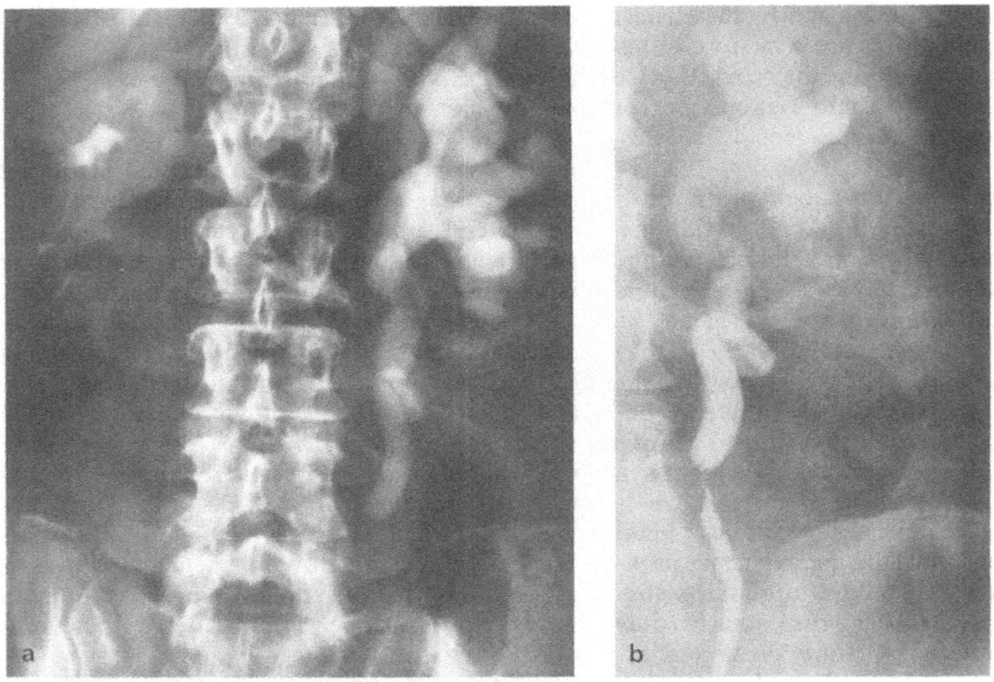

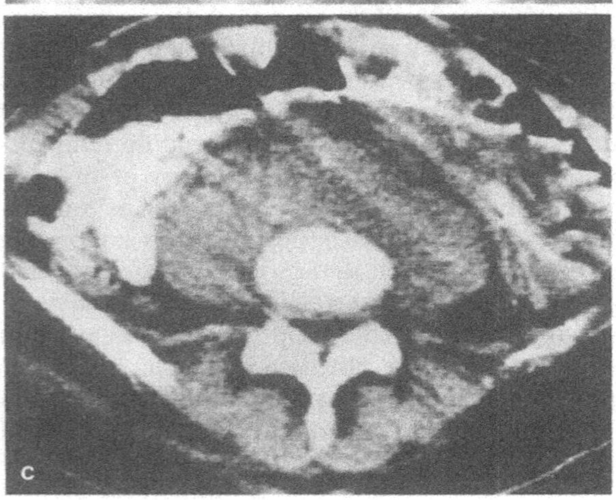

Fig. 1 a – c. A 79-year-old woman who had had carcinoma of the colon 6 years earlier had a bone scan for back pain and hydronephrosis of the left kidney was suggested. **a** Urogram: hydronephrosis of left kidney and dilated upper left ureter is noted, with obstruction at level of iliac crest. **b** Left retrograde pyelogram reveals narrowed segment of left ureter. **c** CT scan at level of ureteral obstruction reveals large mass enveloping retroperitoneal structures consistent with recurrent tumor. Percutaneous needle aspiration biopsy revealed adenocarcinoma consistent with previous colon primary. In most patients with a history of previous malignancy and ureteral obstruction, CT will be more revealing than pyelography. (From [7])

abdominal organs is also seen in these cases, making the diagnosis of metastatic disease obvious.

In an occasional patient with metastatic carcinoma as the etiology of the ureteral obstruction there are false-negative results on CT, no mass being seen at the site of obstruction. Percutaneous needle biopsy at the level of ureteral obstruction, even without a demonstrable mass, might be tried [4] and may occasionally be productive, but a negative result does not rule out malignancy and surgical exploration might be necessary unless disease can be documented elsewhere. False-positive CT results are also possible in those patients who have had radiation therapy, since CT cannot distinguish radiation fibrosis from periureteral fibrosis caused by a metastatic tumor. In these cases, surgical biopsy may be necessary. However, the false-positive and false-negative studies make up less than 5% of the total.

Lymphoma

While retroperitoneal lymphoma frequently causes hydronephrosis, it is rarely the initial manifestation of the disease. Usually, the patient is already known to have the disease and the etiology of the ureteral obstruction is obvious. CT can define retroperitoneal adenopathy and/or an extranodal mass, and needle biopsy can differen-

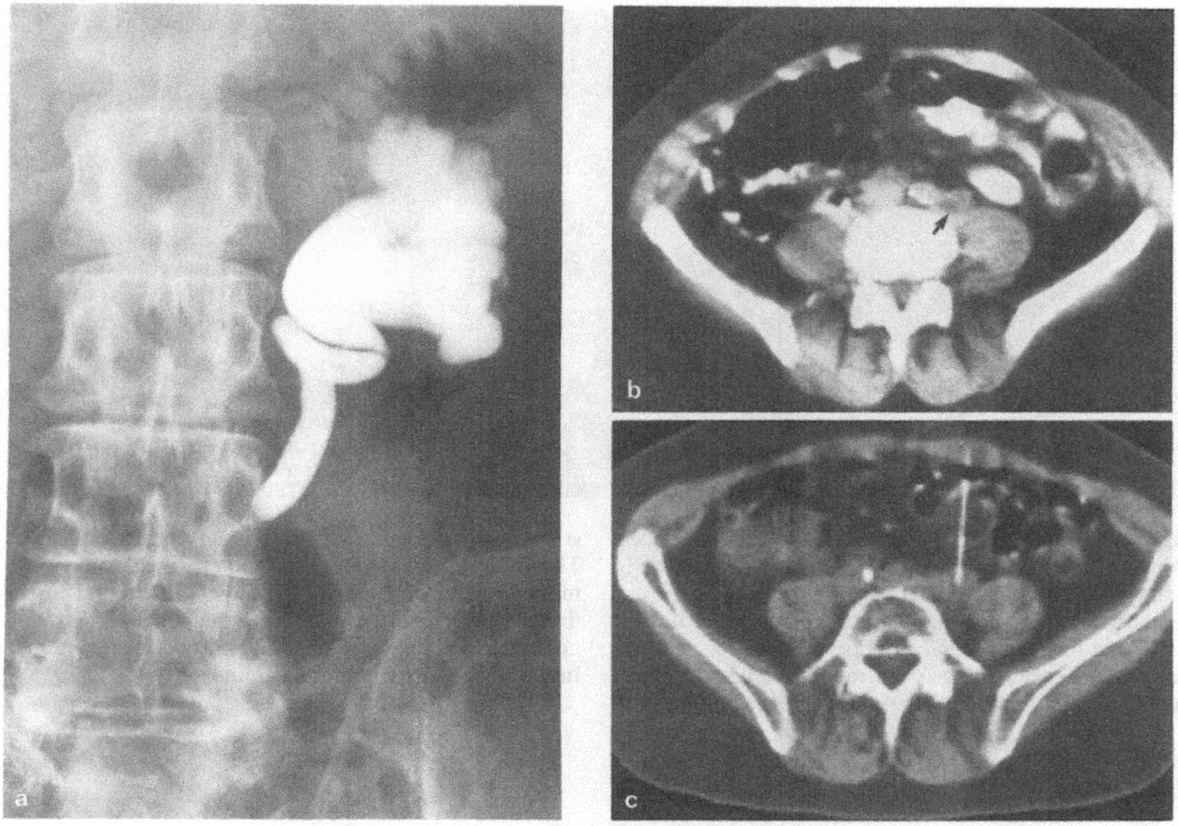

Fig. 2 a – c. A 61-year-old woman complained of back pain. She had had her uterus removed for adenocarcinoma 3 years earlier. Urography did not visualize the left kidney. **a** Delayed film from retrograde pyelogram reveals hydronephrosis with obstruction of the mid-ureter at level of L4. Some medial deviation of the ureter is noted. **b** CT scan performed at the level of the ureteral obstruction reveals a soft tissue mass (*arrow*) adjacent to the aorta suggestive of metastatic tumor. **c** CT scan at the time of aspiration biopsy, showing the needle in the tumor mass. Cytologic evaluation indicated metastatic adenocarcinoma consistent with uterine primary

tiate lymphomatous adenopathy from metastatic disease in those cases in which the etiology of retroperitoneal lymph nodes is unknown.

Primary Ureteral Tumors

Primary ureteral neoplasms are usually readily identified by urography and pyelography, and it is rare that CT is needed to help establish the diagnosis. However, in the occasional case where the etiology of ureteral obstruction is unclear and it is difficult to differentiate nonopaque calculus from intraluminal tumor or intrinsic from extrinsic tumor, CT can be very accurate in making the distinction. In a patient with an intraluminal defect, if CT fails to demonstrate the increased attenuation seen with calculus disease, the diagnosis is likely to be primary ureteral neoplasm [5]. CT can also clearly define the ureteral obstruction as being intraluminal vs extrinsic by showing the intraluminal lesion and the periureteral tissues (Fig. 3).

Ureteral Obstruction Due to Benign Conditions

Calculus Disease

On occasion, a radiolucent or faintly calcified obstructing ureteral stone cannot be diagnosed by urography and/or pyelography, particularly in the portion of the ureter overlying the pelvic bones. It is in this setting that CT can be particularly helpful. Calculi have increased attenuation on CT, whether or not they contain calcium. Nonopaque

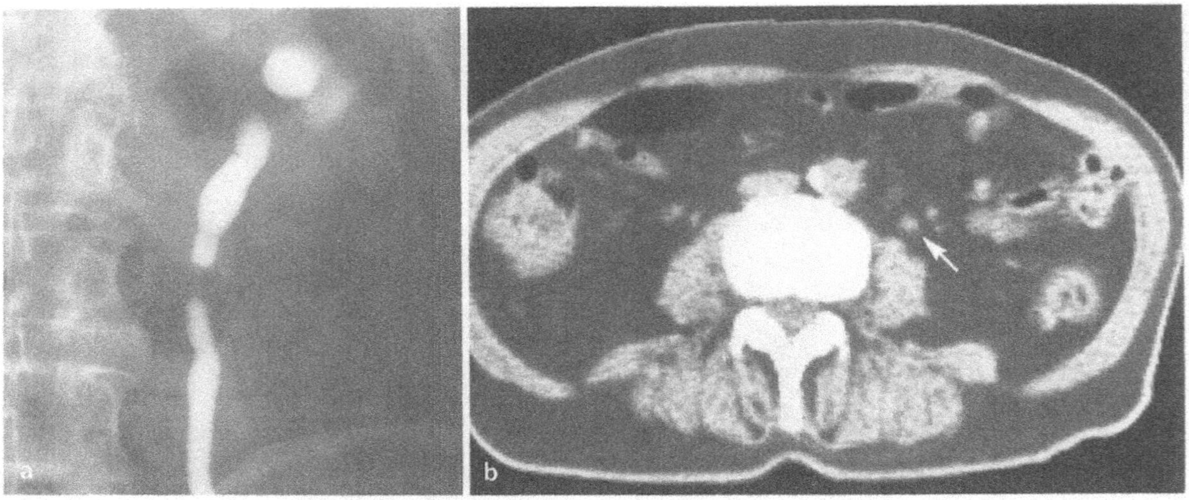

Fig. 3a, b. A 70-year-old man had some left-sided back pain. An intravenous urogram revealed hydronephrosis with mid-ureteral narrowing. **a** Retrograde pyelography demonstrates the short narrowed segment of the ureter. **b** CT scan through the narrowed segment shows a small soft tissue density (*arrow*) indicated localized thickening of the ureteral wall. The increased attenuation of a stone is not present, and there is no periureteral mass. These films indicate that the lesion is likely to be a primary ureteral carcinoma. Note that just lateral to the ureter is a structure representing the gonadal vein. Left nephrectomy and ureterectomy was performed for an invasive, anaplastic ureteral carcinoma

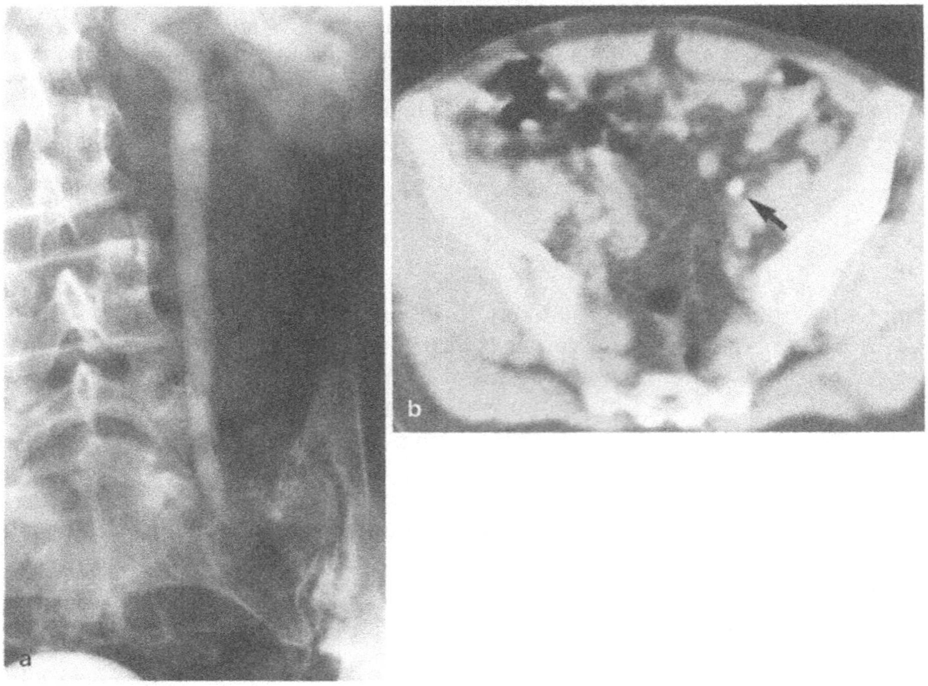

Fig. 4a, b. A 50-year-old man had left flank pain. **a** Urogram reveals obstruction of the ureter at the level of S1. On the preliminary film no opaque calcification could be seen. Retrograde pyelogram could not be performed. **b** CT scan at level of ureteral obstruction was performed without oral or intravenous contrast. An area of increased attenuation is noted (*arrow*), indicating a calculus. The patient eventually had to have surgical removal of a uric acid calculus. (From [16])

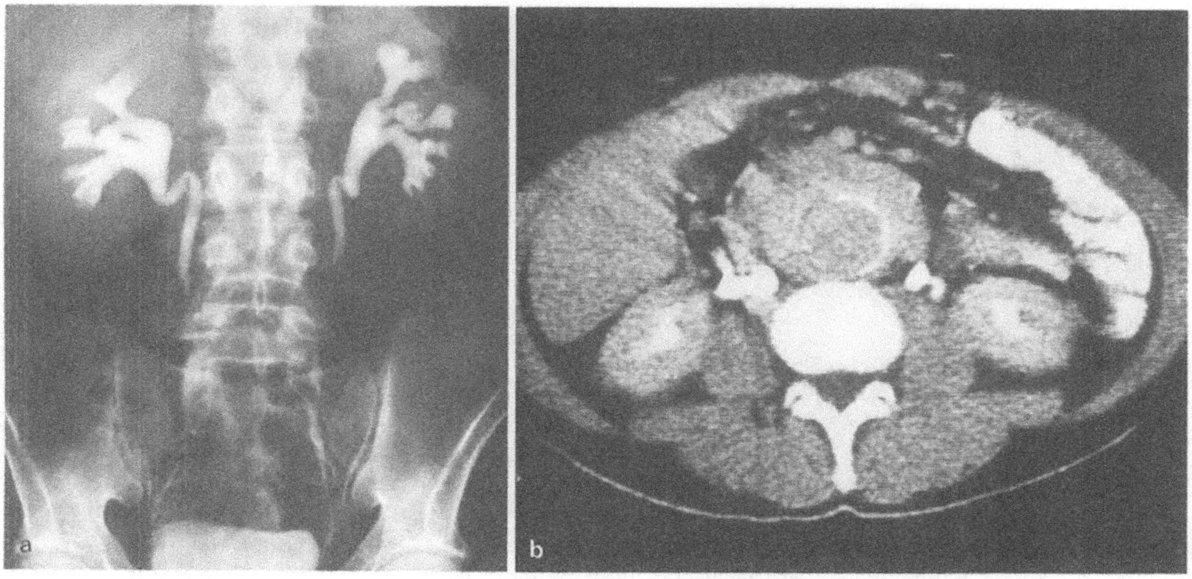

Fig. 5a, b. A 61-year-old man had low back pain. **a** Urography revealed mild bilateral hydronephrosis with obstruction seen at the mid-ureters. Some slight medial deviation of the ureters is present. **b** CT scan at level of ureteral obstruction reveals an aneurysm of the abdominal aorta. A cuff of fibrotic tissue is seen surrounding the aneurysm encasing and obstructing the adjacent ureters. At surgery, an inflammatory aneurysm of the abdominal aorta was resected and the encased ureters were dissected free. (From [17])

stones (uric acid, cystine) show increased attenuation compared to surrounding tissues [1, 12, 18]. CT identification of this increased attenuation at the point of ureteral obstruction is diagnostic of calculus, and while the problem is not common, this information can be very important in patient management (Fig. 4).

Retroperitoneal Fibrosis

Retroperitoneal fibrosis is caused by both malignant disease (as described earlier) and a number of benign conditions [3]. Whereas it is generally impossible to distinguish benign from malignant fibrosis on CT, the pattern of involvement and the clinical history can be very revealing. For instance, methysergide maleate, used for vascular headache relief, has been implicated in causing retroperitoneal fibrosis, and a history of the use of this drug would be almost diagnostic as to etiology.

Perianeurysmal Fibrosis

Inflammatory perianeurysmal fibrosis that can trap adjacent ureters and cause hydronephrosis is an entity that is being increasingly recognized [8, 17, 19, 21]. CT can detect this process by visualizing the aneurysm, the large perianeurysmal fibrotic mass, and the involved ureters (Fig. 5).

Radiation Fibrosis and Postsurgical Fibrosis

It is a limitation of CT that it is unable to distinguish benign fibrosis from malignant fibrosis. Fortunately, it is not common for radiation or surgical fibrosis to cause ureteral obstruction, but when this does occur it can be impossible to distinguish the condition from malignancy.

Idiopathic Retroperitoneal Fibrosis

The CT findings in retroperitoneal fibrosis have been well described [10, 11]. In most instances, the smooth fibrotic encasement of retroperitoneal structures is quite characteristic. In other instances, differentiation from malignant retroperitoneal fibrosis cannot be made by CT. If a patient has not had a previous malignancy, has not had radiation or retroperitoneal surgery, has not been taking methysergide, and has the characteristic urographic, pyelographic, and CT findings

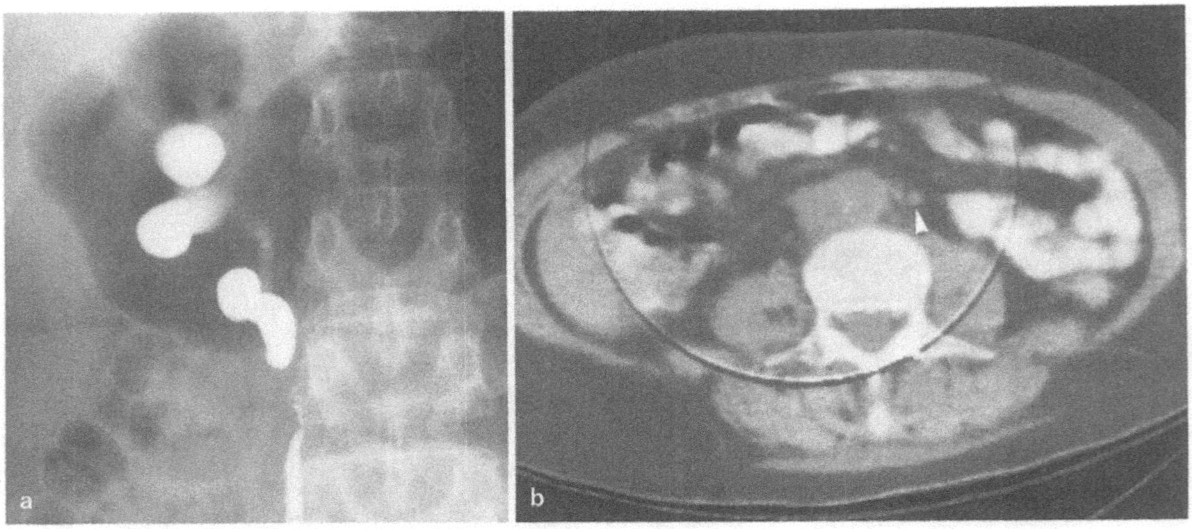

Fig. 6a, b. A 67-year-old woman entered the hospital for workup of hypertension. There was no history of prior malignancy. Urography did not visualize the right kidney. **a** Retrograde pyelography reveals a markedly narrowed, somewhat medially placed segment of the upper ureter with severe hydronephrosis. **b** CT scan performed at site of obstruction reveals loss of the usual tissue planes about the aorta and inferior vena cava. No discrete mass is present, but the right ureter is caught up in this perivascular density. Note that the left ureter (*arrowhead*) is somewhat medially placed and is just outside the fibrotic mass. The findings are quite characteristic of idiopathic retroperitoneal fibrosis. Artifactual ring density is superimposed on image. At surgery, the right ureter was freed from the fibrotic mass. No evidence of malignancy was found. (From [16])

of retroperitoneal fibrosis, the diagnosis of idiopathic retroperitoneal fibrosis can be made with considerable certainty (Fig. 6). However, with a history of prior malignancy, histologic confirmation of this diagnosis is necessary.

Miscellaneous Conditions

Other less common conditions in which CT has been valuable in determining the etiology of unexplained obstruction are noted in Table 1. The list is long, showing the importance of the technique in determining the etiology of obstruction in a wide variety of instances. In many of our cases, the treatment approach to the patient was changed because of the CT findings. This was particularly true in the cases of inflammatory bowel disease, abscess, and hematoma, where a surgical approach was changed to medical treatment, or to percutaneous drainage in the case of abscess. One noteworthy example of the value of the technique was seen in a case of inflammatory bowel disease. In the workup for suspected neoplasm, CT revealed thickened loops of bowel adjacent to the obstructed ureter. Since no solid mass was present in the area of ureteral obstruction, the diagnosis of inflammatory bowel disease was suggested. Small bowel series revealed Crohn's disease of the ileum, the first suggestion of that condition, and the subsequent clinical course confirmed the diagnosis [15].

Conclusion

It is clear that CT can be extremely helpful in evaluating the etiology of ureteral obstruction when this information is not clear from urography and pyelography. Because CT can visualize the periureteral tissues, it can help define metastatic neoplasm and clearly distinguishes between intrinsic and extrinsic ureteral disease. Since it can appreciate the increased attenuation of a calculus, it can differentiate stone from ureteral tumor. It makes a major contribution by outlining periureteral disease processes for percutaneous needle biopsy, which can eliminate exploratory laparotomy for tissue diagnosis. In our experience, the use of CT has been helpful in defining the etiology of ureteral obstruction in over 95% of cases. The major limitation of the technique is that it cannot distinguish between radiation fibrosis and malignant fibrosis and will miss those cases when tumor recurs without a distinctive mass. However, this accounts for only a small proportion of cases. The use of CT contributes greatly to less invasive diagnosis and treatment. We believe that CT should replace pyelography in the evaluation of many cases and will make surgical exploration unneccessary for diagnosis in almost all instances.

References

1. Alter AJ, Peterson DT, Plautz AC Jr (1979) Non-opaque calculus demonstrated by computerized tomography. J Urol 122:699–700
2. Ambos MA, Bosniak MA, Megibow AJ, Raghavendra B (1979) Ureteral involvement by metastatic disease. Urol Radiol 1:105–112
3. Arger PH, Stolz JL, Miller WT (1973) Retroperitoneal fibrosis. An analysis of the clinical spectrum and roentgenographic signs. AJR 119:812–821
4. Barbaric ZL, MacIntosh PK (1981) Periureteral thin-needle aspiration biopsy. Urol Radiol 2:181–185
5. Baron RL, McClennan BL, Lee JKT, Lawson TL (1982) Computed tomography of transitional cell carcinoma of the renal pelvis and ureter. Radiology 145:743–747
6. Blaufox MD, Kalika V, Scharf S, Milstein D (1982) Applications of nuclear medicine in genitourinary imaging. Urol Radiol 4:155–164
7. Bosniak MA, Megibow AJ, Ambos MA, Mitnick JS, Lefleur RS, Gordon R (1982) Computed tomography of ureteral obstruction. AJR 138:1107–1113
8. Brock J, Soloway MS (1980) Retroperitoneal fibrosis and aortic aneurysm. Urology 15:14–16
9. Cohen WM, Freed SZ, Hasson J (1974) Metastatic cancer to the ureter. A review of the literature and case presentations. J Urol 112:188–189
10. Dalla Palma L, Rocca-Rossetti S, Pozzi-Mucelli RS, Rizzatto G (1981) Computed tomography in the diagnosis of retroperitoneal fibrosis. Urol Radiol 3:77–83
11. Fagan CJ, Larrien AJ, Amparo EG (1979) Retroperitoneal fibrosis. Ultrasound and CT features. AJR 133:239–243
12. Federle MP, McAninch JW, Kaiser JA, Goodman PC, Roberts J, Mall JC (1981) Computed tomography of urinary calculi. AJR 136:255–258
13. Feun LG, Drelichman A, Singhakowinta A, Vaitkevicius VK (1979) Ureteral obstruction secondary to metastatic breast carcinoma. Cancer 44:1164–1171
14. Geller SA, Lin CS (1975) Ureteral obstruction from metastatic breast carcinoma. Arch Pathol 99:476–478
15. Megibow AJ, Bosniak MA, Ambos MA, Redmond PE (1981) Crohn's disease causing hydronephrosis. J Comput Assist Tomogr 5:909–911
16. Megibow AJ, Mitnick JS, Bosniak MA (1982) The contribution of computed tomography to the evaluation of the obstructed ureter. Urol Radiol 4:95–104
17. Megibow AJ, Ambos MA, Bosniak MA (1980) Computed tomographic diagnosis of ureteral obstruction secondary to aneurysmal disease. Urol Radiol 1:211–215
18. Segal AJ, Shapiro RF, Linke CA, Frank IN, Rabinowitz R (1978) Diagnosis of non-opaque calculi by computed tomography. Radiology 129:447–450
19. Saxton HM, Allibone GW (1980) The association of aorta-iliac aneurysms with ureteral obstruction. Urol Radiol 1:205–210
20. Usher SM, Brendler H, Ciavarra VA (1977) Retroperitoneal fibrosis secondary to metastatic neoplasm. Urology 9:191–194
21. Vint VC, Usselman JA, Warmath MA, Dilley RB (1980) Aortic perianeurysmal fibrosis. Computed tomographic density enhancement and ureteral obstruction. AJR 134:577–580
22. Whittaker RH (1981) Percutaneous upper urinary tract dynamics in equivocal obstruction. Urol Radiol 2:187–189

Radiologic Management of Adult Traumatic Renal and Pelvic Hemorrhage

H. Schmoller, R. Kloss, and T. Irnberger

Blunt Renal Trauma

To evaluate a blunt renal trauma we have nowadays the following diagnostic methods: (a) plain film of the urogenital tract, (b) excretory urography with zonography, (c) sonography, (d) CT, and (e) angiography. We demand from all these procedures that they can be performed rapidly, do not harm to the patient, and permit a precise and unmistakable statement about the injury and its extent, thus leading to the appropriate therapy. In blunt renal trauma we can distinguish acute direct lesions from late traumatic lesions. The classification of the blunt renal trauma according to Hodges [1] is commonly accepted (Table 1). The diagnostic sequence generally followed is shown in Fig. 1. The sequence must be modified, however, with regard to interventional therapy. Angiography is then carried out before sonography and CT, immediately after urography, or immediately after CT. A decision to this effect will be made in the presence of massive life-threatening hematuria, since as much renal parenchyma as possible should be preserved. Arterial catheter embolization has been employed since 1973, first being used in the cerebral region. In blunt renal trauma it was first employed by Richman et al. in 1977 [5].

The reason for the efficiency of transcatheter embolization in a bleeding blunt renal trauma lies in the anatomic structure of the kidneys. Renal arteries are end-arteries. Blockage of a renal arterial branch stops the arterial bleeding and also the venous backflow. In principle one should use the angiographic technique which one also practises for conventional angiography and the embolization material with which one is familiar. It is recommended to block as selectively as possible in order to preserve as much renal parenchyma as possible.

Grave complications are not usual. Reflux into lumbar arteries must be guarded against, and uninjured segmental arteries should be preserved. Complications of infection are avoided by using an appropriate technique. One must reckon with the side effect of hypertension, although no cases are described in the literature. The application of transfemoral catheter embolization must always be adapted to the individual circumstances and arranged in a flexible manner. It should be performed when massive life-threatening bleeding is present which cannot be controlled except with nephrectomy.

Traumatic Pelvic Hemorrhage

Transfemoral angiographic occlusion by embolization in massive traumatic bleeding in the pelvis was first reported by Ring et al. in 1973 [6].

In the past, about 60% of pelvic trauma deaths were from loss of blood. The effect of a central ligature is questioned by several authors because of the possibility of peripheral collaterals. In addition, hemorrhage in severe pelvic trauma is partly caused by rupture of venous branches and therefore cannot be stopped by arterial embolization.

Hemorrhage is sometimes caused by removal of a tamponading and therefore therapeutic hema-

Table 1. Classification of blunt renal trauma according to Hodges

Group I	Mild injury: normal urogram, temporary hematuria
Group II	Severe injury: rupture of the renal capsule, rupture of the parenchymal as far as the collecting system, injured collecting system, perineal hematoma, urinary, severe, urographic changes
Group III	Critical injury: partial or total organ destruction with vessel or renal hilus disruption, nonfunctioning kidney in the urogram, severe bleeding

toma during surgery. Motsay et al. [3] stated that especially veins lead to bleeding, but Reinold et al. [4] showed that in a series of 25 bilateral pelvic venograms after severe trauma, just one bleeding vein could be found.

So it seems that massive hematomas arise from bleeding of major arterial branches. Certain types of fractures of the pelvis lead to disruption of special vessel branches.

Catheter embolization in the pelvis is, for the reasons mentioned, limited to individual cases. The angiographic technique is in principle the same as in the management of renal trauma. A precondition is exact localization of the source of bleeding. The superselective blockage of the vessel must of course be optimal. Complications may arise related to the angiographic technique, and there may be ischemia with claudication of the buttocks if the tip of the catheter is not distal to the origin of the superior gluteal artery. Furthermore, the risk of impotence in men and also bladder gangrene after embolization of the internal iliac artery are reported.

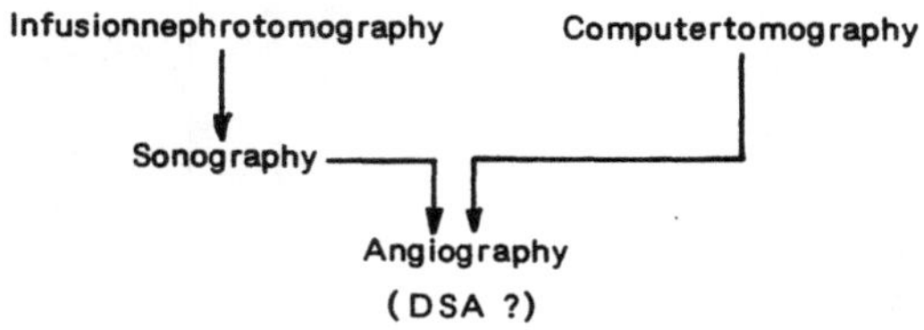

Fig. 1. Diagnostic sequence in blunt renal trauma

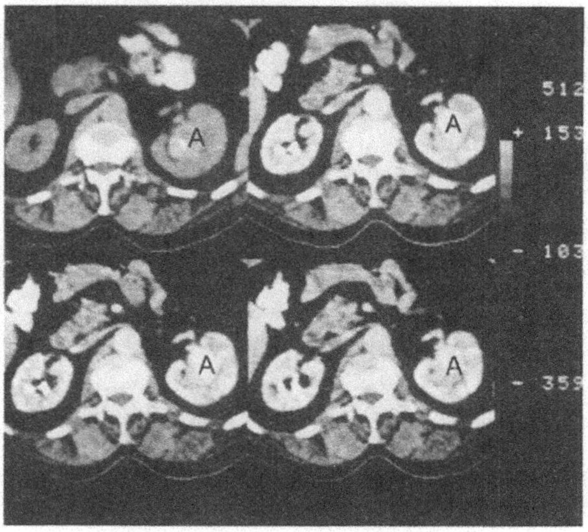

Fig. 2. Arteriovenous aneurysm in the left kidney (*A*) demonstrated by contrast dynamic CT

Late Effects of Renal Trauma

Late consequences of renal trauma can have general effects on the organism, e.g., chronic hematuria, hypertension, and, in the case of big arteriovenous fistulas, right heart failure.

If late changes after trauma are suspected, angiography should be performed first, or possibly after CT. Late angiography can demonstrate arteriovenous fistulas, post-traumatic aneurysms, stenoses, and parenchymal changes in form of defects and scars [2]. The angiographic demonstration is important, since it may lead directly to interventional therapy.

Case Report

A 64-year-old man suffered from severe, painless, intermittent hematuria 6 weeks after a blunt flank trauma. Urography revealed a normal right kidney. On the left, there was delayed nephrographic effect and no excretory function. Sonography also revealed a normal right kidney. On the left side there was found an approximately 3-cm cystic lesion in the upper pole of the kidney. Contrast dynamic CT and contrast flow curves showed that this was no usual cyst, confirming the suspicion of post-traumatic arteriovenous aneurysm which had arisen on routine CT. This was proven with the characteristic flow curves of aorta and vena cava (Fig. 2).

The results of CT could now be confirmed by angiography. The films showed a plumsized aneurysm fed by an enlarged interlobar artery. The venous backflow was early via a great venous vessel (Fig. 3). The evaluated high shunt volume and the hematuria demanded active therapy.

Operative ligation of the feeding artery for obliteration of the fistula involves partial renal resection, and in unfavorable circumstances may lead to nephrectomy, and therefore transcatheter embolization was performed after superselective angiography of the feeding arterial branch. Collagen and cyanacrylate was made radiographically visible with contrast medium and used for embolization.

To prevent antegrade washout of the embolization material along the venous pathway, a balloon catheter was inserted in the renal vein. In this way we succeeded in obtaining complete filling of the aneurysm, which thrombosed (Fig. 4). The blood supply of the remaining renal parenchyma was in no way disturbed.

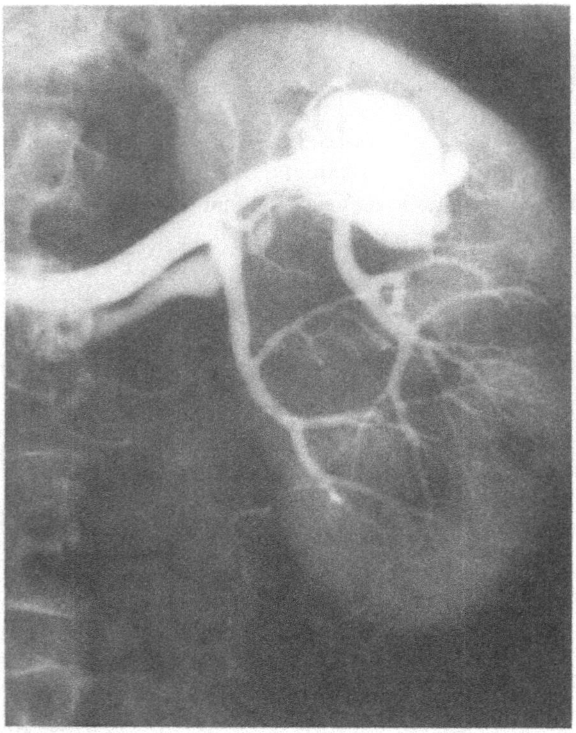

Fig. 3. Arteriovenous aneurysm in the left kidney demonstrated by selective angiography

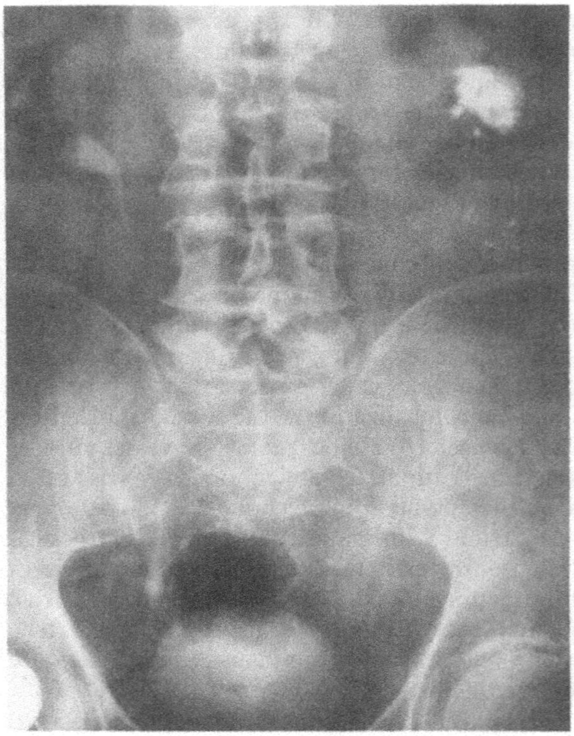

Fig. 4. The thrombosed aneurysm in the left kidney

A control study by means of excretory urography and angio-CT showed an improvement of the excretory function. The renal collecting system was now visible and the hematuria had stopped.

Summary

The radiologic management of blunt renal trauma is possible because renal arteries are end-arteries. It is also possible to stop the venous backflow after arterial embolization. The application is limited to cases in which there is massive hemorrhage from segmentary arteries, and as much renal parenchyma as possible should be preserved. Embolization of pelvic arteries is problematic in a trauma, because the amount of bleeding from the iliac veins cannot be estimated, and venous bleeding in this region cannot always be stopped by means of arterial embolization. This procedure is limited to individual cases.
Interventional management is helpful in posttraumatic lesions of the kidneys, especially in arteriovenous fistulas and aneurysms.

References

1. Lutzeyer W (1981) Traumatologie des Urogenitaltraktes. Springer, Berlin Heidelberg New York
2. Maranta E, Schnauder A (1964) Angiographie und Nierentrauma. Schweiz Med Wochenschr 94:1484–1490
3. Motsay GJ, Manlou C, Perry JF (1969) Major venous injury with pelvic fracture. J Trauma 9:343–346
4. Reynolds BM, Balsano NA (1971) Venography in pelvic fractures: a clinical evaluation. Ann Surg 173:104–106
5. Richman DST, Green WM, Kroll R, Casarella JW (1977) Superselective transcatheter embolisation of traumatic renal hemorrhage. AJR 128:843–844
6. Ring JE, Athanasoulis CH, Waltman CA, Margolis NM, Baum S (1973) Arteriographic management of hemorrhage following pelvic fracture. Radiology 109:65–70

Examinations of the Female Lower Urinary Tract and Ureter

G. Egender, H. Frommhold, and A. Furtschegger

The conventional radiologic methods (excretory urogram, retrograde and anterograde pyelography, urethrocystography, miction cystogram) are undisputed as the standard methods of determining morphologic and functional, pathologic alterations in the urinary tract. They provide direct and indirect evidence on the location, form and extent of a lesion. However, in some respects – cause of an obstruction, displacement of the ureter, pathological changes in the area surrounding the urinary tract, alterations in the walls of the bladder – there are limits to the information that conventional radiology can supply, and it has been supplemented by other imaging methods.

As an alternative to CT examination, ultrasonography is now increasingly being used as a diagnostic supplement to the usual conventional methods of examining the lower urinary tract. Noninvasiveness and the absence of radiation exposure are the advantages of this method that are of special value when examining children, juveniles, patients of child-bearing age, and pregnant women.

In pregnant patients and those of child-bearing age the possibilities offered by ultrasonographic diagnostics are exhausted in full to avoid radiation exposure, while for older patients ultrasonography takes second place to conventional radiologic methods, providing no more than supplementary information.

Table 1. Indications for ureteral sonography

Pathomorphologic	Functional
Obstruction	Vesicourethral reflux
Malformations	(pre- or postoperative)
Ectopic opening	
Ureterocele	
Ureteral diverticulum	
Prune Belly syndrome	

However, the quality of ultrasound images of structures of the female lower urinary tract is restricted by superimposed gas, fresh wounds, scars, and bone. Although the evidence provided by ultrasonography is sufficient in some diagnostic respects, particularly in the area of the ureters and the urethra, the image quality does not compare with that of conventional radiologic methods. Ultrasound examination is time-consuming for the examiner and requires him to have considerable experience in echo diagnostics.

Examination of the Ureters

Only a dilated ureter can be shown by ultrasonography, therefore the most important indication is obstruction (Table 1).

The sonographic image of the ureter can be divided into three methodologic sections related to the anatomical structures concerned [5]. The first ranges from the pyeloureteral transition to the lower renal pole and is examined in frontal section.

The second reaches from the caudal renal pole to the intersection of the iliac artery and vein. The ultrasound image is obtained from the ventral direction. The ureter is shown running in a straight or curving line parallel to the aorta and crossing the iliac artery and vein ventrally.

In the third section, from the vascular intersection to the ostium in the bladder the ureter is seen from a transverse direction as a ventral, oval, vascular structure with the iliac artery and vein running longitudinally. If the transducer is used in the direction of the ureter, the above-mentioned vessels are seen in cross section. The ureter runs from ventral to caudal into the small pelvis, where the intestinal gas above a short prevesical section makes it hardly visible. The ureter can be seen well somewhat pre- and retrovesically through the full bladder. The intramural ureter is also easily accessible through transurethral sonography.

Table 2. Obstructions of upper ureter ($n = 24$)

Stone proven	12 (57%)
No stone proven	9 (43%)
Aneurysm	1
Pregnancy	2

Table 3. Obstructions of middle ureter ($n = 26$)

Proof of stone	4 (36%)
Tumor	1
Pregnancy	2
Proof of obstructed passage	44%
No proof of stone	7 (64%)
Retroperitoneal fibrosis	1
Postoperative stricture	1
No proof of obstructed passage	56%

Table 4. Obstruction of lower ureter ($n = 43$)

Direct proof of obstructed passage	
Concretions	5
Tumor	5
Ureterocele	6
Megaloureter	6
Infravesical obstruction	11
Total	33 (76%)
No direct proof of obstructed passage	
Concretions	5
Tumor	3
Megaloureter	1
Stricture	1
Total	10 (24%)

The dilation can be caused by any one of several pathologic changes. Obstruction can be due to concretion, tumor, fibrosis, pregnancy, trauma, malformation, or afflictions of the bladder, prostate, or urethra.

Obstructions Caused by Concretions

Tables 2–4 show our own results for the upper, middle, and lower parts of the ureter in cases, where ultrasound was used primarily. An obstruction due to a concretion can be determined by ultrasonography in 36%–56% of cases. Proving the existence of a concretion depends on the extent of the obstruction, the size and position of the concretion, and the individual ultrasonography characteristics of the patient. The size of concretions found by ultrasound examination ranges from 4 mm to 15 mm. They are most easily recognized retrovesically and intramurally, where they can be seen more than 50% of the time.

Obstructions Caused by Tumors

Ultrasonographic examination can also be employed to diagnose a tumorous obstruction of the ureter, whereby it is also possible to determine the tumor's size and origin (Fig. 1) [2, 14]. In borderline cases, ultrasonography can be used to guide a fine-needle puncture as a quick means of clearing any doubts. The ultrasonography-guided percutaneous nephrostomy with anterograde pyeloureterography has given ultrasonography a further indication in settling the question of obstructions.

Differential Diagnosis of Obstruction During Pregnancy

Ultrasonographic conditions are improved by the enlargement of the uterus during pregnancy and post partum, the intestines being pushed cranially. By having the patient change position during examination, compression of the uterus is achieved in different body positions, and the most favorable position for passing urine can be recommended to the patient. Once the existence of a concretion during pregnancy has been proved by ultrasonography, it is no longer necessary to perform the conventional urogram.

Malformations

Malformations such as megaloureter, faulty opening (Fig. 2) [3, 6, 16], and ureterocele can be seen in part. Ureterocele can be observed in an ultrasound examination as a circular echo band in the bladder adjoining the bladder wall in the trigonum zone.

Reflux Test

Cystography is still the preferred method for determining reflux [9]. Filling the bladder with a physiological saline solution permits observation

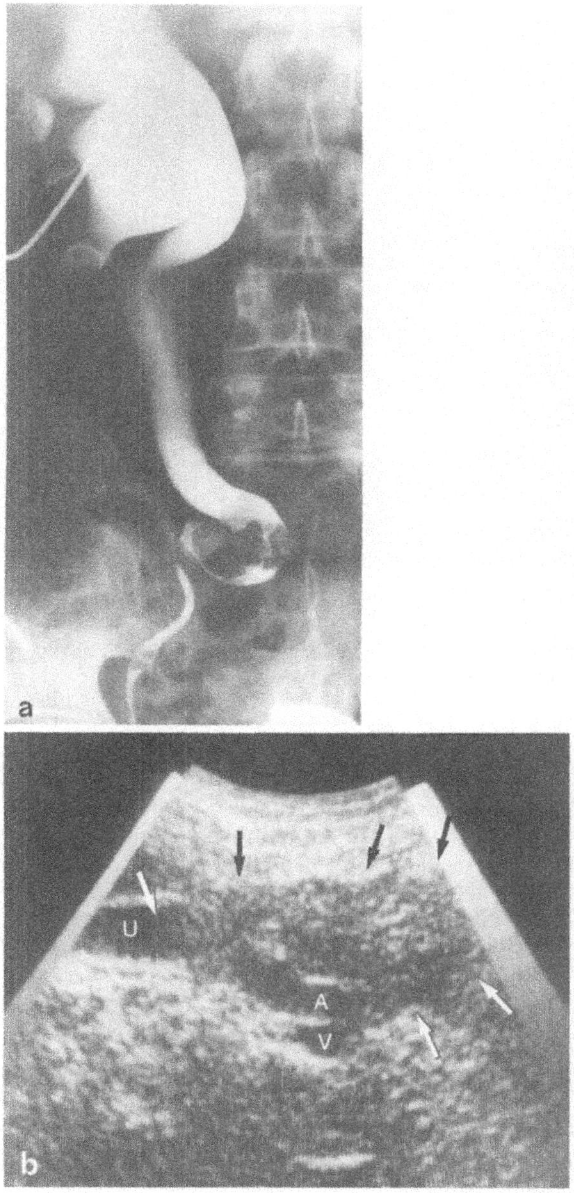

Fig. 1 a, b. Tumor obstruction of the ureter (*U*) at the level of the vascular junction. **a** Antegrade pyelography. The *line* shows the plane of ultrasonography. **b** Ultrasonography. *T*, tumor ventral to the vessels; *A*, common iliac artery; *V*, common iliac vein. The *arrows* show the external boundaries of the tumor

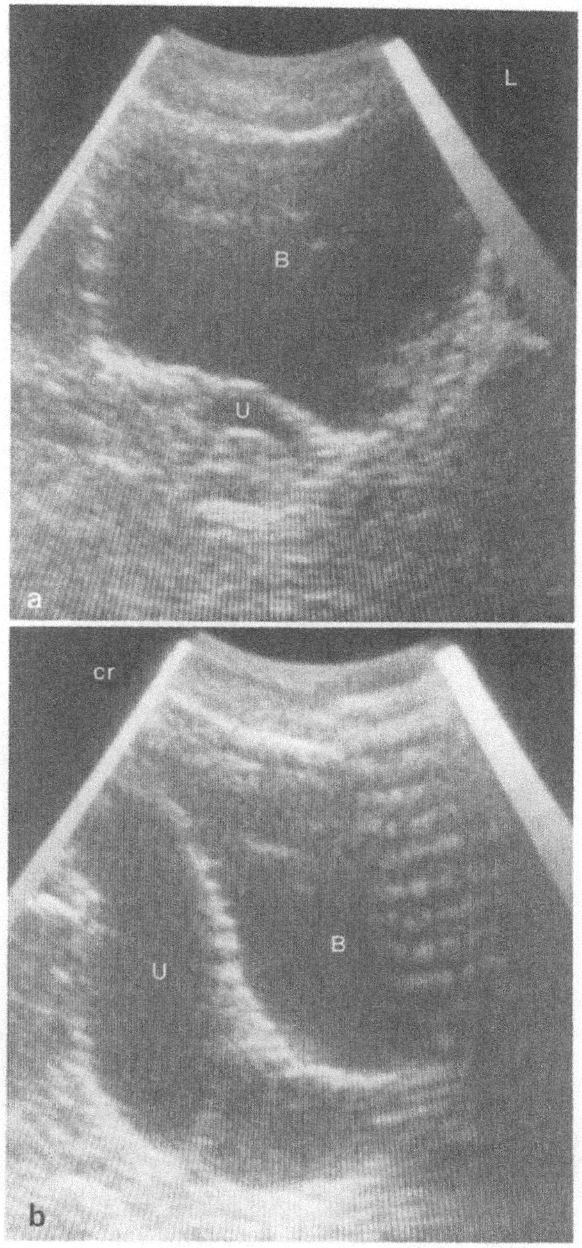

Fig. 2 a, b. Abnormal opening of the ureter. The dilated ureter opens blind dorsomedially in the bladder (*B*). **a** Transverse section through the pelvis. **b** Longitudinal section through the pelvis

of the vesicoureteral and the vesicorenal reflux. However, this method is not used very frequently. Provided the examiner has the necessary experience, ultrasonography can be applied to an increased number of cases.

The implications of the results of sonography in obstruction of the ureter are demonstrated in Fig. 3.

Examination of the Bladder

Diagnosis of the inflammatory illnesses of the bladder is reserved for clinical and conventional radiologic procedures. CT and ultrasonography have opened up new possibilities in the diagnosis of tumors in the bladder and the surrounding area. The indications for bladder sonography are

Obstruction

known → *Ultrasonography* ← unknown

Controls of stone discharge vesical (bladder tumors) Infravesical obstruction	1. Extent of obstruction 2. Type of obstruction 3. Localization of obstruction
↓	↓
Reduction of urograms	Further procedure depending ultrasonography results

1. *Sonographically proven concretion*

↓

Abdominal plane

↓

Diuresis function scintiscan
(urogram not acute)

2. *Sonographically proven tumor*

Ultrasonographically guided fine-needle puncture	Urogram, retro- and anterograde-pyelography, CT, Diuresis function scintiscan

3. *Sonographically proven malformation*

↓

Urogram
Diuresis function scintiscan

4. *No sonographic information on the type of obstruction*

Urogram, antero- and retrograde pyelography, CT,
Diuresis function scintiscan

Fig. 3. Algorithms for investigations of obstructions of the ureter. *BPH,* benign prostatic hypertrophy

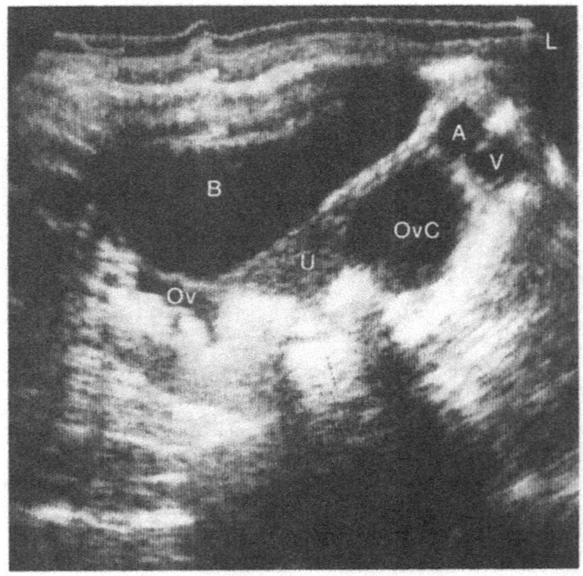

Fig. 4. Relationship of adnexa to bladder: transverse section through the bladder. A left ovarian cyst (*OvC*) is pressing on the bladder (*B*). *U,* uterus; *Ov,* right ovary; *A,* common iliac artery; *V,* common iliac vein

Table 5. Indications for bladder sonography

Pathomorphologic	Functional
Bladder tumor	Bladder convulsions
Pelvic tumors	Neurogenic bladder
Intestines	Measurement of residual urine
Adnexa	Vesicoureteral reflux
Retroperitoneum	Incontinence
– Tumor of soft parts	
– Metastases	
– Fibrosis	
Trauma	
Malformations	

shown in Table 5. The prerequisite for ultrasonographic examination is a well-filled bladder, ensuring on the one hand that the bladder wall is smooth and free of wrinkles, and on the other hand that the movable intestinal loops are forced out of the small pelvis, thus facilitating a sonographic image.

The ultrasonographic approaches available for bladder examination are the suprapubic transcutaneous, endovesical transurethral, and transrectal methods.

Normal Anatomy of the Female Pelvis

The uterus and ovaries can be easily visualized through the filled bladder, which is triangular in its longitudinal section and round to oval in its cross section. In its usual position, the normal-sized uterus is pressed against the bladder dorsal in a flat-arched curve. The ovaries are generally easy to locate near the iliac artery and vein (Fig. 4). Echographically, the bladder wall is a 5-mm-wide, dense echo band whose interior and exterior borders are easily discernible. In the area of the trigonum its external contours are not readily distinguished because of the differing muscular composition and the muscle fibers emanating into the pelvic floor. The vagina is visible as a three- layered band dorsal to the bladder [4].

Diagnosing and Staging a Bladder Tumor

A bladder tumor can be diagnosed, and particularly staged, by ultrasonography and CT with an accuracy of up to 90%, depending on the stage of development. For the purposes of sonographic diagnosis it has been found practical to divide the stages as follows [4, 7, 8, 11, 15]:

Stage I (Superficial). T_1 T_2 T_{3a}: tumors well defined from the inner bladder wall (Fig. 5).
Stage II (Wall-Infiltrating). T_{3b}: outer bladder wall defined, inner bladder wall not defined, wall thickened.
Stage III (Pervesical). T_4: tumor structures protruding beyond bladder contours.

In Stages I and II transurethral ultrasonography brings the best results, but in Stage III CT and suprapubic transcutaneous ultrasonography are superior. CT shows no differentiation in Stages I and II, while in Stage III it is the best method for showing the infiltration and the relationship to the neighboring organs.
In the case of a tumor having penetrated from the exterior (uterine cervix, ovaries, rectum), transcutaneous ultrasonography and in particular CT can be used to obtain definite information.

Inflammatory Illnesses of the Bladder and the Lower Urinary Tract

The inflammatory illnesses that occur in the area of the bladder with and without spreading to the bladder itself can be observed by ultrasonography. Examples of these are the inflammatory infiltrate with transmitted cystitis following appendectomy, and abscess following appendectomy without cystitis.

Alterations in the Bladder Following Blunt Trauma

After a blunt trauma, ultrasonography supplies quick information on the conditions in the lower urinary tract and the area of the bladder.
Free intra-abdominal liquid and irregular bladder contour can indicate a ruptured bladder, especially when the bladder is catheterized and the volume of free intraabdominal liquid increases. In the case of a pelvic hematoma, a good picture can be obtained of the impression or deformation of the bladder. Coagulated blood in a normal-shaped bladder points to a trauma in the upper urinary tract.
Urograms and urethrocystograms are necessary here in all but exceptional cases.

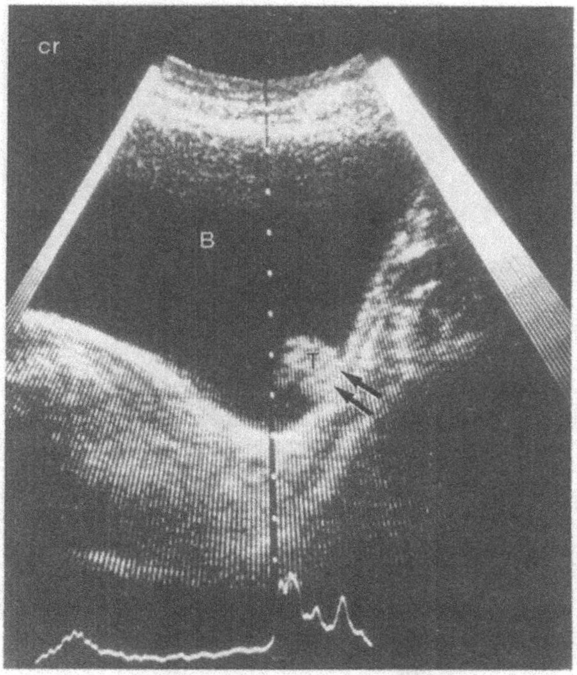

Fig. 5. Stage I bladder tumor (*T*): longitudinal section through the bladder. The internal contour of the bladder wall (*arrows*) can be differentiated from the tumor

Examination of the Urethra

The cross-sectional ultrasound image shows the urethra as a round zone giving off poor echoes. Along its longitudinal axis it shows a band 1 cm in diameter giving off poor echoes, that is clearly visible dorsal to the symphysis and ventral to the vagina. The urethra runs in a straight line craniocaudally and ventrodorsally, and can be observed along its entire length.
Suspicion of any of the following conditions indicates ultrasonography: *Morphologic alterations that cause functional disturbances with and without repercussions on the rest of the urinary tract, and also purely functional disturbances.* A thickened bladder wall points to the existence of a urethral stenosis, particularly a urethral valve (Fig. 6). Ul-

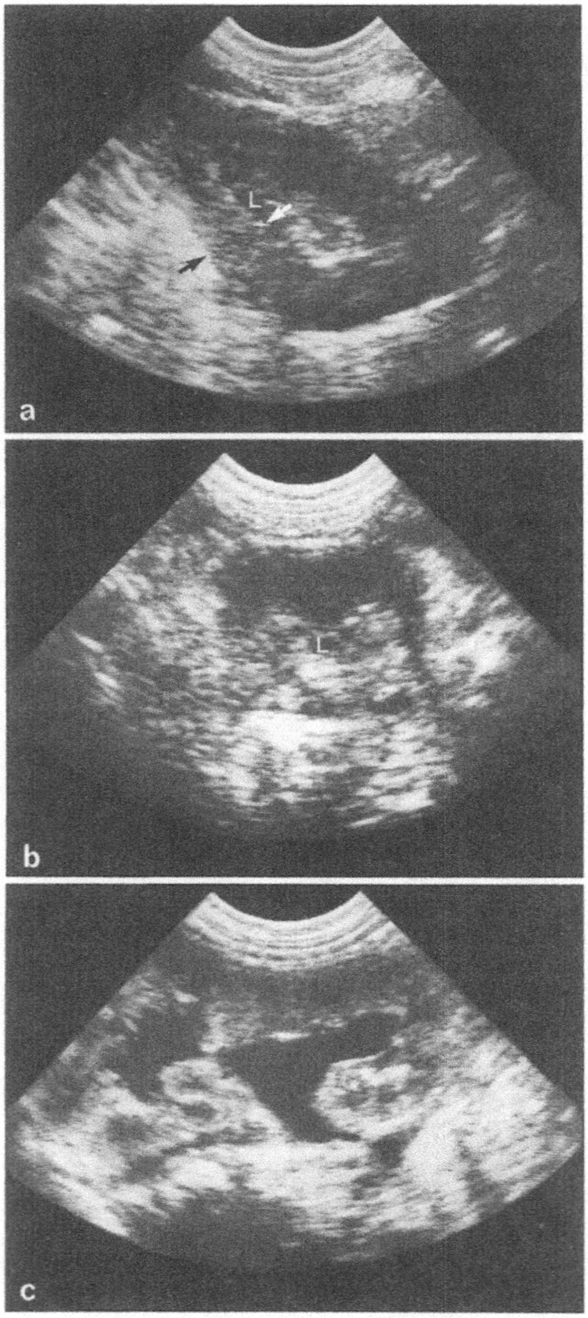

Fig. 6a–c. Urethral valve. **a** Longitudinal section through the bladder. **b** Transverse section through the bladder: the wall (*arrows*) is considerably thickened, the lumen (*L*) very small. **c** Frontal section through the kidney during dilation of the renal cavities

trasound examination will be able to provide a direct image of the urethral valve. Residual urine can be measured with sufficient accuracy [13]. In the case of purely functional disturbances, such as incontinence, the preferred examination methods are miction cystogram and urodynamic examinations. However, the most recent examination forms (observation of urethral function by means of transrectal ultrasonography) lead us to expect increased use of ultrasonography [10, 12]. Sonography for measurement of the vesicovaginal angle is already a clinically practiced method [1].

Alterations in the bladder involving the urethra: In descensus uteri, ultrasonography can be employed to show the displacement of the urethra with a convex curve running ventral. Used for cystorectocele, ultrasonography reveals the corresponding changes in bladder shape. Following cystocele surgery, the bladder shows a V-shaped imprint dorsally.

Purely morphologic periurethral changes: paraurethral and vaginal cysts can be shown by ultrasonography. Proving the existence of urethrovaginal fistulas is the domain of conventional radiologic procedures.

Summary

Ultrasonography can be put to advantageous use in examining the female lower urinary tract. The ureters, bladder, and the urethra are accessible to pulse-echo diagnosis. Depending on the indication, the conventional radiologic methods and CT procedures are supplemented by additional information. In some cases, however, these methods can be replaced by diagnostic ultrasonography. This is especially true for those patients for whom examination with ionizing rays poses a risk.

References

1. Bernaschek G, Spernol R, Wolf G, Kratochwil A (1981) Vergleichende Bestimmung des Urethra-Blasenwinkels bei Inkontinenzfällen mittels Ultraschall und lateralem Urethrozystogramm. Geburtshilfe Frauenheilk 41:339

2. Crone-Munzebrock W, Brockmann WP, Brassow F, Meyer WH (1983) Computerized tomography and sonography in ureter tumors. Fortschr Rontgenstr 138:19
3. Dholakia S, Bejjani B, Elist J, Edson M (1983) Ureteral seminal vesicle anomaly. Gross hematuria as presenting symptom. Urology 21:604
4. Egender G, Goidinger K, Jakse G (1982) Klassifikation der Harnblasentumoren durch Sonographie. Fortschr. Rontgenstr 136:359
5. Egender G, Helweg G, Frommhold H (1983) Sonographie des unteren Harntraktes. Radiologe 23:121
6. Griffin J, Jennings C, MacErlean D (1983) Ultrasonic evaluation of simple and ectopic ureteroceles. Clin Radiol 34:55
7. Gualdi GF, Di Natale G, Liberti M, Di Biasi C, Iannicelli E (1982) Ultrasound and computed tomography in staging of bladder tumours. Eur J Radiol 2:296
8. Jaeger N, Radeke H-W, Adolphs HD (1983) T-Klassifizierung des Harnblasen-Karzinoms durch transurethrale Sonographie. In: Otto RCH, Jann FX (eds) Ultraschalldiagnostik 82. Thieme, Stuttgart, p 455
9. Kessler RM, Altmann DH (1982) Real-time sonographic detection of vesicoureteral reflux in children. AJR 138:1033
10. Lorraine GS, Friedland GW, Perkash I (1983) Transrectal sonographic voiding cystourethrography: studies in neuromuscular bladder dysfunction. AJR 141:83
11. McLaughlin IS, Morley P, Deane RF, Barnett E, Graham AG, Kyle KF (1975) Ultrasound in the staging of bladder tumors. Br J Urol 47:51
12. Nishizawa O, Tsuchida S, Harada T, Morita T, Moriya I, Satoh S, Ohya A, Nakamura H, Fukuda T, Kin N (1983) Improved technique of combined ultrasonotomographic and urodynamic monitoring: simultaneous displaying and videotaping of ultrasonotomography and urodynamic data in color. Neurourol Urodynamics 2:201
13. Rageth JC, Langer K (1983) Sonographische Restharnbestimmung. Urologe 22:87
14. Roemer CE, Pfister RC, Brodsky G, Sacknoff EJ (1980) Primary leiomyosarcoma of ureter. Urology 16:492
15. Schüller J, Walther V, Schmiedt E, Staehler G, Bauer HW, Schilling A (1982) Intravesical ultrasound tomography in staging bladder carcinoma. J Urol 128:264
16. Sumner TE, Crowe JE, Resnick MI (1980) Diagnosis of ectopic ureterocele using ultrasound. Urology 15:82

Evaluation of the Male Lower Urinary Tract

P. Reindl and P. Carl

The lower urinary tract comprises the bladder and the urethra. Although the two parts form a unity, they display differences from a clinical point of view as far as tumors or urinary disorders are concerned. Therefore, they have to be considered separately. In male patients, the following possible causes for pain, hematuria, disturbed or painful urinary flow, or incontinence have to be considered: stone; inflammation; displacement; trauma; tumor (bladder); prostatic disease. The diagnostic imaging modalities available are: X-ray; intra-venous pyelogram (IVP); cystourethrogram (CUG); direct and indirect lymphography; transabdominal and transrectal sonography; CT; and magnetic resonance (MR).
From a radiologic point of view, progress has been made mainly in diagnosis of the prostate. Any more than brief discussion of the other points would exceed the frame of reference of this paper.

Stone

Conventional X-rays, IVP, and CUG are the main diagnostic procedures for the detection of urinary disorders.

Inflammation

Inflammatory diseases of the bladder and urethra are – apart from special types like cystitis bullosa – only radiologically demonstrable in their chronic stage, when contraction of the bladder or stricture of the urethra occurs. With this in mind, the method of choice is IVP, followed by CUG and (with considerable limitations) conventional X-rays.

Displacement and Trauma

Displacement diagnosed radiologically may be due to any one of the following [12]: enlargement of the prostate; tumors of the sigmoid and rectum; enlargement of lymph nodes, aneurysm of the pelvic vessels; osseous tumors; tumors of the soft tissue; inflammatory processes; hematoma (traumatic and postoperative). In all cases, changes in the bladder contour and the urethra demonstrated on IVP or CUG and CT are guides to diagnosis.
Sufficient filling of the bladder is a prerequisite. The so-called tear-drop bladder [9] is pathognomonic for bladder rupture or pelvic hematoma. Filling is especially important for conventional X-ray views of the bladder, e.g., oblique and lateral, in trauma cases. Insufficient filling results in failure to visualize any suspected rupture [11].
Pelvic injuries are associated in up to 12% of cases with ruptures of the urethra, the male/female ratio being 60:1 [8].
From a radiologic point of view, knowledge of staging from type 1 to 3 is significant in cases with fractures with central urethral rupture [3].

Tumor of the Bladder

IVP, CUG, and CT are relevant diagnostic measures in all cases of recess or contour irregularity of the filled bladder. The former may be due to tumor pressure, the latter to infiltration into the muscles of the bladder wall. Independent of infiltration depth, a tumor may cause displacement of the ostium with urinary obstruction. CT can demonstrate the perivesical tissue and gives marked improvement in staging. Transurethral sonography is one of the invasive diagnostic methods and will not be discussed here.

Diseases of the Prostate

Diseases of the prostate are high in frequency among the diseases of the lower urethra in males. The primary diagnosis of the prostate and staging have been improved by intracavitary sonography and by CT.

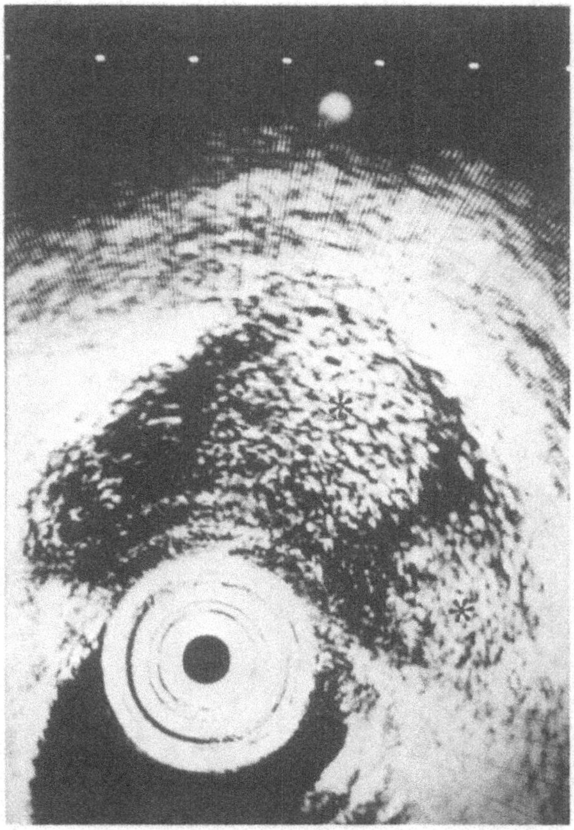

Fig. 1. Transrectal sonography of the prostate, showing adenomatous nodules (*asterisks*)

Table 1. Accuracy of transrectal ultrasonography in carcinoma of the prostate: survey of the literature

Year of publication	Author(s)	Histology (*n*)	Correct *n*	Correct %
1980	Harada [5]	21	18	86
1981	Brooman et al. [1]	99	91	90
1981	Brooman et al. [2]	30	28	93
1981	Watanabe [14]	57	54	94.7
1982	Frentzel-Beyme [4]	89	75	84.2
1984	Reindl [10]	129	112	87

Table 2. Accuracy of transrectal ultrasonography of the prostate

Histology		Correct *n*	Correct %
Benign prostatic	177	164	93
Chronic prostatitis	104	93	89
Carcinoma of prostate	129	112	87
Total	410	369	90

All the imaging modalities listed above have been applied to diagnosis of the prostate. IVP and CUG help only indirectly, direct diagnosis of the prostate being exclusively achieved by transrectal sonography of the prostate, sometimes with transperineal, echo-guided biopsy using the Tru-Cut needle, as well as – with certain limitations – by CT.

With the help of transrectal sonography, the size and shape of the organ may be assessed exactly and information gained on the inner structure [10]. Measurement of anterior-posterior diameter as well as right-left diameter is possible. The distance between apex and base can also be measured by determination of the longitudinal shifting of the probe. In this way, the volume and weight of the organ can be determined with accuracy of up to 98% [10].

Circumscribed adenomatous transformation and organ enlargement can be demonstrated (Fig. 1). In normal cases and in cases of benign hyperplasia of the prostate, the echo structure is homogeneous. In additional isolated middle lobe enlargements growing into the bladder and in circumscribed adenoma nodes, a homogeneous increase in structural density occurs. Difference in structure may also indicate inflammatory changes, with temporary enlargement in an acute state and inhomogeneous echo structure in chronic states. Here, however, may lie the diagnostic difficulty in differentiation from carcinomas, particularly in stages T_1 and T_2. This is especially true in cases of granulomatous prostatitis.

Incidental carcinomas (T_0) cannot be identified sonographically, but diagnostic accuracy increases with the stage. According to the literature it varies from 84% to 94% (Table 1) [1, 2, 4, 5, 10, 14] and in our patient material (1600 examinations, 129 carcinomas of the prostate) lies at 87% (Table 2; 72% for T_2 tumors). In simple differentiation between carcinoma and noncarcinoma, sensitivity and specificity are 88% and 91% respectively (Table 5) [7].

Sonographic diagnosis of the seminal vesicle has to be considered as supplementary to diagnosis of the organ. The vesicles are normally demon-

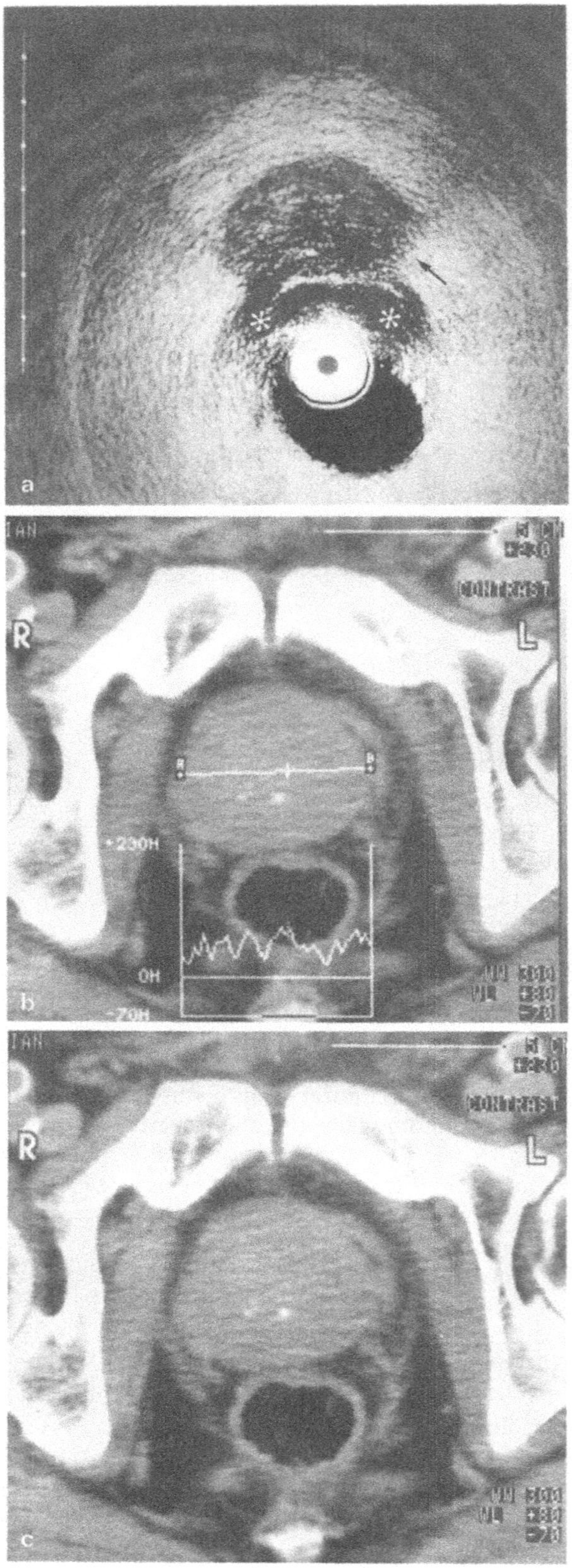

◂ **Fig. 2. a** Transrectal sonography of the prostate, showing carcinoma in the left lobe (*arrow*), seminal vesicles (*asterisks*). **b** Density profile gives no differentiation of inner structure of the prostate. **c** CT of the prostate (6 mm slice thickness): good delineation of the periprostatic tissue

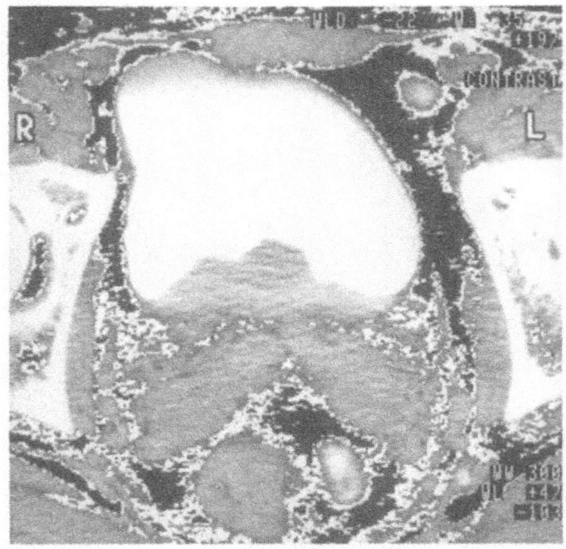

Fig. 3. Better delineation of the periprostatic tissue by "level detection"

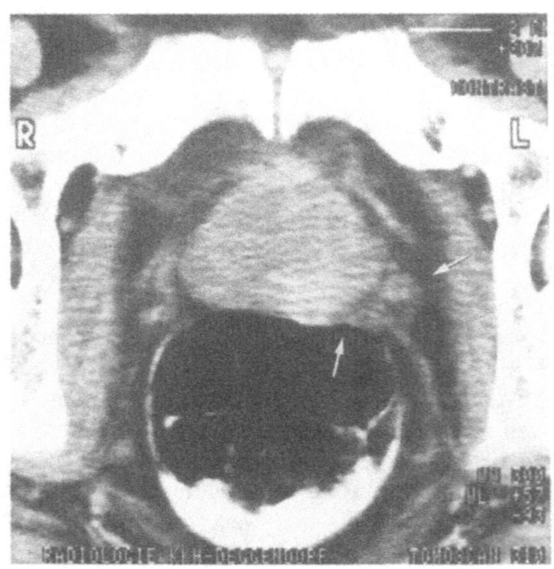

Fig. 4. CT of the prostate with carcinoma in the left lobe (*dorsal*) and histologically proved infiltration of periprostatic tissue (*arrows*)

Table 3. Sensitivity and specificity (%) of various ultrasonographic techniques in 75 cases (from Malzacher [7])

Method	Sensitivity	Specificity
Transrectal	88	91
Transvesical real time	69	95
Transvesical compound	65	93

strated as symmetrical in structure and echo-poor. They may, however, be enlarged by a compressive or infiltrating process which cannot be delineated. Within the framework of staging, inclusion of the lymph nodes is essential, as nodes are involved in 25% of stage T_2 and 45% of stage T_3 cases [6]. Transrectal sonography is, however, limited to the prostate and the seminal vesicles. In staging, diagnosis is improved by CT. Although CT does not contribute to differentiation of structures (Figs. 2a, b), it allows better delineation of the periprostatic tissues (Figs. 2c, 3, 4). Layer thickness of 6 mm seems sufficient. At layer thickness of 3 mm, we could not find any diagnostic advantages. Despite thinner layers and changes in scanning geometry, diagnosis of the lymph nodes remains to be investigated. Direct lymphography covers only the superior lymph nodes of the pelvis and the first filter station (inguinal nodes). The paravesical, pararectal, parasacral, and hypogastric lymph nodes are not visualized on pedal lymphography [13]. Experiments with indirect lymphography using oily and water-soluble contrast media have given no satisfactory results so far.

References

1. Brooman PJ, Griffiths GJ, Roberts EE, Peeling WB, Evans K (1981) Transrectal ultrasonography in the evaluation of cancer of the prostate. In: Schulman CC (ed) Advances in diagnostic urology. Springer, Berlin Heidelberg New York, p 158
2. Brooman PJ, Peeling WB, Griffiths GJ, Roberts E, Evans K (1981) A comparison between digital examination and perirectal ultrasound in the evaluation of the prostate. Br J Urol 53:617
3. Colapinto V, McCallum RW (1977) Injury to the male posterior urethra in fractured pelvis: a new classification. J Urol 118:575–580
4. Frentzel-Beyme B, Schwarz J, Aurich B (1982) Das Bild des Prostataadenoms und -karzinoms bei der transrektalen Sonographie. ROFO 137:261–268
5. Harada K, Takahashi Y, Igari D, Numata I, Orikasa S (1980) Clinical evaluation of inside echo patterns in gray scale prostatic echography. J Urol 124:216
6. Klosterhalfen H, Altenähr E, Franke HD (1982) Das Prostatakarzinom, Pathologie-Diagnostik-Therapie. Thieme, Stuttgart, p 56
7. Malzacher F (1984) Vergleichende Untersuchungen zur transrektalen und suprapubisch-transvesikalen echographischen Darstellung der Prostata. Inaugural-Dissertation, Ruprecht-Karls-Universität, Heidelberg
8. Pokorny MJ, Edson-Pointes, Pierce JM (1979) Urological injuries associated with pelvic trauma. J Urol 121:455–457
9. Prather GC, Kaiser TF (1950) The bladder in fracture of the bone pelvis. Significance of "tear-drop bladder". J Urol 63:1019
10. Reindl P (1984) Die transrektale transversale Sonographie der Prostata. Springer, Berlin Heidelberg New York Tokyo
11. Rieser C, Nicholas E (1963) Rupture of the bladder: unusual features. J Urol 90:53
12. Schreyer H (1974) Erkrankungen der unteren Harnwege und Genitalorgane. In: Vogler E (ed) Radiologische Diagnostik der Harnorgane. Thieme, Stuttgart
13. Viamonte M Jr, Rüttimann A (1980) Atlas of Lymphography. Thieme, Stuttgart, p 271
14. Watanabe H (1981) Prostatic cancer. In: Watanabe H, Holmes JH, Holm HH, Goldberg BB (eds) Diagnostic ultrasound in urology and nephrology. Igaku-Shoin, Tokyo, p 130

Low-Osmolality Contrast in Urography

H. M. Saxton

Introduction

The choice of a contrast agent for urography depends on four factors: (1) urographic quality; (2) side effects; (3) safety; and (4) cost.

Until recently, there has been little choice. The standard, tri-odinated, ionic contrast agents (SICA) developed in the 1950s have similar side effects and mortality levels. The quality of urogram produced is also similar, with a slight but definite improvement when sodium rather than meglumine salts are used [5, 27].

The low-osmolality contrast agents (LOCA), though principally developed for vascular use, now offer an alternative for urography, and radiologists may ask themselves whether they should change to these more expensive media. In this paper, after a brief discussion of their molecular structure, LOCA will be considered in relation to the headings outlined above, and alternative policies suggested for their use in urography.

Contrast Structure and Osmolality [15, 16]. Conventional contrast media are ionic; as a result, each molecule consists of *two* osmotically active particles, so that the ratio of iodine atoms to osmotic particles is 1.5:1 (Fig. 1). LOCA achieve a lower osmolality in one of two ways. Some, e.g., iopamidol and iohexol, have a tri-iodinated benzene ring molecule, with a non-ionic structure (Fig. 2). The ioxaglate molecule, on the other hand, is dimer-like with two tri-iodinated benzene rings linked together (Fig. 3). There is one sodium or meglumine ion in the whole molecule. Thus the ratio of iodine atoms to ionic particles is 3:1 for both types of structure. More surprisingly, the measured osmolality of LOCA is one-third that of SICA, rather than one half as would be expected [15]. The reduction in vascular discomfort is well recognised, but recent work by Dawson and his colleagues, discussed below, has shown that many other side effects are also reduced.

Urographic Quality

The factors affecting the quality of an intravenous urogram (IVU) are contrast concentration and pelvicaliceal filling.

Contrast Concentration. This will be highest with normally functioning kidneys in a well-dehydrated subject given an adequate dose of contrast. Increasing doses of SICA produce an increasing osmotic diuresis and a point is reached when further contrast doses do not improve contrast density [6, 30, 35]. Clearly, this effect will be reduced with LOCA, and there is evidence of improved contrast concentration in the urine of experimental animals given LOCA [13, 31].

Pelvicaliceal Filling. This depends on urine flow, on pelvicaliceal distensibility and on ureteric compression or obstruction. The osmotic diuresis produced by SICA is an advantage in normal subjects, and it has been suggested that the use of LOCA, by diminishing this effect, might in fact worsen the overall urographic quality. So far, the

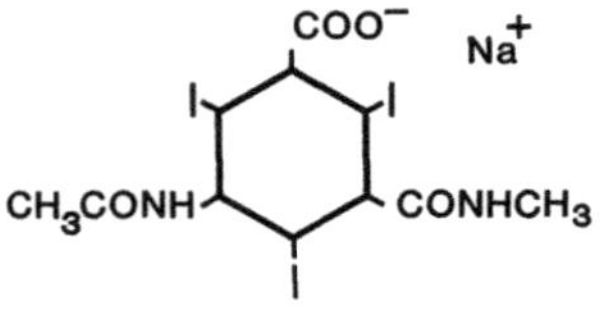

Sodium Iothalamate
('Conray 420')

Fig. 1. Molecular structure of sodium iothalamate, a representative SICA. Three iodine atoms are attached to the benzene ring. The hydrogen ion originally present on the carboxyl group in iothalamic acid has been replaced by a sodium ion (in other SICA a meglumine ion is used, in some there is a mixture of sodium and meglumine). In solution, ionic dissociation is virtually complete, so that in this, as in other SICA, the ratio of iodine atoms to osmotic particles is 1.5:1

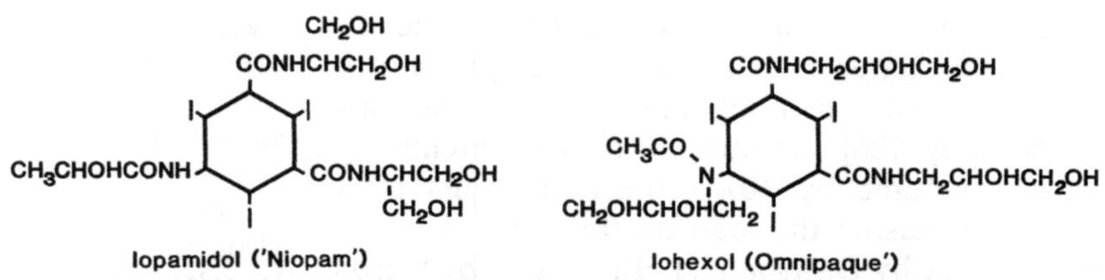

Fig. 2. Molecular structures of iopamidol and iohexol. Both have three iodine atoms, but an amide group is present instead of the carboxyl group in standard media. No ionisation therefore occurs and the ratio of iodine atoms to osmotic particles is 3 : 1

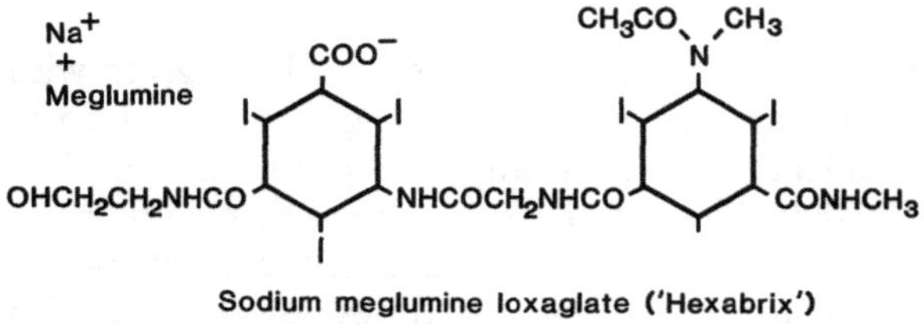

Fig. 3. Molecular structure of ioxaglate. Two similar tri-iodinated benzene ring derivatives are linked to form a dimer. Only one acid radical is present, and the hydrogen ion is replaced by a sodium or meglumine ion. Again, the ratio of iodine atoms to osmotic particles is 3:1

clinical evidence is that urographic quality is maintained, particularly if compression is used [7, 12].

LOCA in Renal Failure

The improved concentration of contrast in experimental animals given LOCA led to the suggestion that LOCA might improve the contrast concentration in subjects with renal failure. In clinical [7] and experimental work [34, 35], this expectation has not been realised, apparently because the overwhelming osmotic diuresis produced by the urea load in renal failure prevents any significant increase in contrast concentration.

Urographic Indications for LOCA

It is clear that there are few urographic indications for LOCA, because SICA given in adequate doses usually produce satisfactory urograms. Two possible indications may be considered:

1. In the normal subject who has been inadvertently hydrated, a larger total dose of contrast could safely be given with LOCA.
2. In neonates and young children, renal tubular immaturity makes it harder for the kidney to concentrate contrast adequately. There is some clinical evidence [29, 33] that better results are obtained in this age group with LOCA than with SICA.

Side Effects

The incidence and mechanisms of contrast side effects have been extensively investigated, but although many aspects have been clarified, no comprehensive explanation of all these effects is available. Some reactions are inconvenient but harmless, others are potentially life threatening. Many side effects are reduced with LOCA, though reactions still occur.

Possible Mechanisms

Psychogenic. Lalli [19] suggested that the majority of side effects have a psychogenic basis. Undoubtedly, anxiety can aggravate side effects, and Heron et al. [17] have suggested that the infrequency of disturbing sensations with LOCA may help to reduce anxiety.

Hyperosmolality [15, 16]. In urography, the hyperosmolar effects include arm pain, and probably also the warmth, metallic taste, other strange sensations and the nausea and vomiting. All these are reduced or abolished with LOCA [12, 17]. High osmolality is also a possible mechanism for the occurrence of cardiac dysrhythmias, occurring after bolus injection of SICA [32, 28]. These potentially dangerous changes have been shown to occur less frequently or not at all after iohexol [17].

Another effect of SICA is vasodilatation, which can lead to hypotension, particularly if the cardiac output is fixed, e.g. in patients with a cardiac pacemaker. Vasodilatation has not been specifically investigated in relation to urography, but it is diminished when iopamidol is used for arteriography [26]. Expansion of the circulating plasma volume by 10%–20% [18] occurs after SICA, increasing the load on the heart. Unpublished work by Dawson and Hine (cited by Heron et al. [17]) shows that LOCA diminish this effect.

Histamine Release. This can occur with contrast. There are several mechanisms; among others, contrast agents can stimulate release of histamine from human basophils in vitro by a non-immune effect [14, 24]. Assem et al. [4] showed that LOCA caused much less histamine release from basophils than SICA.

Cholinesterase Inhibition. This effect of contrast is linked to its protein-binding capacity [21]. The resulting augmentation in cholinergic activity could explain many contrast effects – peripheral vasodilatation, bronchospasm, urticaria, disturbances of cardiac rhythm. This effect, too, is less pronounced with LOCA: ioxaglate shows a smaller improvement over iothalamate than do iopamidol and iohexol [8].

Complement Activation. Contrast agents can activate complement both in vitro and in vivo [20, 22, 25], though the significance for contrast reactions has been uncertain. Dawson et al. [11] have confirmed in vitro that the anaphylatoxin C3a is released from C3 by contrast. There was no significant difference between different contrast media. Other mechanisms have also been proposed, but their place in relation to the newer contrast agents is still under study. It will be seen that in the majority of cases, the LOCA would tend to reduce unpleasant or harmful side effects.

Safety

The LD_{50} in mice is widely used as an index of relative contrast toxicity. Aspelin and Almen [3] showed that metrimazide has a higher LD_{50} in mice than metrizoate, and also that rapid injection significantly lowers the LD_{50} for both contrast agents. Table 1 shows that in mice, the new contrast agents have an LD_{50} of up to three times that found with Urografin (Renografin) and Conray. This is borne out by the available data on humans. A generally accepted figure for mortality from urography with standard contrast media is 1 in 40 000 examinations. Some four million injections of sodium ioxaglate have been given with eight reported deaths (Grainger, personal communication), a mortality of 2 per million or 1 in 500 000. Even if there has been some under-reporting of deaths, it seems that the death rate is likely to be five or ten times lower than with SICA. The evidence therefore suggests that the newer contrast agents are safer than standard media.

Table 1. Relative mortality rates in mice given intravenous contrast medium (after Dawson et al. [9])

Contrast medium	LD_{50} (gI/kg)
Conray 420	8.0
Urografin 370	7.6
Ioxaglate (Hexabrix)	12.5
Iopamidol (Niopam)	21.8
Iohexol (Omnipaque)	24.2

Cost

The current cost of LOCA is at least four times that of SICA. In the UK, exclusive use of LOCA would add between £ 4 million and £ 7 million to the annual bill for contrast.

Policies for the Use of LOCA in Urography

If it is accepted that the mortality from urography would be substantially reduced by a change to routine use of LOCA, there are, broadly, three possible approaches (Table 2). Policy A would accept that LOCA are safer and would involve their exclusive use regardless of cost. The second and third Policies B and C would involve using SICA as a routine except in categories known to be at increased risk. Policy B would use LOCA in the majority of such high-risk cases; Policy C would employ SICA after appropriate precautions in most such patients, and LOCA would only be used when there seemed to be no alternative means of reducing risk. In all high-risk cases, the need to consider alternative imaging modalities should be stressed. The table shows the application of these policies to the various high-risk groups discussed below.

Infants and Small Children. The main risk is from excessive rise in plasma osmolality during rapid

Table 2. The three possible approaches to the use of LOCA

Patient category	Policy A	Policy B	Policy C
Infants/small children	LOCA	LOCA	Slow injection (3–5 min) SICA
Heart disease	LOCA	LOCA	Slow injection (3–5 min) SICA
Over 60	LOCA	LOCA	Slow injection (3–5 min) SICA
Asthma/chronic bronchitis	LOCA	LOCA	Severe cases, LOCA Mild or moderate cases, LOCA. Avoid meglumine [1]
Other allergies	LOCA	LOCA	Prior steroids. SICA
Previous severe contrast reaction	LOCA	LOCA	LOCA
Long-term diabetes (if other modalities inconclusive)	LOCA	LOCA	LOCA, avoid dehydration
Renal failure (if other modalities inconclusive)	LOCA	LOCA	SICA, avoid dehydration
Myeloma (if other modalities inconclusive)	LOCA	LOCA	SICA, avoid dehydration
Indians	LOCA	LOCA	SICA, avoid dehydration
Anxiousness	LOCA	LOCA	Reassurance and SICA
All others	LOCA	SICA	SICA

injection or from overdose due to careless computation. The use of LOCA would reduce risks and would improve urographic quality [29].

Patients with Heart Disease. These show increased mortality, particularly in congestive failure [2]. Three possible mechanisms are known; first, the danger of inducing a disorder of cardiac rhythm; second, a fall in blood pressure resulting from vasodilatation after contrast; and third, an increase in circulating blood volume following SICA. These effects are reduced or abolished with LOCA. The first two are also reduced by slow injection of contrast.

Older Patients. Mortality from urography is three times greater in patients over 60 [2]. This may reflect the higher incidence of heart disease in this group. Routine use of LOCA in this group would almost certainly diminish mortality, as would routine slow injection of SICA.

Patients with Asthma or Chronic Bronchitis. Many normal subjects develop subclinical bronchospasm during urography [24], and asthmatics not uncommonly develop frank asthma after contrast. Iopamidol produces less bronchospasm in normal subjects than SICA [10]. It seems reasonable to assume that routine use of LOCA would reduce asthma attacks in susceptible individuals, and that patients with severe chronic bronchitis should also be given LOCA. Alternatively, the protective effect of prior steroids could be used [23].

Patients with Other Forms of Allergy. There is a fourfold risk of serious reaction [2]. The work quoted on histamine release and cholinesterase inhibition suggests that routine use of LOCA would reduce risk here: prior steroid medication is a valid alternative.

Previous Reactors to Contrast. Severe reactions are increased tenfold in this group [2]. Routine use of LOCA appears rational.

Diabetic Subjects. Diabetics of long standing are at risk of developing renal failure or of worsening existing mild renal failure after contrast has been given. So far, there is no clinical evidence to prove that LOCA are safer, but this seems likely.

Renal Failure and Myeloma. Urography has proved remarkably benign in subjects with chronic renal failure and/or myeloma: the main risks are from inadvertent dehydration. The use of ultrasound and nuclear medicine has also reduced the need for urography. The indications for LOCA remain uncertain.

Ethnic Groups. Ansell et al. [2] have shown an eightfold increase in severe reactions among Indians and some increase among Mediterranean subjects. The mortality rate was not increased, and in the absence of confirmatory evidence, it is difficult to know how seriously to take this point.

Anxious Patients. The significance of anxiety [19] is hard to assess, and a precise definition and grading of anxiety would be impossible. Any decision here must be arbitrary.

Comment

It is impossible to give dogmatic advice on the use of LOCA in urography, and these policies illustrate how different approaches can be logically sustained. My personal inclination is for policy C, accepting that as further work is done, the positive indications for use the LOCA will broaden.

References

1. Ansell G (1970) Adverse reactions to contrast agents. Scope of problem. Invest Radiol 5:374–384
2. Ansell G, Tweedie MCK, West CR, Price Evans DA, Couch L (1980) The current status of reactions to intravenous contrast media. Invest Radiol 15: 532–539
3. Aspelin P, Almen T (1976) Studies on the acute toxicity of ionic and non-ionic contrast media following rapid intravenous injection. An experimental study in mice. Invest Radiol 11:309–314
4. Assem ESK, Bray K, Dawson P (1983) The release of histamine from human basophils by radiological contrast agents. Br J Radiol 56:647–652
5. Benness GT (1970) Urographic contrast agents. A comparison of sodium and methylglucamine salts. Clin Radiol 21:150–156
6. Cattell WR, Fry IK, Spencer AG, Purkiss P (1967) Excretion urography. I. Factors determining the excretion of Hypaque. Br J Radiol 40:561–571
7. Dalla Palma L, Rossi M, Stacul R, Agostini R (1982) Iopamidol in urography. A comparison between ionic and non-ionic contrast media in patients with normal and impaired renal function. Urol Radiol 4:1–3
8. Dawson P, Edgerton D (1983) Contrast media and enzyme inhibition. I. Cholinesterase. Br J Radiol 56:653–656
9. Dawson P, Grainger RG, Pitfield J (1983) The new low osmolar contrast media: a simple guide. Clin Radiol 34:223–226
10. Dawson P, Pitfield J, Britton J (1983) Contrast media and bronchospasm: a study with iopamidol. Clin Radiol 34:227–230
11. Dawson P, Turner MW, Bradshaw A, Westaby S (1983) Complement activation and generation of C 3a anaphylatoxin by radiological contrast agents. Br J Radiol 56:447–448
12. Dawson P, Heron C, Marshall J (1984) Intravenous urography with low-osmolality contrast agents: theoretical considerations and clinical findings. Clin Radiol 35:173–175
13. Evill CA, Benness GT (1978) Urographic excretion studies: preliminary results with a six-iodine, singly-ionizing sodium salt – P 286. Invest Radiol 13:325–327
14. Findlay SR, Dromk AM, Kagey-Sobotka A (1981) Hyperosmolar triggering of histamine release from human basophils. J Clin Invest 67:1604–1613
15. Grainger RG (1980) Osmolality of intravascular radiological contrast media. Br J Radiol 53:739–746
16. Grainger RG (1982) Intravascular contrast media – the past, the present and the future. Br J Radiol 55:1–18
17. Heron CW, Underwood SR, Dawson P (1984) Electrocardiographic changes during intravenous urography. A study with sodium iothalamate and iohexol. Clin Radiol 35:137–142
18. Huet Y, Wirquun H, Loiret J (1981) Effects of contrast material on blood volume. In: Amiel H (ed) Contrast media in radiology: appraisal and prospects. Springer, Berlin Heidelberg New York
19. Lalli AF (1974) Urographic contrast media reactions and anxiety. Radiology 112:267–271
20. Lang JH, Lasser EC, Kolb WP (1976) Activation of serum complement by contrast media. Invest Radiol 11:303–308
21. Lasser EC, Lang JH (1970) Contrast protein interactions. Invest Radiol 5:446–451
22. Lasser EC, Kolb WP, Lang JH (1974) Contrast medium activation of the serum complement system. Invest Radiol 9:6
23. Lasser EC, Lang J, Sovak M, Kolb W, Lyon S, Hamilton AE (1977) Steroids: theoretical and experimental basis for utilisation in prevention of contrast media reactions. Radiology 125:1–9
24. Littner RM, Rosenfield AT, Ulreich S, Putnam C (1977) Evaluation of bronchospasm during intravenous urography. Radiology 124:17–21
25. Neoh SH, Sage MR, Willis RB, Roberts Thomson P, Bradley J (1981) The in vitro activation of complement by radiologic contrast materials and its inhibition with ε-aminocaproic acid. Invest Radiol 16:152–158
26. Padayachee TS, Reidy JF, King DH, Reeves M, Gosling RG (1983) Femoral artery flow and pain during lumbar aortography: comparison of ionic and non-ionic contrast media. Clin Radiol 34:79–85
27. Pearson MC, Gilkes R, Hall JH, Boultbee JE, Saxton HM (1971) Sodium or methylglucamine? A comparison of iothalamates in urography. Br J Radiol 44:55–57
28. Pfister RC, Hutter AM, Newhouse JH, Yoder IC, Travers E (1983) Contrast-medium induced electrocardiographic abnormalities. AJR 140:149–153

29. Robey G, Reilly BJ, Carusi PA, Nguyen KB (1984) Pediatric urography: comparison of metrizamide and methylglucamine diatrizoate. Radiology 150: 61 – 63
30. Saxton HM (1969) Urography (review article). Br J Radiol 42:321 – 346
31. Sjöberg S, Almén T, Colman K (1980) Excretion of urographic contrast media. Iohexol and other media during free urine flor in the rabbit. Acta Radiol Supplement 362
32. Stadalnik RC, Vera S, Da Silva O, Davies R, Kraus JF, Mason DT (1977) Electrocardiographic response to intravenous urography: prospective evaluation of 275 patients. AJR 126:825 – 830
33. Stake G, Borgens J, Monn E (1979) Urography in children. A double blind study of metrizamide and metrizoate. Ann Radiol 22:202 – 203
34. Webb JAW, Fry IK, Cattell WR, Cummack B, Jewell SE (1978) The effect of osmotic diuretics on urinary iodine concentration using contrast media of different osmolality. Br J Radiol 51:106 – 110
35. Webb JAW (1984) The role of the distal nephron mechanism in the concentration of contrast medium in the urine. Br J Radiol 57:381 – 386

RETROPERITONEAL AND PELVIC MASSES

Retroperitoneal Masses

H. Schreyer, G. H. Schneider, and E. Tölly

The aim of investigation methods in the diagnosing of retroperitoneal diseases is to confirm their existence and to determine their location, extent, and consistency. The retroperitoneum is difficult to evaluate with conventional radiographic methods. Intravenous urography and, in some cases, barium studies provide only indirect evidence based on organ displacement, and lesions may grow to a considerable size before being detected. It was not until advances were made in abdominal angiography that progress in visualizing retroperitoneal mass lesions became possible. Lymphography made the visualization of some of the retroperitoneal lymph nodes feasible. When ultrasound and CT were introduced direct imaging of retroperitoneal lesions became possible. These methods enable determination of retroperitoneal pathology and its relationship to other retroperitoneal structures.

Retroperitoneal diseases may be divided into neoplastic and non-neoplastic conditions. Neoplastic conditions are subdivided into primary and secondary (metastatic) tumors, non-neoplastic conditions into hematomas, inflammatory lesions, and retroperitoneal fibrosis. Most of these diseases have their specific diagnostic problems.

Primary Retroperitoneal Tumors

Primary tumors of the retroperitoneum are rare. In order of frequency, they may develop from mesenchymal, neural, epithelial (urogenital ridge), or embryonic remnant tissues. They may be either malignant or benign, but malignancies predominate (70%–80%). Clinical symptoms develop late, and for this reason the tumors are usually very large at the time of discovery.

Investigation Methods

Plain Film. The findings are positive in 44%–50% of cases [8, 9]. A mass of soft tissue density displacing the kidney or altering its configuration, as well as obliterating the psoas contour, may frequently be observed. Displacement of the bowels is common. Calcifications may occur in teratomas or neurogenic tumors.

Urography. Kidney and ureter may be displaced by large tumors. Additionally, an obstruction of the ureter with urinary stasis may develop. In these cases, urography frequently reveals positive findings (85% according to Duncan and Evans [9]) (Fig. 1 a). However, accurate differential diagnosis between renal and extrarenal tumors on the basis of urography may be problematic. Furthermore, large intra-abdominal tumors may cause a displacement of urinary organs similar to that caused by retroperitoneal tumors. In intraperitoneal tumors, however, urinary stasis is rarely observed, a fact which may be used as a differential diagnostic criterion.

Ultrasound. Sonography enables differentiation between cystic and solid lesions, but not between benign and malignant growth (Fig. 1 b) [5]. Differential diagnostic problems between intrarenal and extrarenal lesions may arise in cases where the kidney has been infiltrated by a retroperitoneal tumor or when renal carcinoma has developed extensively into the retroperitoneal space. In very large masses, differential diagnosis between intraperitoneal and retroperitoneal tumors may be a further problem.

Computed Tomography. CT provides highly accurate and clinically important information about retroperitoneal tumors. The location of the tumor is usually correctly identified; however, retroperitoneal tumors may resemble primary tumors of the organs which they infiltrate. Conversely, primary tumors of the retroperitoneal organs may extend far into the retroperitoneum and mimic primary retroperitoneal tumors. CT displays the size of the tumor very accurately and

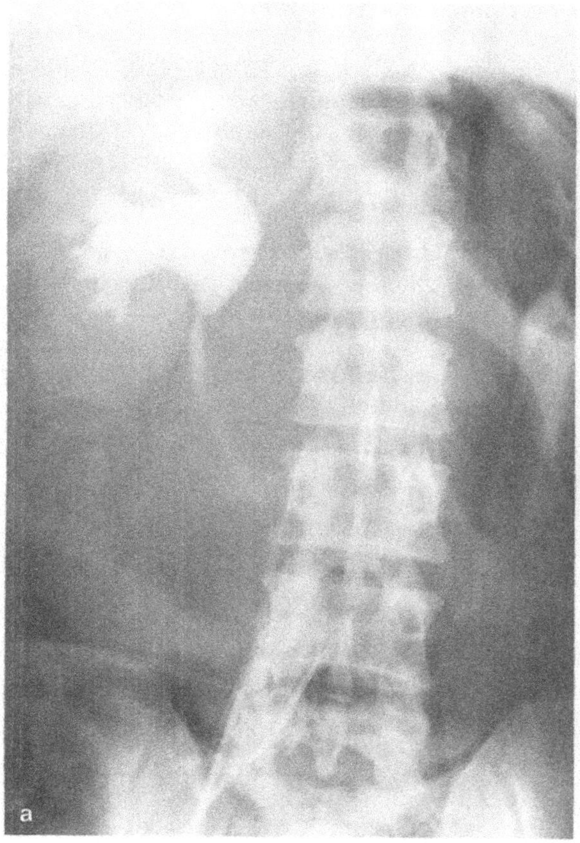

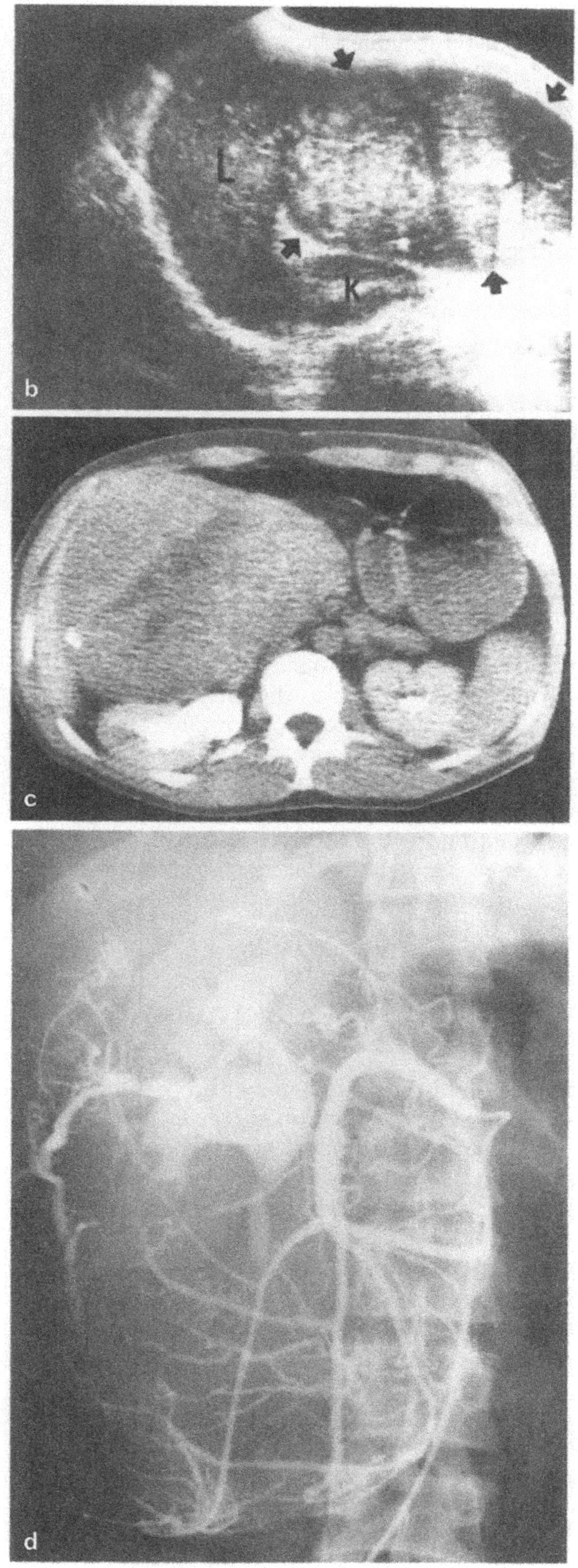

Fig. 1a–d. Retroperitoneal sarcoma. **a** Urography: cranial displacement of right kidney by mass in right upper abdomen. **b** Sonography: solid and partly necrotic extrarenal tumor (*arrows*) displacing and compressing right kidney (*k*). *L*, liver. **c** CT: solid and partially necrotic extrarenal tumor compressing right kidney. **d** Angiography: highly vascularized retroperitoneal tumor, visualized by injecting a lumbar artery at the level of L1/L2

provides important information concerning the effect of tumors on adjacent anatomic structures. Invasion of muscles and the spine may be detected as representing symptoms of malignant growth. The measurement of attenuation values enables differentiation between solid, necrotic, and cystic components of a tumor, and differentiation between lipomatous and nonlipomatous tumors is also possible [26] (Fig. 1c). All this makes CT invaluable, not only for primary diagnosis, but also for therapy planning and follow-up studies, helping to assess tumor progression and response to all types of therapy.

Angiography. Since ultrasound and CT are widely used in the detection of retroperitoneal tumors, angiography is no longer employed as a primary diagnostic procedure. Localization of lesions and exclusion of primary visceral tumors is possible when using selective techniques. Tumor enhancement on angiography of lumbar arteries is a characteristic indication of a retroperitoneal tumor [19]. In large retroperitoneal tumors, a range of other arteries, such as the intercostal, renal, adrenal, inferior phrenic, superior and inferior mesenteric, and celiac, may contribute to the blood supply. In addition to determining the degree of tumor vascularity, such findings supply important information for the surgeon. Differential diagnosis is between benign and malignant lesions based on the patterns of neovascularity is not possible (Fig. 1d) [7, 17].

Diagnostic Approach

Plain film of the abdomen and urography are still the primary investigation methods for these tumors. Depending on the clinical symptoms and signs, ultrasound may be employed prior to urography or as an additional method to reveal localization and composition of the tumor. CT is the chosen method in planning any kind of therapy. Angiography is used preoperatively and for resolving differential diagnostic problems.

Secondary Retroperitoneal Tumors

There are several possibilities in secondary involvement of the retroperitoneum by malignant tumors: involvement of lymph nodes by lymphomas, cancer metastasis to lymph nodes, or direct spread of cancer of adjacent organs.

Investigation Methods

Plain Film. As a study itself the plain film is of little value, but it is important in connection with other studies. It will show a mass only if the latter is sufficiently large. Calcifications are rare except after irradiation.

Urography. Urography has proved to be a nonspecific study which shows enlarged retroperitoneal lymph nodes except in cases of extensive enlargement of the nodes or when they are close to the urinary organs. The kidney and upper ureter may be displaced laterally, the lower ureter and bladder medially.

Ultrasound. The sonographic criterion of a diseased lymph node is enlargement of the node. It is possible to detect lymph nodes of 2 cm in size or more, also in sites where such nodes are not shown by lymphography. There are no criteria for distinguishing between small tumor-infiltrated nodes and normal nodes. Other, non-neoplastic causes of lymph node enlargement may give false-positive results. Intestinal gas and overlying bone may limit the effectiveness of ultrasound in the lower and mid-abdomen [3] (Fig. 2a).

Computed Tomography. As in ultrasound the diagnostic criterion of neoplastic lymph node disease is an enlargement of the node (Fig. 2b). Diseased but nonenlarged lymph nodes may give false-negative results. CT does not differentiate between benign and malignant enlargement, but lymph nodes of 3 cm and more in diameter are unusual in benign, reactive, and inflammatory conditions. Enlarged lymph nodes may appear as bulky masses in which individual nodes are not recognizable, a sign indicating malignant lymph node disease. CT displays lymph nodes in areas which are not visualized by lymphography. Furthermore, CT has been found to be superior to lymphangiography in demonstrating metastatic lymph nodes which are not opacified, because lymphangiography does not visualize nodes completely infiltrated by tumor. This is an important point in radiotherapy planning. Bone and gas are no obstacle for adequate imaging [18].

Lymphangiography. Lymphangiography shows the size, shape, and position of the nodes along the external and common iliac artery as well as those along the aorta and vena cava. The nodes cranial to the renal arteries, those in the mesentery, and the hepatic, splenal, and hypogastric

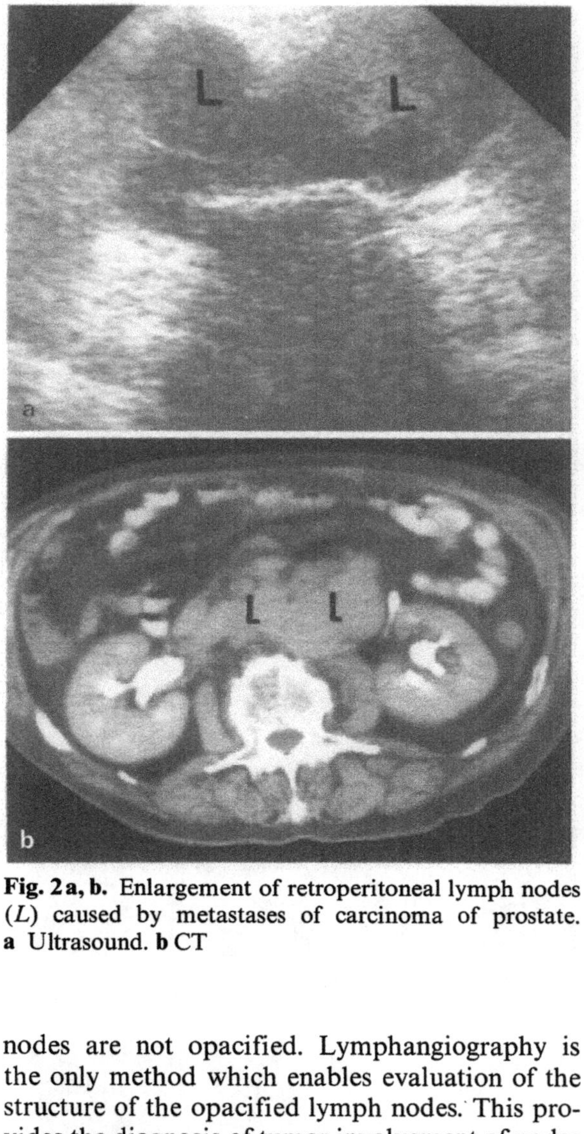

Fig. 2 a, b. Enlargement of retroperitoneal lymph nodes (*L*) caused by metastases of carcinoma of prostate. **a** Ultrasound. **b** CT

nodes are not opacified. Lymphangiography is the only method which enables evaluation of the structure of the opacified lymph nodes. This provides the diagnosis of tumor involvement of nodes that are not enlarged [6]. Differentiation between reactive enlargement and enlargement by tumor is possible. In the diagnosis of metastatic disease, diagnostic problems associated with lymphography are the inability to detect small (microscopic) metastases and the lack of differentiation between malignant and nonmalignant peripheral filling defects of the lymph nodes. Lymph nodes totally replaced by tumor cannot be visualized by lymphography. Fine-needle biopsy will help to obtain an accurate diagnosis [29–30].

Diagnostic Approach: Lymphomas

The primary method of choice in diagnosing retroperitoneal lymph nodes in a known lymphoma is CT. Its results are fundamental for any therapy planning [15]. The major cause of false-negative CT in the staging of lymphomas is the inability to detect tumor in normal sized lymph nodes (5%–10% of the cases of Hodgkin's disease). In such cases lymphography should be performed. In non-Hodgkin's lymphoma a higher incidence of enlarged lymph nodes occurs both in the retroperitoneum and in other abdominal sites [15]. Ultrasound has about the same diagnostic value as CT, but has its specific limitations. It is useful as a screening method and follow-up study. Urography is performed in clinically suspicious or sonographically diagnosed urinary stasis due to ureteral obstruction, a condition which is rare in lymphomas, occurring in only about 6% of cases [21], mainly after radiation therapy.

Diagnostic Approach: Metastases

As in lymphomas, CT is the primary method used in diagnosing retroperitoneal lymph node metastases. Provided that the conditions for ultrasound are ideal, this investigation method has about the same diagnostic value as CT. In metastases of pelvic cancer the size of the lymph nodes often remains normal, and thus lymphography plays a role in diagnosing metastatic disease [29]. One exception are the metastases of testicular tumors (seminomas), in which the lymph nodes are usually more enlarged and therefore more easily detectable by ultrasound and CT [20].

In contrast to lymphomas, in metastases and in direct tumor spread, urinary stasis due to ureteral obstruction occurs frequently. Depending on clinical symptoms and signs, urography is performed either as a primary procedure or as a secondary procedure following an ultrasound study. However, urography may not demonstrate the cause of the obstruction. In this cases CT is the method of choice to display the lesion in the retroperitoneum (Fig. 3a and b). In some cases further exploration of the lesion by means of needle biopsy is necessary, as tumor and fibrosis may have a similar appearance [2].

Non-neoplastic Diseases

Hemorrhage

Spontaneous retroperitoneal hematomas are found in three main locations: Pararenal hematomas are caused by a bleeding lesion of the kidney; the psoas muscle is the main site of

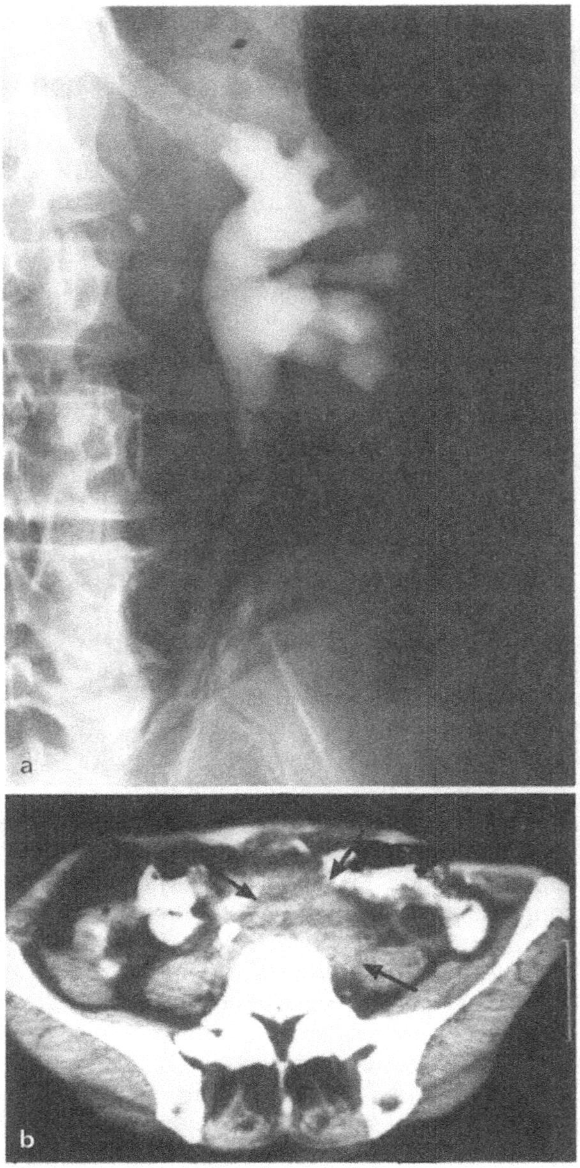

Fig. 3a, b. Lymph node metastases from colon carcinoma. **a** Urography: obstruction of ureter at level of sacroiliac joint developed after surgery of colon carcinoma. **b** CT: retroperitoneal lymph node metastases (*arrows*) causing ureteral obstruction

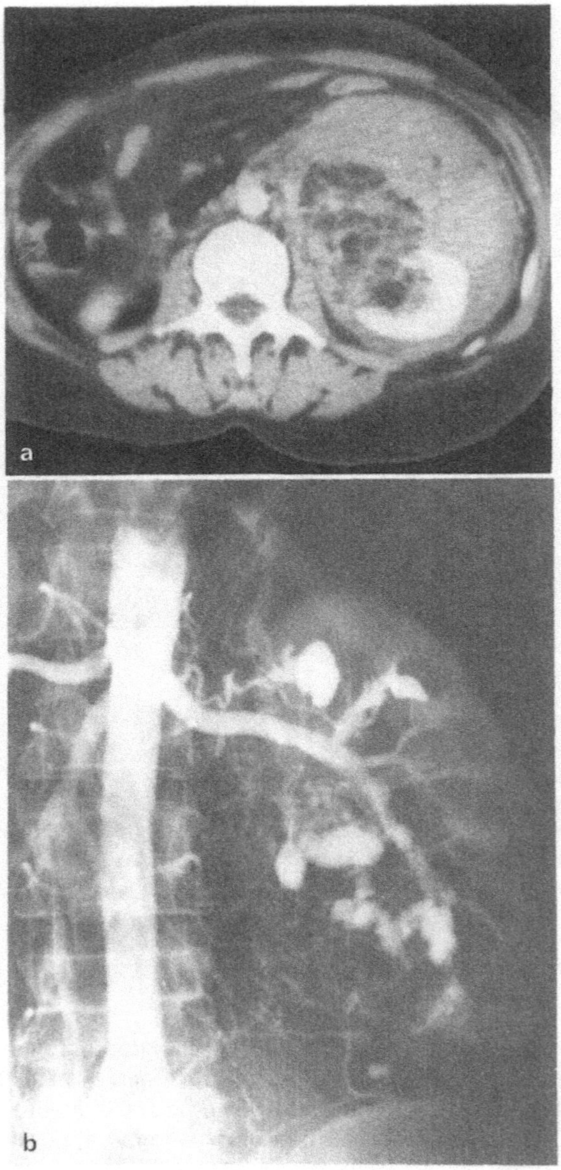

Fig. 4a, b. Peri- and pararenal hematoma in bleeding angiomyolipoma of left kidney. **a** CT: angiomyolipoma. Kidney and tumor surrounded by large peri- and pararenal hematoma. **b** Angiography: highly vascularized tumor with multiple aneurysms of tumor vessels. Kidney had to be removed because of tumor extent. (Urography: nonexcreting left kidney, mass lesion)

hemorrhage in bleeding disorders; hematomas in the rest of the retroperitoneal space are most frequently due to a ruptured aortic aneurysm.

Investigation Methods

Plain Film and Urography. The detection of retroperitoneal hemorrhage by conventional radiographic methods is limited to indirect signs and is therefore insensitive. The loss of the psoas shadow caused by a mass of soft tissue density and displacement of retroperitoneal organs (kidney and ureter) and/or the bowels are signs of a mass lesion in the retroperitoneum due to hematoma. Calcification of the aortic wall may point to an aneurysm. Isolated enlargement of the psoas muscle may be due to psoas hematoma. Urography is important in evaluating pararenal hematoma for signs of renal pathology.

Ultrasound. Ultrasound has proved to be a reliable method for detecting fluid collections in the retroperitoneum; however, it cannot differentiate between various fluids, such as blood, urine, or pus [16, 22, 27]. The etiology of hematoma, e.g., aortic aneurysm or neoplastic disease of the kidneys or adrenals, may be detected.

Computed Tomography. Retroperitoneal hemorrhage is detectable by CT, appearing as a mass of soft tissue density. The hematoma can be accurately localized and quantified by this method, which is also valuable as a noninvasive follow-up study. CT may also provide an etiologic explanation of hematoma by displaying aortic aneurysms [4, 10, 24] or neoplastic disease of the kidneys and adrenals (Fig. 4a).

Angiography. Angiography is essential in demonstrating vascular lesions within the kidney as the cause of pararenal hematomas (Fig. 4).

Inflammatory Lesions: Psoas Abscess

Alongside pararenal abscess, the psoas muscle is a frequent site of abscess formation in the retroperitoneum. Psoas abscesses develop mainly as sequelae of inflammatory diseases of adjacent organs; however, the cause of abscess formation is not always known.

Investigation Methods

Plain Film and Urography. Conventional radiologic methods frequently fail to detect psoas abscess. Yet enlargement of the psoas, as well as kidney and ureter displacement, may be observed. Destruction of the vertebrae by osteomyelitis is visualized on plain films, pointing to the etiology of the abscess.

Ultrasound. Abscess formation is directly displaced by ultrasound in an enlarged psoas muscle [27]; however differentiation from blood is not possible.

Computed Tomography. CT visualizes an abscess in the psoas muscle as an enlargement of the muscle with centrally localized hypodense areas due to necrosis or gas collection caused by *E. coli.* A hematoma or a tumor of the muscle also may not be differentiated from an abscess [13] (Fig. 5a–c).

Diagnostic Approach in Retroperitoneal Hemorrhage and Psoas Abscess

Ultrasound and CT will display both hemorrhage and abscess formation. They are the chosen methods for primary exploration, also showing adjacent organs which are useful in explaining the etiology of these disorders. CT provides additional information on pathology of the spine. Urography is performed in renal disease.

Retroperitoneal Fibrosis

The etiology of retroperitoneal fibrosis is not known in the majority of cases (idiopathic fibrosis). There are, however, a number of diseases that cause secondary retroperitoneal fibrosis, and some of these can be diagnosed by means of imaging methods [1, 23, 25, 28]: inflammatory disease of the gastrointestinal tract (pancreatitis, Crohn's disease, etc.); tumors (lymphoma, metastases); hemorrhage; urinoma; aortic aneurysm. Other causes of fibrosis may be drugs (ergot compounds), autoimmunization diseases, radiation therapy, and operations. The fibrotic lesions are usually located in the area between L4 and the sacral promontory. They may effect the ureters through shrinkage or extrinsic compression, causing obstruction and urinary stasis. Obstructive nephropathy and renal failure may develop.

Investigation Methods

Plain Film and Urography. Urography is an efficient diagnostic method, visualizing typical displacement, obstruction of the ureter, and urinary stasis.

Ultrasound and Computed Tomography. Ultrasound and CT display both fibrous lesions and diseases which may be the cause of fibrosis (Fig. 6a, b) [11, 12].

Diagnostic Approach

While urography is the initial investigation method, in renal failure ultrasound is the best way

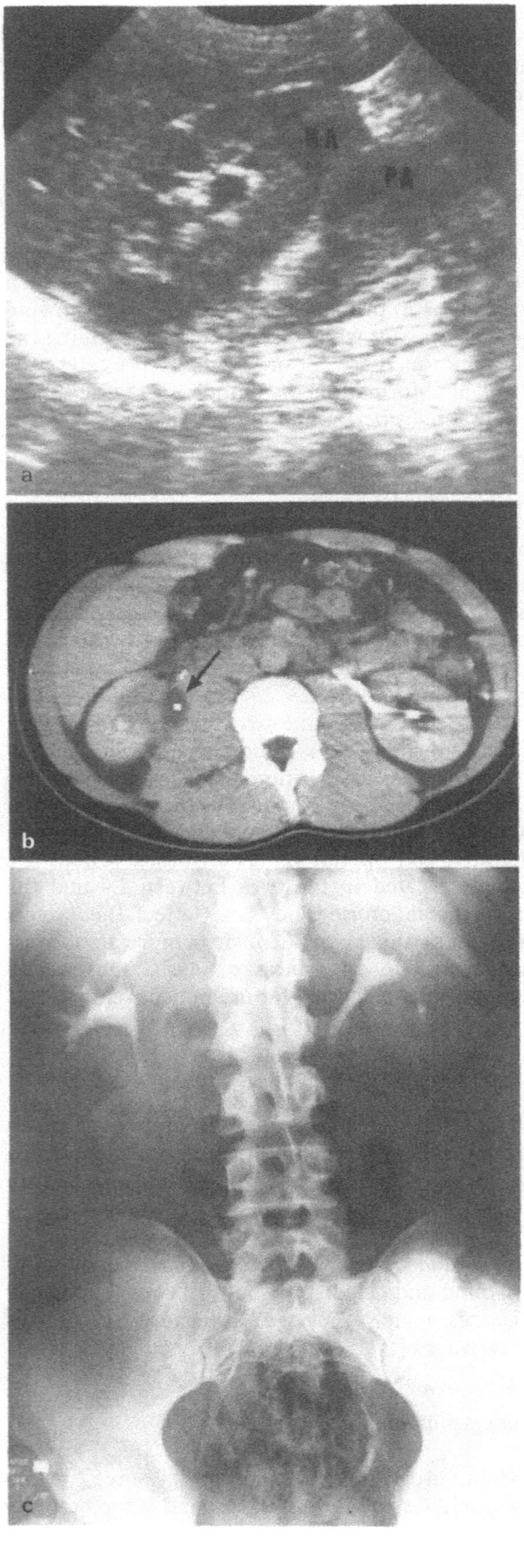

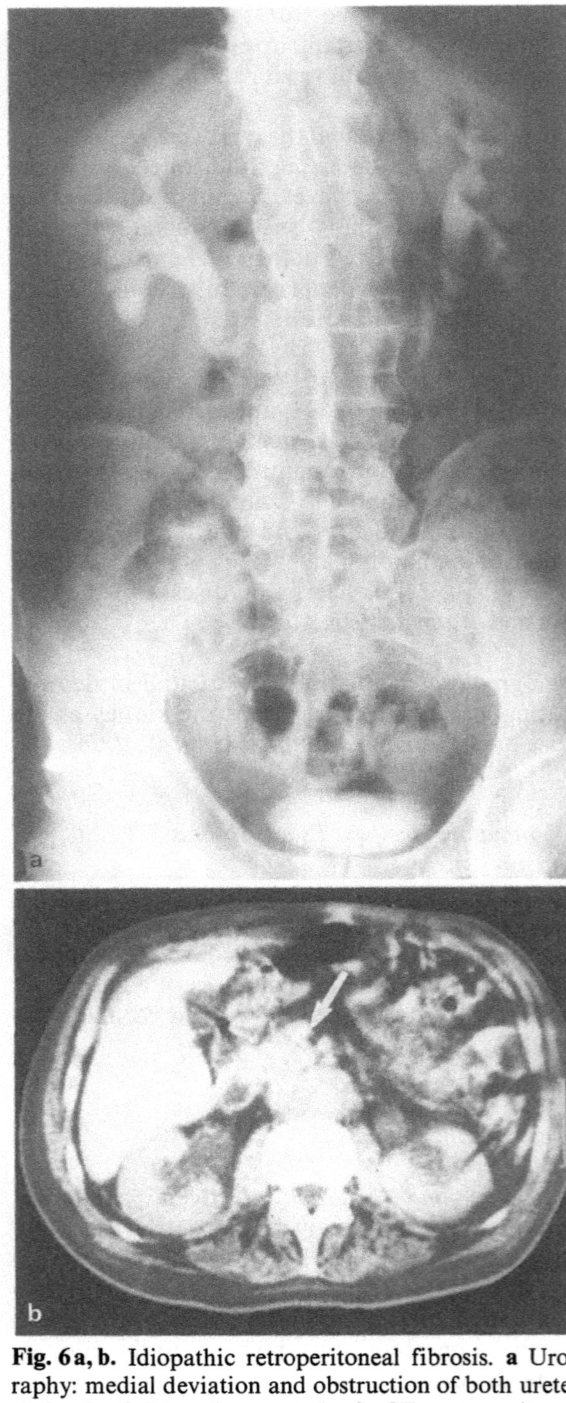

Fig. 6a, b. Idiopathic retroperitoneal fibrosis. **a** Urography: medial deviation and obstruction of both ureters at level of L4, urinary stasis. **b** CT: retroperitoneal fibrotic tissue with a tumor-like appearance (*arrow*)

◂ **Fig. 5a–c.** Renal abscess and psoas abscess. **a** Sonography. *RA*, renal abscess, lower pole of right kidney. *PA*, anechoic lesion in enlarged psoas muscle caused by abscess formation. **b** CT: renal abscess and psoas abscess (hypodense area in enlarged muscle; *arrow*). **c** Urography: slight displacement of right kidney and ureter, enlarged but well-defined psoas muscle of evaluating bilateral urinary stasis and will also help to display the cause of obstruction. CT of the retroperitoneum will visualize extrinsic lesions and display more distinctly conditions causing retroperitoneal fibrosis without the limitations of ultrasound.

References

1. Allibone GW, Saxton HM (1980) The association of aorto-iliac aneurysms with ureteral obstruction. Urol Radiol 1:205–210
2. Bosniak MA, Megibow AJ, Ambos MA, Mitnick IS, Lefleur RS, Gordon R (1982) Computed tomography of ureteral obstruction. AJR 138:1107–1113
3. Brascho DJ, Durant JR, Green LG (1977) The accuracy of retroperitoneal ultrasonography in Hodgkin's disease and non-Hodgkin's lymphoma. Radiology 125:485–487
4. Brecht G, Lackner K, Brecht Th, Thurn P (1979) Das Aortenaneurysma im Computertomogramm. Fortschr Rontgenstr 130:162–171
5. Bree RL, Green B (1978) The gray scale sonographic appearance of intraabdominal mesenchymal sarcomas. Radiology 128:193–197
6. Castellino R, Marglin St, Blank N (1980) Hodgkin's disease, non-Hodgkin lymphomas and leukemias in the retroperitoneum. Semin Roentgenol. 15:288–301
7. Damascelli B, Musumeci R, Botturi M, Petrillo R, Spapuloi I (1975) Angiography of retroperitoneal tumors. A review. AJR 124:565–670
8. Daniels V, Brünner H (1979) Primäre retroperitoneale Tumoren. Dtsch Med Wochenschr 104:1202–1207
9. Duncan RE, Evans AT (1977) Diagnosis of primary retroperitoneal tumors. J Urol 117:19–23
10. Erikson I, Hemmingsson A, Lindgren PG (1980) Diagnosis of abdominal aortic aneurysms by aortography, computed tomography and ultrasound. Acta Radiol 21:209–214
11. Fagan ChI, Larrieu AJ, Amparo FG (1979) Retroperitoneal fibrosis. Ultrasound and CT features. AJR 133:239–243
12. Haertel M, Bollmann J, Vock P, Zingg E (1979) Computertomographie und retroperitoneale Fibrose. Fortschr Rontgenstr 131:504–507
13. Jeffrey RB, Calen PW, Federle MP (1980) Computed tomography of psoas abscesses. J Comput Assist Tomogr 4:639–641
14. Jing BS, Wallace S, Zornoza I (1982) Metastases to retroperitoneal and pelvic lymph nodes. Computed tomography and lymphangiography. Radiol Clin North Am 20:511–530
15. Kaplan HS (1980) Essentials of staging and management of the malignant lymphoma. Semin Roentgenol 15:219–228
16. Laing FC, Jacobs RP (1977) Value of ultrasonography in the detection of retroperitoneal inflammatory masses. Radiology 123:169–172
17. Lamarque IL, Triby X, Bruel MJ, Ronanet JP, Lopez P (1981) The results of angiographic studies of abdominal masses. Eur J Radiol 1:24–29
18. Lee IK, Stanley RI, Sagel SS, McClennan BL (1978) Accuracy of CT in detecting intraabdominal and pelvic lymph node metastases from pelvic cancers. AJR 131:675–679
19. Lowman RM, Gruja V, Peck DR, Osborn D, Love L (1972) Angiographic patterns of the primary retroperitoneal tumors: the role of the lumbar arteries. Radiology 104:259–268
20. Marchal G, Coenen Y, Wilms G, Baert AL (1978) The accuracy of CT scan in the diagnosis of retroperitoneal metastases of malignant testicular tumors. Fortschr. Rontgenstr 128:746–753
21. Martinez Moldano M, Romirez de Avellon G (1962) Renal involvement in malignant lymphoma. Am J Med 32:184–187
22. McCullough DL, Leopold GR (1976) Diagnosis of retroperitoneal fluid collections by ultrasonography: a series of surgically proved cases. J Urol 115:656–659
23. Persky L, Kursh ED, Feldman ST (1978) Extrinsic obstruction of the ureter. In: Campell's urology, 4th ed, vol 1. Saunders, Philadelphia
24. Raskin MM, Cunningham JB (1978) Comparison of computed tomography and ultrasound for abdominal aortic aneurysms: a preliminary study. J Comput Tomogr 2:21–23
25. Scott T, Cerny JG (1971) Non-idiopathic retroperitoneal fibrosis. J Urol 105:49–55
26. Stephens DH (1977) Computed tomography of the retroperitoneal space. Radiol Clin North Am 15:377–390
27. Triller I, Haertel M (1978) Zur sonographisch radiologischen Diagnostik abdominaler Abszesse. Fortschr Rontgenstr 128:739–745
28. Usher SM, Brendler H, Ciavarra VH (1977) Retroperitoneal fibrosis secondary to metastatic neoplasm. Urology 9:191–194
29. Wallace S, Jing BS (1977) Carcinoma. In: Clause ME (ed) Clinical lymphography. Williams and Wilkins, Baltimore
30. Zornoza I, Wallace S, Goldstein GH (1977) Transperitoneal percutaneous retroperitoneal lymph node aspiration biopsy. Radiology 122:111–115

Imaging of Adrenal Masses

L. Ekelund

In many aspects, the various methods of adrenal imaging reflect the evolution of diagnostic radiology over the years. Starting with retroperitoneal pneumography, moving on to selective arteriography and adrenal phlebography, and more recently taking advantage of less invasive imaging techniques like scintigraphy, ultrasound, CT, and eventually magnetic resonance imaging (MRI), the diagnostic accuracy has continued to improve. The purpose of the present overview is to discuss the role of adrenal imaging techniques available today and to suggest a proper sequence for the investigation of adrenal masses.

Scintigraphy

Although ^{131}I-19-iodocholesterol is not in widespread use and not commonly available, reports have appeared demonstrating the usefulness of this radioisotope in the evaluation of patients with various adrenal diseases [12]. Following intravenous administration, scans are performed with a gamma camera after 2 to 14 days, the delay being due to the fact that the isotope must be incorporated into the synthesis of the adrenal steroids. The relatively long period that a patient must be followed and scanned is a major drawback, and the procedure has not gained widespread use.

Another, potentially more interesting scintigraphic technique that has been used for the diagnosis of pheochromocytoma was recently described by Francis et al. [8]. ^{131}I-metaiodobenzylguanidine (MIBG), an adrenergic tissue-localizing radiopharmaceutical, was used in 32 patients with pathologically proved primary, metastatic, or recurrent pheochromocytoma, and the results were compared to those obtained by CT. Scintigrams were obtained with a gamma camera 24, 48, and 72 h after intravenous injection of the tracer, thus providing a much faster scanning procedure than the aforementioned technique with iodocholesterol. In all 12 patients with primary adrenal tumors, both MIBG scintigraphy and CT were positive (sensitivity = 100%). The smallest adrenal pheochromocytoma imaged was 1 cm in diameter, but most of the tumors were larger than 3 cm. In all four cases of recurrent pheochromocytoma, the tumor was demonstrated by both methods. Of the nine extra-adrenal tumors, five were in the thorax (intrapericardial) and both CT and MIBG were positive. Seven cases of metastatic pheochromocytoma, most involving the axial skeleton, were studied; in each patient lesions were confirmed by both methods.

MIBG scanning specifically identifies an adrenal mass as a pheochromocytoma because the radiopharmaceutical localizes adrenergic tissues. The authors' experience suggested complementary roles for ^{131}I-MIBG scintigraphy and CT, and in patients with biochemical evidence of pheochromocytoma, an MIBG scan was recommended as a logical initial study. Even though this new technique seems most promising the present limited availability of the radiopharmaceutical is a problem, and therefore radioisotope scanning of the adrenals is only used in a few centers where evaluation and clinical testing continue.

Angiography

Angiography has been used extensively in the investigation of adrenal disease. With the advent of ultrasound and especially CT, its use as an imaging diagnostic modality has rapidly decreased. However, CT is still not available in all institutions. Adrenal arteriography is often more rewarding in the patient with a large mass, and the demonstration of the blood supply to such lesions may provide important preoperative information. When performing adrenal arteriography one has to be aware that the adrenal arterial system is complex, rendering most examinations to some degree incomplete. A complete arteriographic ex-

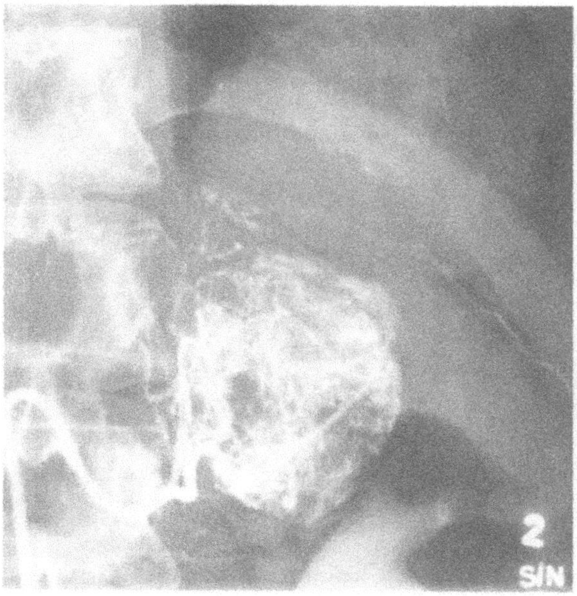

Fig. 1. Pheochromocytoma. Selective angiography of the left middle adrenal artery showing hypervascular tumor. The angiographic appearance is not specific, however, and the same finding can be seen in an adrenal metastasis, for example

amination should therefore include abdominal aortography as well as selective injections into the celiac, renal, and adrenal arteries. A comprehensive description of adrenal and related arteries in normal and pathologic conditions was given by Madsen [13].

It must be strongly emphasized that any patient suspected of having a pheochromocytoma should have adrenergic blockade prior to angiography to avoid complications, as the injection of contrast medium into the tumor may induce the release of catecholamines and result in a hypertensive crisis followed by shock and death.

The angiographic findings in adrenal masses have been reported by several investigators [2, 10, 11]. Adrenal angiography in eight patients with pheochromocytoma associated with Sipple's syndrome was reported by Ekelund and Hoevels [5]. The diagnosis of an adrenal tumor can usually be made at angiography, which, however, does not provide any reliable information as to the nature of the lesion (Fig. 1). Metastases cannot be distinguished from primary adrenal tumors, and often it is not possible to differentiate by means of arteriography between various benign and malignant tumors. Angiographic features typical of adrenal pheochromocytoma do not seem to exist, and adrenal hyperplasia may be present even when angiography does not demonstrate enlargement of the gland. As always in diagnostic radiology, clinical correlation is necessary, and therefore when an adrenal tumor is demonstrated by arteriography in a patient with biochemical evidence of pheochromocytoma, the differential diagnosis should not be too complicated.

If arteriography is no longer routinely used in the investigation of adrenal lesions, *adrenal vein catheterization* for blood sampling continues to be a most important means of establishing adrenal pathology. However, a thorough knowledge of adrenal vein anatomy and its variations is a prerequisite for these procedures. Valuable information about the venous communications of the adrenal glands has been provided by Mikaelsson [15] and El-Sherief [6], among others. One has to be especially aware of the variations in the anatomy of the right adrenal vein; certain patterns of the lower hepatic veins may mimic the adrenal veins, and the adrenal vein may join a lower hepatic vein, opening via a common trunk into the inferior vena cava. Due to the varying anatomy, the right adrenal vein is usually somewhat more difficult to catheterize selectively, and most investigators report a success rate of 70%–80%. Because of the small dimensions of the adrenal vein, aspiration of blood may be difficult. This problem can be solved by making a side-hole very close to the tip of the catheter.

Venous sampling with hormone assays has been shown to be useful in a variety of hormonally active lesions, especially in patients with primary aldosteronism (Conn's syndrome). Dunnick et al. [3] recently reported their results in the localization of functional adrenal tumors by CT and venous sampling. Twenty-eight patients had primary aldosteronism, 20 had Cushing's syndrome, and 10 had pheochromocytoma. Adrenal venous sampling was correct every time it was undertaken, and reliably distinguished adrenal tumors from hyperplasia. It was recommended that adrenal venous sampling should follow a negative CT scan in patients suspected of having functional adrenal pathology. Furthermore, El-Sherief et al. [7] evaluated the diagnostic accuracy of CT, venous sampling, and angiography in 50 patients with proven adrenal pathology, including hyperplasia, adrenal cortical masses and pheochromocytomas. Sampling was 100% accurate in those cases where it was performed.

Catheterization of the adrenal veins with blood catecholamine determinations is also a very sensitive method for the localization of pheo-

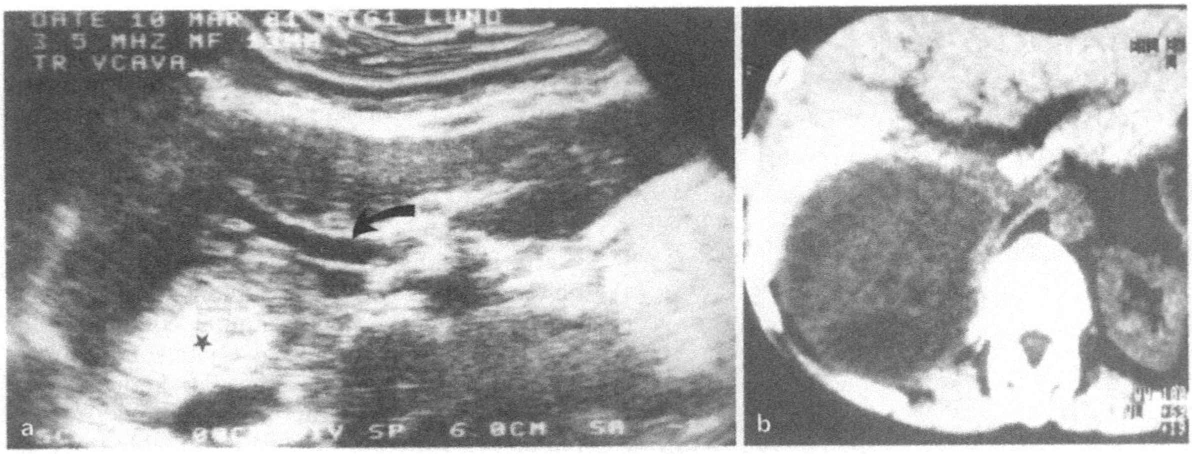

Fig. 2. **a** Transverse ultrasound scan in a patient with pheochromocytoma showing large echogenic mass in the right adrenal (*star*) with an area of necrosis posteriorly. The portal vein is seen anteriorly (*arrow*). **b** Corresponding CT scan in the same patient

chromocytomas. By the use of this technique three adrenomedullar neoplasms were detected which were too small to be visualized with CT [19].

Ultrasound

Sonography has been advocated as a useful screening test for the identification of adrenal tumors [20, 23]. Both normal glands and tumors may be identified (Fig. 2). According to Yeh the accuracy for detecting adrenal masses is very high, with a false-negative rate of only 3%. However, the demonstration of a normal adrenal gland or small adrenal mass is technically complex and intimately related to the experience and skill of the ultrasonographer. Furthermore, in obese patients (e.g., Cushing's disease) the image is degraded and the examination less reliable.

The data on the sensitivity and specificity of ultrasound are less complete than are those for CT, but generally they suggest a lower sensitivity. Few comparative studies of the two methods have been undertaken. Therefore, the results of a recently published prospective study of the accuracy of CT and ultrasound in 112 consecutive patients with suspected adrenal disease are important [1]. CT had a sensitivity of 84% (47/56), a specificity of 98% (55/56), and an accuracy of 90%. Ultrasound had a sensitivity of 79% (22/28), a specificity of 61% (14/23), and an overall accuracy of 70%. Receiver operating characteristic curves differed for CT and ultrasound, and strongly suggested the diagnostic superiority of CT. However, if CT is not available, sonography can be a useful screening test for many patients who are suspected to have adrenal masses. Complementary studies (angiography, venous sampling) are usually indicated.

Computed Tomography

The value of CT in the diagnosis of adrenal pathology has been convincingly documented in the literature. Since less operator effort and skill are required, this imaging technique has largely replaced ultrasound in departments where both methods are available. Continuous and fast scans have made it possible to identify both adrenals in most cases. An example of normal adrenals by CT is shown in Fig. 3. Although the shape of the gland varies on CT scans, the normal margins are usually straight or concave. The primary diagnostic problem in adrenal studies is the differentiation between a mass, hyperplasia, and a normal gland. If size and contours are normal, an adrenal tumor is unlikely. Hyperplasia, however, cannot be definitely ruled out, and if such abnormality is suggested by biochemical tests, further evaluation with adrenal vein sampling has to be undertaken. Small lesions usually appear as discrete bulges from normal gland contours, while larger masses are more obvious (Fig. 4). The attenuation of an adrenal mass is usually that of soft tissue. Some tumors have low densities due to high lipid content, as in myelolipoma [21]. Others have low attenuation values because of cystic or necrotic degeneration (Fig. 5).

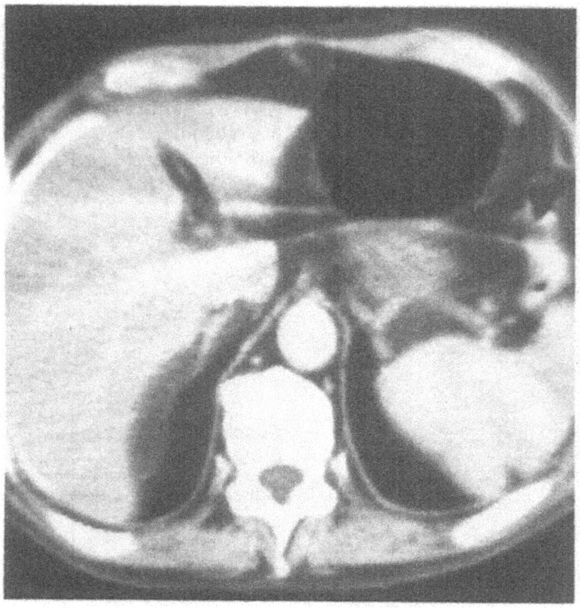

Fig. 3. CT scan showing normal adrenal glands

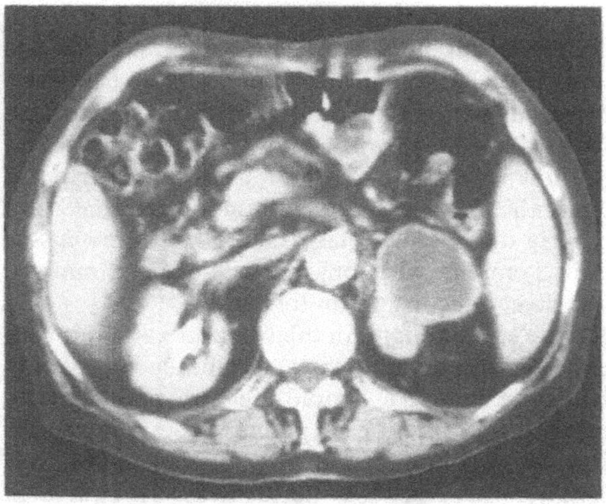

Fig. 5. CT scan in a patient with left-sided partially necrotic pheochromocytoma

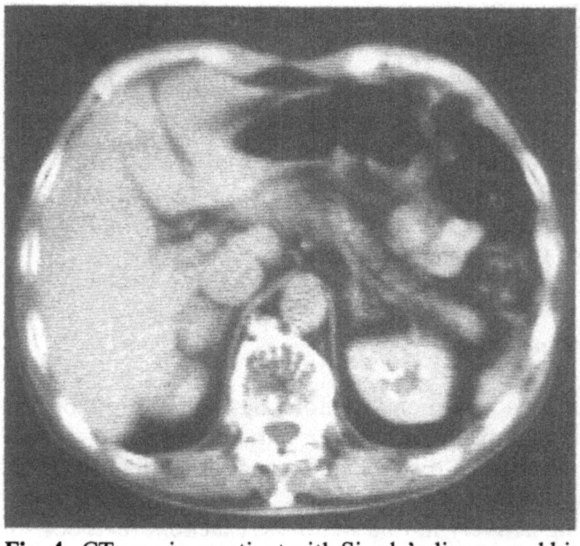

Fig. 4. CT scan in a patient with Sipple's disease and bilateral pheochromocytomas

CT has been shown to be the method of choice for demonstration of pheochromocytomas. A recent review of 60 histologically proved pheochromocytomas confirmed the value of CT [22], which was found to be an accurate means of locating the tumor in 52 patients presenting for the first time, and in eight patients with recurrences.
The size of adrenal tumors demonstrated by CT varies considerably, ranging from 0.5 cm to 12 cm [4]. Smaller tumors are usually not detected.
In another series, CT correctly identified adrenal tumors in 11 (61%) of 18 patients with aldosteronomas, six of six patients with benign cortisol-producing adrenal tumors, and five of six patients with pheochromocytomas [3]. Bilateral adrenal hyperplasia appeared as normal or prominent glands; however, CT was not able to exclude the presence of small adenomas. Adrenal venous sampling, on the other hand, correctly distinguished adrenal tumors from hyperplasia.
Meek et al. [14] used CT in 18 patients with primary aldosteronism. In seven patients, the CT results were verified by operation (six adenomas, one adrenal hypertrophy). However, in one further patient a 2-cm adenoma which had not been predicted by CT was found at operation. In the remaining 10 patients with nonsurgical treatment, results concordant with quadric analysis were obtained in eight cases.
Incidental detection of an adrenal mass on CT is not uncommon. Most of these are nonfunctioning adrenal adenomas. If there is a history of known primary malignancy, however, an adrenal lesion must be regarded metastatic until proved otherwise. Percutaneous fine-needle biopsy under CT guidance may then help differentiate primary lesions from metastatic carcinoma [9]. Mitnick et al. [16] studied 18 patients with unilateral, nonmetastatic, nonfunctioning adrenal masses with

CT. The adrenal lesion ranged from 1.2 to 5 cm. All had a smooth contour; 17 were round and one was oval. Pathological examination in six cases revealed benign adrenal adenoma. The others were followed up with serial CT scans and found to show no change in tumor size over a period of 6 months to 3 years. The authors suggested certain criteria of a benign mass, including diameter less than 5 cm, smooth contour, well-defined margin, and no change in size on follow-up.

Based on the reports in the literature and our own experience, the following recommendations can be suggested. CT should be the initial radiographic examination in patients with aldosteronism. If a tumor is clearly demonstrated, adrenalectomy may be performed. In equivocal cases and if no tumor is seen, adrenal venous sampling has to be performed to localize the adenoma or to distinguish an adenoma from bilateral hyperplasia. Patients with Cushing's syndrome also begin their radiographic evaluation with CT. CT is the first radiographic examination for patients with suspected pheochromocytoma, unless MIBG scintigraphy is available. If no adrenal mass is seen, the examination has to be extended to include the para-aortic tissue down to the bifurcation in the search for extra-adrenal manifestations. If results are still negative, arteriography and/or venous sampling is undertaken to localize the lesion.

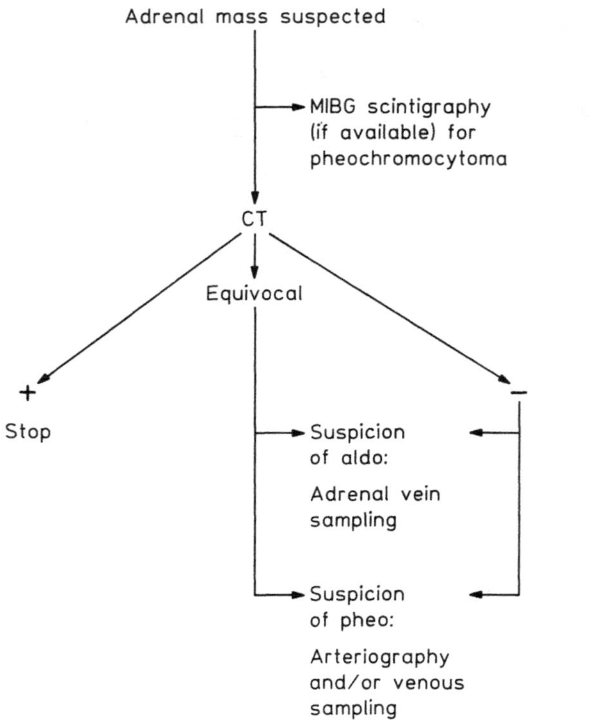

Fig. 6. Suggested diagnostic sequence in patients with suspected adrenal disease

Magnetic Resonance Imaging

Even though this new technique is so far available in only few institutions, a short comment on its potential value as an adrenal imaging modality has to be included. The San Francisco group recently reported their initial experience with MRI characteristics of the normal and abnormal adrenal gland, and comparison was made with CT findings in 42 patients examined [18]. Thirty-six had normal adrenal glands and six had adrenal disease, including three metastatic lesions, one pheochromocytoma, and two adrenal cortical hyperplasias. MRI clearly showed all 42 left adrenals (100%) and 36 right adrenals (86%). An interesting and potentially useful finding was the apparent ability to differentiate the adrenal cortex from the medulla in some patients. All six adrenal lesions were clearly demonstrated by MRI and CT. Metastases appeared as masses of lower intensity than normal adrenal tissue. The pheochromocytoma appeared as a round mass with a low-intensity rim and a high-intensity center. CT demonstrated superior spatial resolution, but MRI provided superior soft tissue contrast. MRI appears to be a promising modality for imaging of the adrenal gland.

Conclusion

It is a common opinion that CT should be the initial examination in a patient suspected of having adrenal disease, and a suggested diagnostic sequence is given in Fig. 6. Finally, to those working actively in this field, the excellent textbook on radiology of the adrenals by Mitty and Yeh [17] is strongly recommended.

References

1. Abrams HL, Siegelman SS, Adams DF, Sanders R, Friberg HJ, Hessel SJ, McNeil BJ (1982) Computed tomography versus ultrasound of the adrenal gland: a prospective study. Radiology 143:121–128
2. Boijsen E, Williams CM, Judkins MP (1966) Angiography of pheochromocytoma. AJR 98:225–232
3. Dunnick NR, Doppman JL, Gill JR, Shott CA, Keiser HR, Brennan MF (1982) Localization of

functional adrenal tumors by computed tomography and venous sampling. Radiology 142:429–433

4. Eghrari M, McLoughlin MJ, Rosen IE, St Louis EL, Wilson SR, Wise DJ, Young HPH (1980) The role of computed tomography in assessment of tumoral pathology of the adrenal glands. J Comput Assist Tomogr 4:71–77
5. Ekelund L, Hoevels J (1979) Adrenal angiography in Sipple's syndrome. Acta Radiol [Diagn] 20:637–647
6. El-Sherief MA (1982) Adrenal vein catheterization: anatomic considerations. Acta Radiol [Diagn] 23:345–360
7. El-Sherief MA, Hemmingsson A, Lörelius LE (1982) Computed tomography and angiography in the evaluation of adrenal diseases. Acta Radiol [Diagn] 23:625–637
8. Francis IR, Glazer GM, Shapiro B, Sisson JC, Gross BH (1983) Complementary roles of CT and ^{131}I-MIBG scintigraphy in diagnosing pheochromocytoma. AJR 141:719–725
9. Heaston DK, Handel DB, Ashton PR, Korobkin M (1982) Narrow gauge needle aspiration of solid adrenal masses. AJR 138:1143–1148
10. Hoevels J, Ekelund L (1979) Angiographic findings in adrenal masses. Acta Radiol [Diagn] 20:337–352
11. Lecky JW, Wolfman NT, Modic CW (1976) Current concepts of adrenal angiography. Radiol Clin N Am 14:309–352
12. Lieberman LM, Beierwaltes WH, Conn JW (1971) Diagnosis of adrenal disease by visualization of human adrenal glands with 131-19-iodocholesterol. N Engl J Med 285:1387–1393
13. Madsen B (1980) Selective adrenal angiography. A study of adrenal and related arteries in normal and pathological conditions. Fadl, Copenhagen
14. Meek DR, Duncan JG, McAreavey D (1981) Computed tomography in the localization of aldosterone-secreting adrenal adenomas. Br J Radiol 54:1039–1043
15. Mikaelsson CG (1970) Venous communications of the adrenal glands. Anatomic and circulatory studies. Acta Radiol [Diagn] 10:369–393
16. Mitnick JS, Bosniak MA, Megibow AJ, Naidich DP (1983) Nonfunctioning adrenal adenomas discovered incidentally on computed tomography. Radiology 148:495–499
17. Mitty HA, Yeh H-C (1982) Radiology of the adrenals with sonography and CT. Saunders, Philadelphia
18. Moon KL, Hricak H, Crooks LE, Gooding CA, Moss AA, Engelsted BL, Kaufman L (1983) Nuclear magnetic resonance imaging of the adrenal gland: a preliminary report. Radiology 147:155–160
19. Nobin A, Karp W, Lunderquist A, Rosengren E, Sandén G, Sundler F (1982) Localization of carcinoids and pheochromocytomas with vein catheterization and amine determination. Brain Res Bull 9:781–797
20. Sample WF (1977) A new technique for the evaluation of the adrenal gland with gray scale ultrasonography. Radiology 124:463–469
21. Vick CW, Zeman RK, Mannes E, Cronan JJ, Walsch JW (1984) Adrenal myelolipoma: CT and ultrasound findings. Urol Radiol 6:7–13
22. Welch TJ, Sheedy PF, van Heerders JA, Sheps SG, Hattery RH, Stephens DH (1983) Pheochromocytoma: value of computed tomography. Radiology 148:501–503
23. Yeh H-C (1980) Sonography of the adrenal glands: normal glands and small masses. AJR 135:1167–1177

Diagnostic Approach to Parapelvic Masses

E. Grabbe and E. Bücheler

Many methods are available for investigation of pelvic masses, including history-taking physical examination, conventional radiologic methods such as plain films, urography, barium enema, lymphography, and angiography, and more sophisticated imaging techniques such as ultrasonography, CT, and nuclear magnetic resonance (NMR). With respect to original of the mass, space-occupying lesions can be generally classified into the following categories: tumors of the genitourinary and intestinal tract; malignant lymphoma; soft tissue masses; bone tumors; metastases; pseudotumors, e.g., hematoma, abscess, aneurysm, lymphocele, urinoma, fibrosis.

This paper will particularly deal with the so-called *parapelvic lesions,* located beside the bladder, the uterus, the rectum, or the pelvic wall. Topographically, they are situated within the retro- and subperitoneal spaces, which are separated by the peritoneum and the muscles of the pelvic floor.

Physical Examination

If a patient has clinical symptoms suspicious of a pelvic mass, after taking the history the next step is a careful digital examination. This gives a rough impression of the localization and structure of the tumor and its relationship to the neighboring organs and the pelvic wall. It is also of interest to know if the tumor is freely mobile or fixed. On the other hand, palpation demands considerable skill and remains subjective. Moreover, it tends to be impossible in high-located tumors and obese patients.

Ultrasonography

In the past decade, ultrasonography has vastly improved as better equipment has been developed and more clinical experience obtained. It has now become an excellent complementary method of clinical examination [2, 4, 7, 9]. Its major advantages are generally well known, especially its noninvasive and nonionizing nature and its relatively low cost when compared to X-ray, CT, and NMR imaging. Ultrasound has proved to be most useful in fine-needle aspiration biopsy. Outside the pelvic organs, it is useful not only in confirming suspicious and high-located masses not detectable by palpation, but also in distinguishing between cystic and solid lesions (Fig. 1). Finally, ascites, hydronephrosis, and liver metastasis can also be demonstrated.

However, certain physical and technological limitations of ultrasound will always restrict its use. Strong reflections of the beam from boundaries between tissue and air within the intestine or from the pelvic bone prohibit its use. Fluid-filled bowel loops may lead to false-positive findings. Another important drawback is the limited spatial resolution, which decreases with increasing penetration depth. Therefore, the dorsal compartment of the pelvis cannot be well visualized by transvesical ultrasonography. Furthermore, ultrasound is unable to demonstrate infiltration of malignant tumors into the muscles and the bone of the pelvic wall, or even to distinguish echogenic masses in more detail.

Computed Tomography

If ultrasound reveals an echogenic mass outside the genitourinary and intestinal tract but the diagnosis remains uncertain, one should go straight on to CT [5, 6, 9, 10]. With respect to the density of a mass, CT can reveal not only fatty tissue and cystic lesions, but also hematoma at an early stage, when the density of the blood has increased, and abscesses in certain cases (Table 1, Fig. 2). While the rim sign of an abscess seems to be characteristic but unspecific, the air bubbles and air-fluid levels visible in more than 40% of

Table 1. Classification of parapelvic masses examined by CT ($n = 224$)

Diagnosis	No.
Abscess	43
Hematoma	51
Aneurysm	17
Lymphocele	15
Neurinoma	6
Myxoma	2
Lipomatosis pelvis	3
Diffuse infiltrating lipomatosis	7
Hemangioma	1
Liposarcoma	19
Fibrosarcoma	17
Leiomyosarcoma	8
Rhabdomyosarcoma	5
Hemangiopericytoma	3
Schwannoma	9
Neuroblastoma	2
Chordoma	4
Malignant histiocytoma	4
Unclassified soft tissue masses	8

our patients are specific. And, of course, puncture can be done: to confirm the diagnosis, to get an antibiogram, or to insert a drainage catheter. One can reply that X-ray imaging can identify pathologic air collections as well. But air bubbles, for example after resection of the rectum, do not alone provide certain proof of an abscess, and therefore an additional imaging method is always necessary. In cases of pelvic lipomatosis it is useful to know the site of these masses: In our experience the only really benign lipomatosis is that which grows inside the perivesical and perirectal fasciae [5]. If it arises outside these fasciae it tends to grow more and more slowly and to penetrate the pelvic wall along the nerves and the blood vessels into other compartiments. After resection, the so-called diffuse infiltrating lipomatosis tends to recur. In addition, we observed two cases of sarcomatous degeneration after 3 and 4 years respectively, which emphasizes that this primarily benign soft tissue mass is a distinct entity, differing in several ways from the so-called lipomatosis pelvis as defined by Engels [1, 3] (Table 2). If an aneurysm or a vascular malformation is suspected, for example on palpation or on ultrasound, a bolus injection of contrast medium leads to final diagnosis. In addition, CT-guided fine-needle aspiration biopsy can be done in supine or prone position in order to check whether a mass is be-

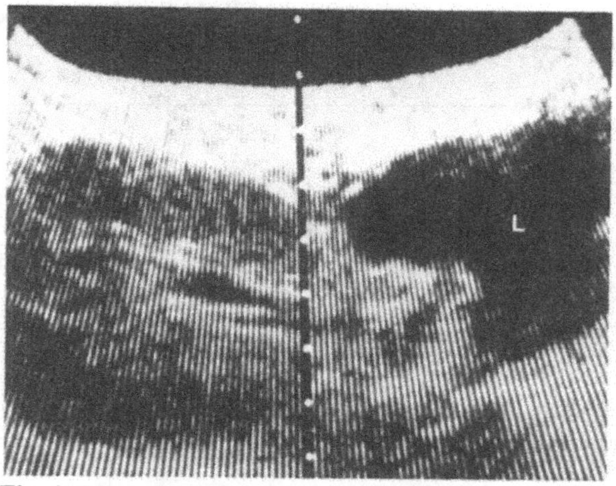

Fig. 1. Ultrasonography, longitudinal section: lymphocele (*L*) after renal transplant

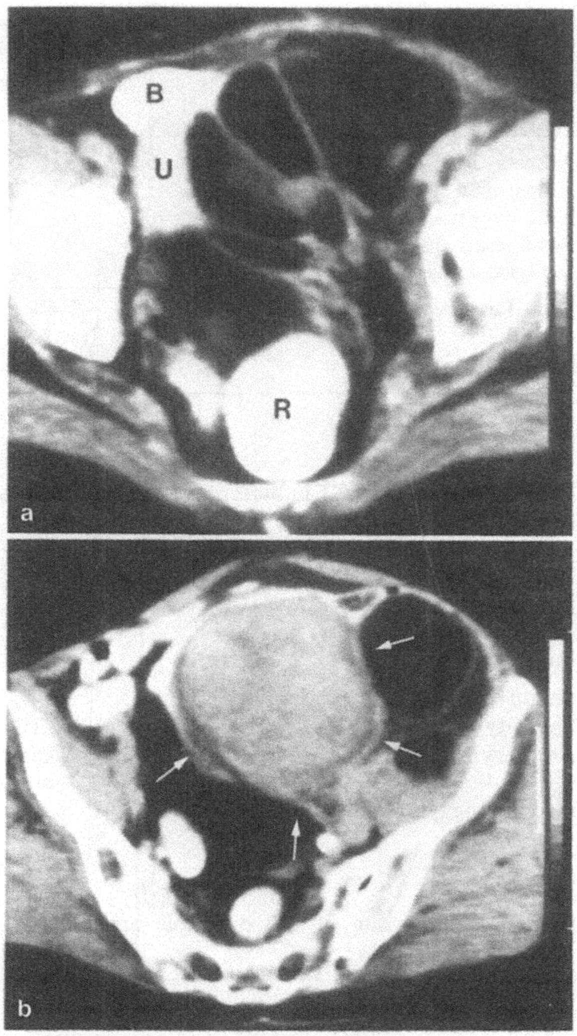

Fig. 2a, b. CT: diffuse infiltrating lipomatosis with malignant degeneration (*arrows*). *B*, bladder; *U*, uterus; *R*, rectum

Table 2. Comparison of characteristics of lipomatosis pelvis ($n = 3$) and diffuse infiltrating lipomatosis ($n = 7$)

Factor	Lipomatosis pelvis	Diffuse infiltrating lipomatosis
Age	35.7 years	47.1 years
Sex	3 M	6 F, 1 M
Localization	Capsula adiposa vesicalis et rectalis	Paravesical, pararectal, retroperitoneal, extension into neighboring compartiments
Histology	Hyperplastic/hypertrophic fat cells	Hyperplastic/hypertrophic fat cells
Therapy	No therapy	Incomplete resection
Follow-up	No progress	Slow progress, recurrence after resection, malignant degeneration (?)
Prognosis	Good	Dubious

Table 3. Accuracy of CT-guided fine-needle aspiration biopsy ($n = 67$)

Lesion	No.	Cytology	
		−	+
Abscess	16	16	0
Hematoma	5	5	0
Cyst, lymphocele	6	6	0
Postoperative scar tissue	9	9	0
Malignant mass	31	7	24
Sensitivity		77.4%	
Specificity		100.0%	
Accuracy		89.6%	

Table 4. Accuracy of CT in detecting parapelvic masses ($n = 224$)[a]

True positive	179
True negative	35
False positive	3
False negative	7
Sensitivity	96.2%
Specifity	92.1%
Accuracy	95.5%

[a] Excluding lymphatic system

Table 5. Comparison of CT diagnosis and final diagnosis ($n = 179$)

	No.	%
Correct	112	62.6
Uncertain and false	67	37.4

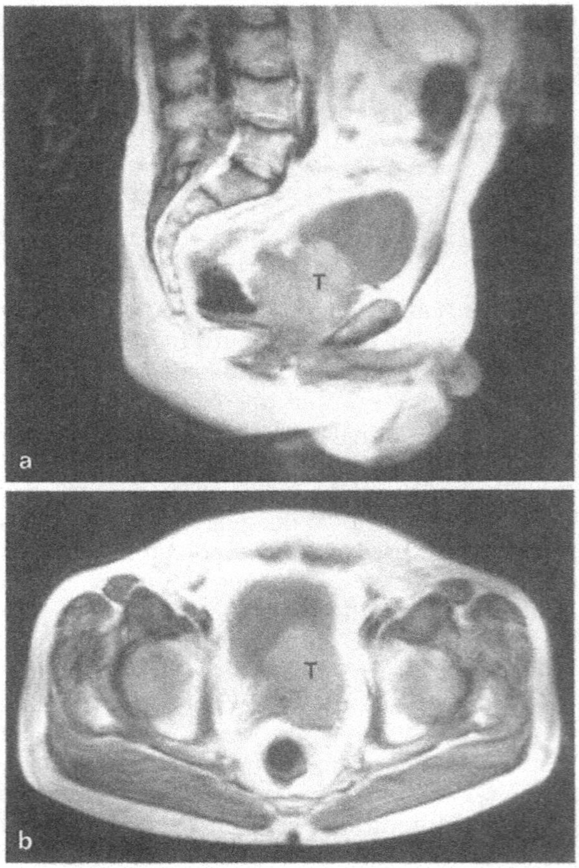

Fig. 3a, b. MR, T1-weighted spin-echo images, transverse and sagittal sections (Philips, Eindhoven): carcinoma of the prostate (*T*) with infiltration of the bladder

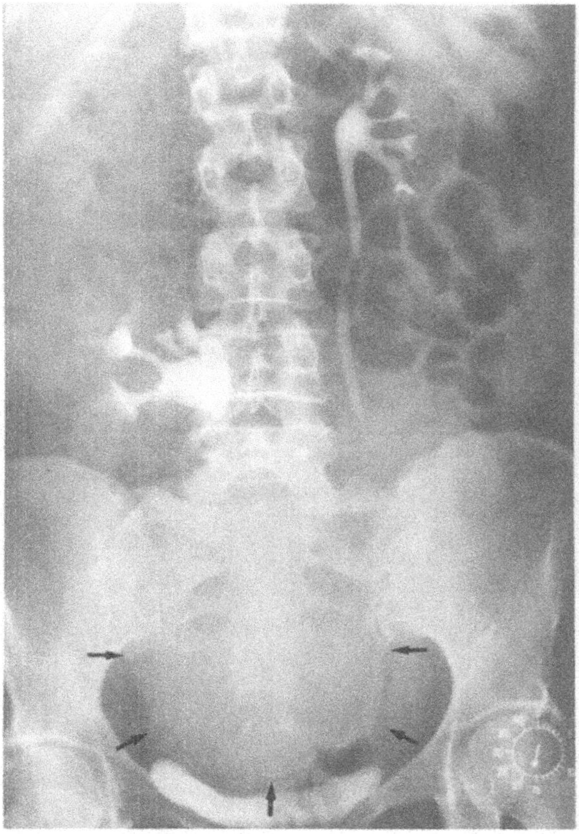

Fig. 4. Urography: leiomyosarcoma with lateral deviation of the ureters and compression of the bladder (*arrows*)

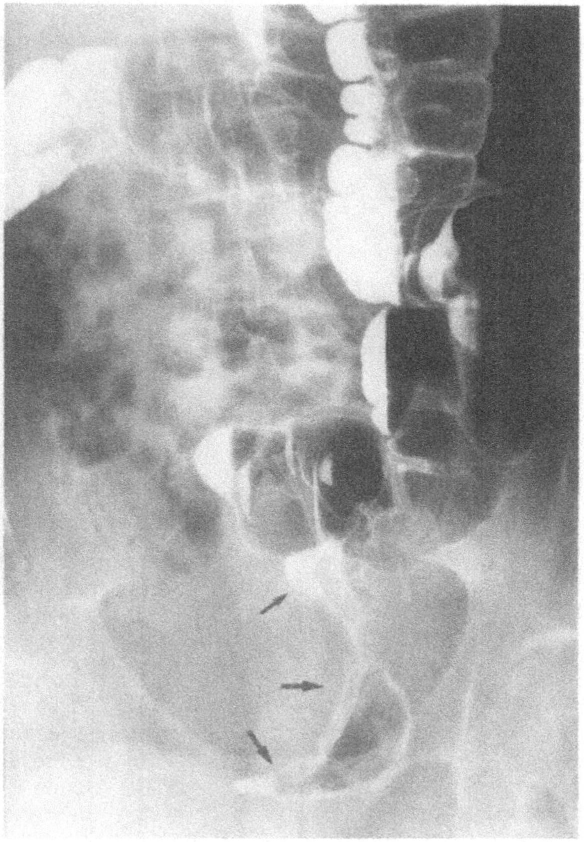

Fig. 5. Barium enema: malignant schwannoma with compression of the rectosigmoid (*arrows*)

nign or malignant [11]. And in fact aspiration cytology is very accurate, especially in metastases and local recurrences (Table 3).

To summarize our findings, CT reached a high accuracy of about 95% in detecting so called "parapelvic" masses, and also led to final diagnosis in about two-thirds of our cases (Tables 4, 5). Moreover, it is generally well known that CT has turned out to be the method of choice, if local recurrence is suspected.

Nuclear Magnetic Resonance

NMR has, of course, obvious advantages in comparison with other noninvasive imaging techniques. Beside the nonionizing nature of the method, three-dimensional images are obtainable which are of significantly better quality than those reconstructed by CT (Fig. 3). The third and most important advantage of NMR, even when compared with CT, is the extremely high contrast resolution due to various kinds of signals resulting from proton density and relaxation times T1 and T2. As we have only been able to work on a high magnetic field strength of 2.0 T at the Philips research center in Hamburg since April 1984, we have as yet little clinical experience and therefore cannot give a statement on its value. In the literature, it has been suggested that NMR might be helpful in detecting and staging carcinoma of the prostate and the uterus. It would also be of interest to know whether NMR can distinguish between scar tissue and local recurrence.

Conventional Radiology

In a parapelvic mass confirmed by ultrasound or CT, conventional radiologic methods, such as urography, barium enema, and angiography give only little additional information with respect to

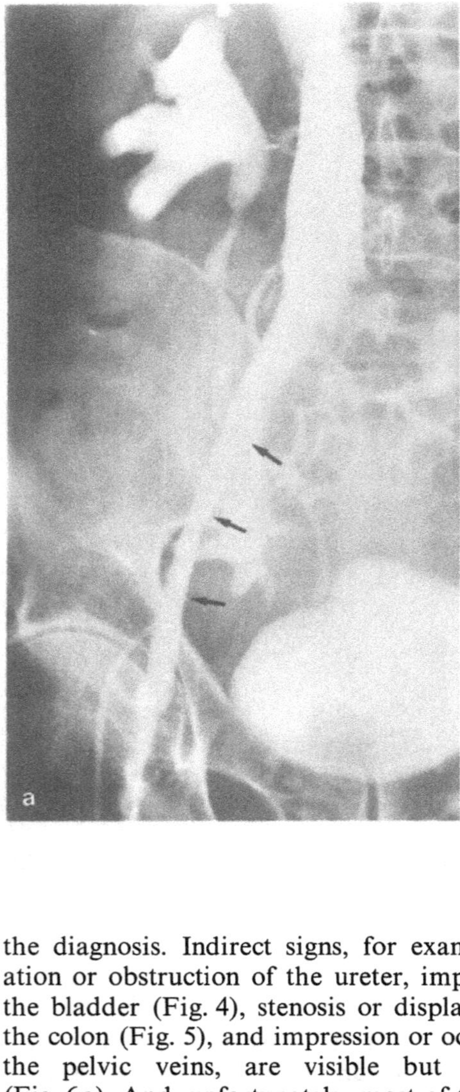

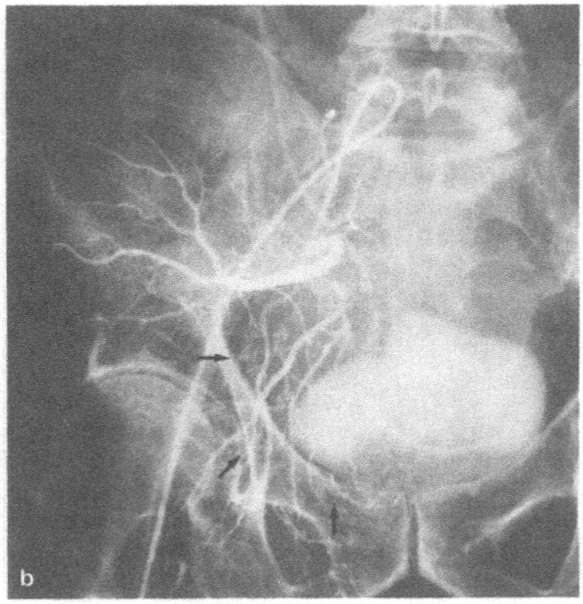

Fig. 6 a, b. Angiography: neurofibroma with obstruction of the right ureter and slight compression of the bladder as well as the iliac vein (**a** *arrows*). The lesion is sparsely supplied with vessels of the internal iliac artery (**b** *arrows*)

the diagnosis. Indirect signs, for example deviation or obstruction of the ureter, impression of the bladder (Fig. 4), stenosis or displacement of the colon (Fig. 5), and impression or occlusion of the pelvic veins, are visible but unspecific (Fig. 6a). And, unfortunately, most of the masses are sparsely supplied with vessels and are therefore poorly visualized on angiography (Fig. 6b). On the other hand, the conventional techniques should always be kept in mind in cases not determinable by noninvasive methods, and also in treatment planning, especially if surgery is contemplated [4, 8].

Conclusion

Beside the history of the patient, clinical investigation combined with ultrasonography is the procedure of choice in detecting so-called parapelvic masses outside the genitourinary and intestinal tracts. Whenever the well-known limitations of ultrasound restrict its use within the pelvis, CT is the next step in the diagnostic procedure. On the other hand, conventional radiologic examinations are more often helpful in patients to be treated surgically. The value of NMR is not yet completely determined.

References

1. Allen PW (1981) Tumors and proliferations of adipose tissue. A clinicopathologic approach. Masson, New York
2. Beyer D, Peters PE (1980) Real-time ultrasonography – an efficient screening method for abdominal and pelvic lymphadenopathy. Lymphology 13:142
3. Engels EP (1959) Sigmoid colon and urinary bladder in high fixation: roentgen changes simulating tumor. Radiology 72:419
4. Fleischer AC, Walsh JW, Jones HW et al. (1982) Sonographic evaluation of pelvic masses: method of examination and role of sonography relative to other imaging modalities. Radiol Clin North Am 20:397
5. Grabbe E, Böcker W, Bücheler E (1984) Die diffus infiltrierende Lipomatosis. Fortschr Rontgenstr 140:645

6. Hidalgo H, Dunnick NR, Rosenberg ER et al. (1982) Parapelvic cysts: appearance on CT and sonography. AJR 138:667
7. Kaude JV, Moccia WA, Wertman DE et al. (1980) Pelvic hemangiopericytoma: ultrasonographic findings and comparison with angiography. Fortschr Rontgenstr 132:347
8. Lang EK (1980) Angiography in diagnosis and staging of pelvic neoplasms. Radiology 134:353
9. Sanders RC, McNeil BJ, Finberg HJ et al. (1983) Prospective study of computed tomography and ultrasound in the detection and staging of pelvic masses. Radiology 146:439
10. Waligore MP, Stephens DH, Soule EH et al. (1981) Lipomatous tumors of the abdominal cavity: CT appearance and pathologic correlation. AJR 137:539
11. Zornoza J, Bernadino ME, Ordonze NG et al. (1982) Percutaneous needle biopsy of soft tissue tumors guided by ultrasound and computed tomography. Skeletal Radiol 9:33

Transrectal and Intrauterine Sonography of Gynecologic Neoplasms

H. Hötzinger

Complementary to bimanual pelvic examination (still the basic procedure), new imaging systems for visualization of the internal genitalia have gained more and more importance in recent years, and for gynecologic cancers they have become a main point in the diagnostic workup. In this connection one has to mention ultrasound, CT, and increasingly, nuclear magnetic resonance (NMR). This work will deal with two newly developed modifications of intracavitary sonography, transrectal sonography (rectosonography) and intrauterine sonography (hysterosonography).

Intrauterine Sonography

The visualization of the fine structure of the myometrium uteri and its pathologic alterations was till now an unresolved problem [1, 6, 7]. However, it is important to know the extent and location of carcinomas when planning operative and radiation therapy. Intrauterine sonography allows the visualization of the normal myometrium, of myomas and carcinomas [5]. We use the ultrasonic equipment SSD 500 and the transurethral scanner ASU 52 (Aloka). The scanner consists of a rotating steel tube with a transducer (frequency 7.5 MHz, diameter 5 mm) on its end.

Over the tip of the scanner we place a plastic cover to prevent lesions of the tissue and standardize the water flow line [8]. The steel tube is inserted into the cervix, and by rotating the transducer 360° a two-dimensional real-time gray-scale scan is produced, showing sectional images of the uterus from the cervix to the fundus. Normally a picture is taken every 0.5 cm.

Intrauterine sonography may be performed before diagnostic curettage or intracavitary radiotherapy. Dilatation of the cervix to Hegar 10 is sufficient.

So far the results of over 200 cases have been histologically verified.

Normal Cervix and Corpus Uteri

In the normal cervix, the contour is round and the myometrium shows homogeneous, diffuse, fine, dotted, medium-strength echoes. The cervix appears well demarcated with capsular echoes from the serosa. Because of the narrow canal the endometrium cannot be seen in most cases.

The normal corpus (Fig. 1) shows the typical oval contour. The cavum is anechoic, the endometrium shows a strong reflection. The appearance of the myometrium does not differ from that of the cervical region. The serosa has a well-defined echo.

Carcinoma of the Cervix

Carcinomas of the cervix are characterized by a less dense echo pattern than normal tissue. In the case illustrated in Fig. 2 the tumor has spread into the left part of the myometrium. It takes up about ⅕ of the whole contour with a maximal diameter of 19 mm. The borders are ill defined without any formation of capsular structures, especially on the right side of the carcinoma. The depth of infiltration can be exactly determined: the carcinoma reaches the serosa, which, however, is preserved without interruption by tumor.

Carcinoma of the Corpus Uteri

Carcinomas of the corpus uteri (Fig. 3) present in a similar manner to those of the cervix. The echo pattern is less dense than that of normal myometrium. There is no formation of capsular structures. The transition to normal tissue is not sharply delineated. This example shows tumor infiltration on the left dorsal side reaching the serosa, and extensive exophytic growth into the uterine cavity with an irregularly defined echo pattern. The ventral portions of the cavity show a well-preserved endometrium.

Table 1. Visualization of the endometrium by intrauterine sonography

Visualized endometrium (%)	Fundus	Corpus	Cervix
100	40	39	4
90–50	55	56	4
50– 0	5	5	92

Two hundred and sixteen cases have been treated surgically and histologically verified. The length of the uterine cavity was correctly measured in 100%, the width of the corpus uteri in 97% and the width of the cervix uteri in 99%. In most cases of false measurement, massive myomas prevented correct determination of uterine size. The quality of the pictures of the fundus was good in 77%, fair in 21%, and bad in 2%, the corresponding figures in the corpus were 78%, 20%, and 2%, and in the cervix 93%, 6%, and 1%. The pictures got worse with increasing size and number of myomas, and artifacts increased with the thickness of the endometrium.

The visualization of the endometrium is shown in Table 1.

Of the 22 carcinomas of the cervix examined, 45% showed no infiltration, 25% showed infiltration within the myometrium, 15% to the serosa, and 15% beyond the serosa. The depth of infiltration was determined correctly in all cases. Of the 16 carcinomas of the corpus uteri examined, 25% showed no infiltration, 50% had an infiltration within the myometrium, and 25% as far as the serosa. Also in this series, the depth of infiltration was correctly determined in all cases.

These results encouraged us to integrate intrauterine sonography into the planning of intracavitary therapy of carcinomas of the corpus uteri in the following manner [4]: Before going ahead with intracavitary radiotherapy we do intrauterine sonography, making a transverse cut of the uterus every 0.5 cm. In this way we are able to determine the size and depth of infiltration of the cancer within the myometrium, i.e., we can exactly define the target volume for intracavitary irradiation. We are able to superimpose the necessary isodose curves on the intrauterine sonographic picture under (Fig. 4) consideration of the depth of infiltration of the carcinoma.

Besides the visualization of carcinomas, intrauterine sonography permits determination of the extent of the uterine cavity and the thickness of the

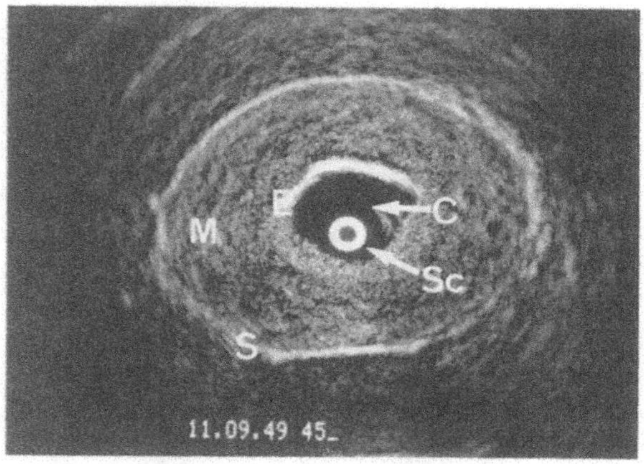

Fig. 1. Intrauterine sonography: normal corpus uteri. *Sc,* scanner; *C,* cavity; *E,* endometrium; *M,* myometrium; *S,* serosa

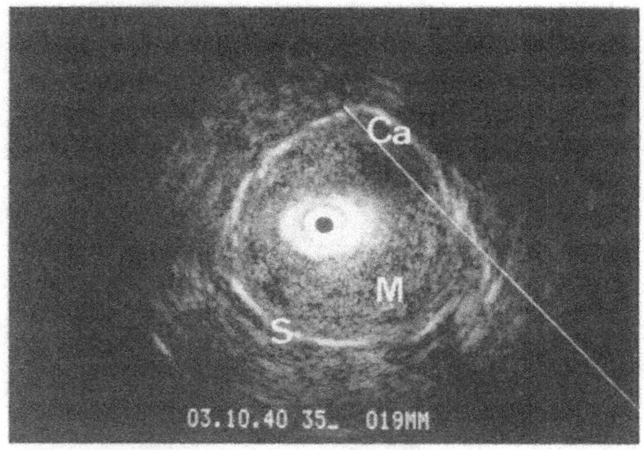

Fig. 2. Intrauterine sonography: carcinoma of the cervix uteri. *Ca,* carcinoma; *M,* myometrium; *S,* serosa

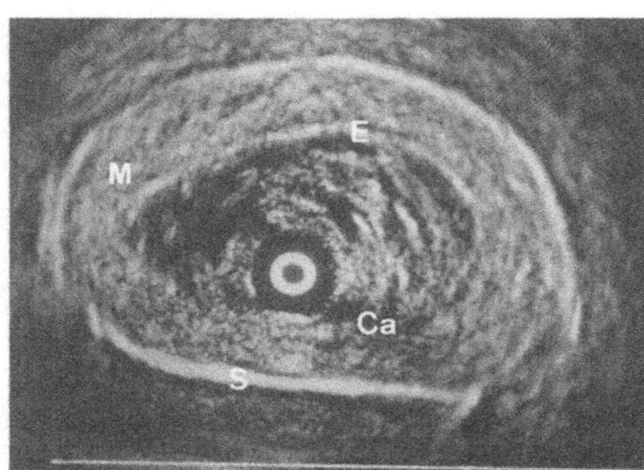

Fig. 3. Intrauterine sonography: carcinoma of the corpus uteri. *Ca,* carcinoma; *M,* myometrium; *E,* endometrium; *S,* serosa

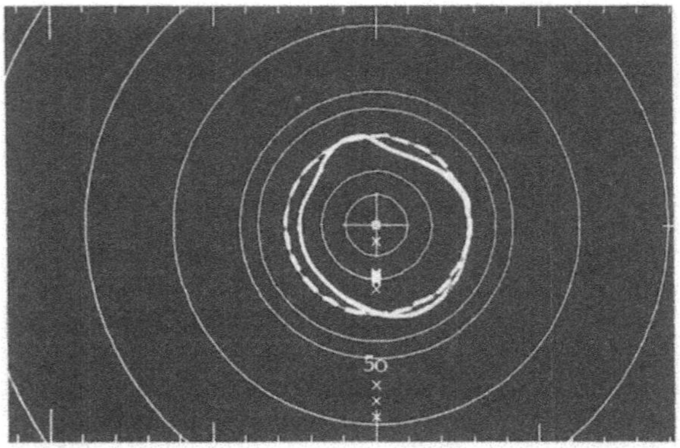

Fig. 4. Isodose curves directly superimposed on an intrauterine sonography scan. ——, contour of the corpus; - - - -, isodose curve wanted for intracavitary irradiation

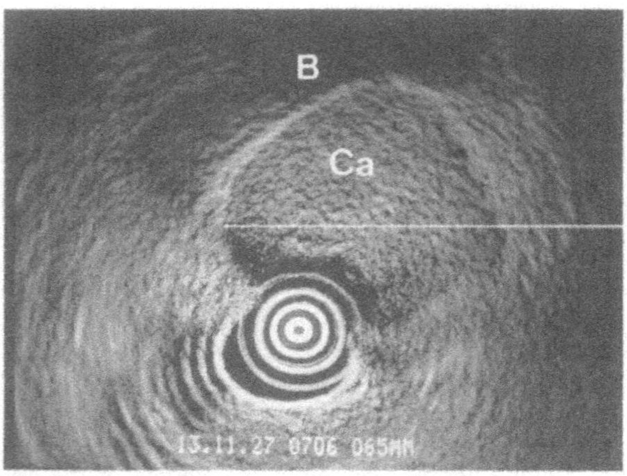

Fig. 5. Transrectal sonography: carcinoma of the cervix uteri stage III. *Ca*, carcinoma; *B*, bladder

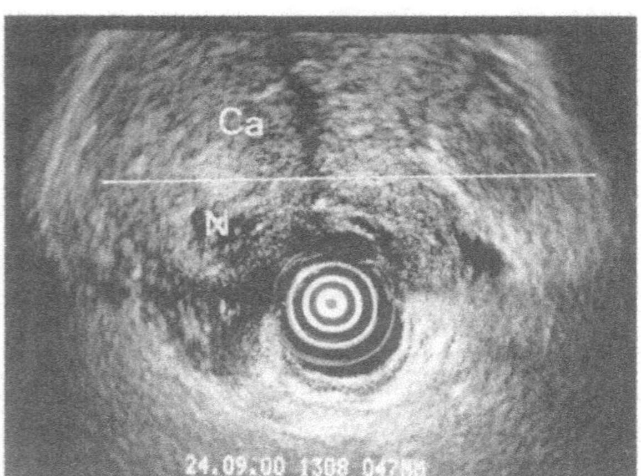

Fig. 6. Transrectal sonography: carcinoma of the corpus uteri. *Ca*, carcinoma; *N*, necrotic areas

uterine wall, and allows immediate recognition of whether one is dilatating the cervix uteri or a via falsa.

Transrectal Sonography

Transrectal sonography is a new diagnostic procedure which allows the visualization of the vagina, the cervix uteri, the corpus uteri, and the paravaginal and paracervical structures [2]. Here again we use the ultrasonic equipment SSD 500, but now in connection with the transrectal scanner ASU 51 (Aloka).
The scanner has a frequency of 5 MHz and a diameter of 10 mm. A rubber balloon is turned over the steel tube before the examination and filled with water, thus producing a constant water flow line. Transrectal sonography is usually done immediately after bimanual pelvic examination. The steel tube is inserted into the rectum, the rubber balloon is filled, and the examination begins at the pelvic floor, ascending parallel to this plane in 0.5-cm steps. Modifications of the direction can be made easily by moving the steel tube. No preparation of the patient is necessary.
So far we have examined over 250 patients [3]. The results have been verified in a few cases by operation, in all cases by comparison with CT, and sometimes by comparison with NMR.

Normal Internal Genitalia

The normal vagina presents as a sickle-shaped area of low echo pattern in front of the steel tube within the rectum. Its sagittal diameter increases at the level of the cervix uteri, which also has a low echo pattern, as does the corpus uteri. Paracervical structures cannot be identified, except for the well-delineated bladder in front.

Carcinoma of the Cervix

Superficial carcinomas of the cervix cannot be identified. The diagnosis of cancer demands modification of the contour, shape, and sometimes the structure of the cervical region. The first sign of an infiltration into the cardinal ligaments is an asymmetric picture of the cervix uteri. Higher stages (Fig. 5) show bulky masses of tumor. In the case presented here the cancer has infiltrated the left cardinal ligament and also shows spread anteriorly. Ventrally lies the partially filled echo-free bladder. The carcinoma has a less dense echo pattern than the normal parametrium on the right. The borders of the tumor are relatively well defined. In contrary to CT images, the pelvic wall cannot be visualized by transrectal sonography.

Carcinoma of the Corpus Uteri

In most cases transrectal sonography is successful in imaging the normal corpus uteri. Often, however, even determination of the shape and size is not without problems, because the scanner cannot be put into contact with every segment of the corpus uteri (especially in strong anteflection). Corpora which are massively enlarged by tumor infiltration (Fig. 6) are often very difficult to demarcate. The echo pattern in this example is inhomogenous because of necrotic areas within the tumor which are less echogenic than growing tumor tissue. The borders on both sides are ill defined.

Carcinoma of the Ovaries

Tumors of the ovaries can be detected when they have a diameter of 4 cm or more. The echo pattern is not as dense as that of carcinomas of the cervix uteri. Benign cysts sometimes show a strong capsular echo, whereas malignant ovarian tumors often present an irregular echo pattern. In most cases, large carcinomas cannot be visualized in the cranial portions.

Therapy Control

Transrectal sonography delivers good information about the course of radiotherapy in carcinomas of the cervix uteri. Normally, the tumor's size decreases with the course of radiation, the echo pattern becoming more irregular with echo-free necrotic areas. Recurrent local carcinoma, which appears like untreated tumor, can be easily differentiated from scars after radiotherapy, which look like normal parametrium.

So far 52 patients with carcinoma of the cervix stage IIb and 60 patient with carcinoma of the cervix stage III have been examined and had the results compared with CT findings. The tumor showed a less dense echo pattern than normal tissue in 97%. The extension of the tumor into the cardinal ligament was classified correctly in correlation to CT in 95%. Forty patients with massive scarring of the parametrium after combined radiotherapy were scanned. No abnormalities were seen by transrectal sonography. In contrast, all 34 local recurrences had the appearance of fresh tumor masses. On CT, all patients with scarring of the parametrium showed at least some degree of thickening of the cardinal ligaments. Of the 34 recurrences, 29 were identified, whereas CT could not decide in the remaining five cases whether the enlarged cervical region consisted of tumor or of scar tissue. Fifty-four patients with cancer of the corpus uteri were examined. In 49% of the cases the image quality was good, i.e., every part of the corpus uteri could be identified. No decision on the stage was possible, because transrectal sonography does not allow a distinction between cancer and normal myometrium. An enlarged corpus was classified as stage III.

Only 23 patients with a malignancy of the ovaries were examined. No reliable correlation could be established between the sonographic picture and the histologic type, except that malignant tumors showed a more irregular echo pattern. Even the tumor extension could be correctly determined in only 43% of the cases in correlation to CT.

Summary

Intrauterine sonography is a method which allows the visualization of the structure of the myometrium and its pathologic alterations. With this information it is possible for the first time to define the exact target volume for intracavitary irradiation of carcinomas of the corpus uteri.

Transrectal sonography is able to visualize the extension of tumor masses into the cardinal ligaments in carcinomas of the cervix uteri. It is a useful help in controlling the course of radiotherapy. The method seems to be promising in distinguishing scars after radiotherapy from local recurrences. In carcinomas of the corpus uteri and of the ovaries, and in general in situations where the scanner cannot be directly put into contact with the mass to be examined, the method seems to be of little value.

References

1. Hämlin PJ, Burgener FA, Beecham JB (1981) CT of intramural endometrial carcinoma: contrast enhancement is essential. AJR 137:551–554
2. Hötzinger H, Willgeroth F, Pfändner K, Atzinger A, Ries G (1982) Erste Mitteilungen über transrektale

Ultraschalluntersuchungen zur Beurteilung des inneren weiblichen Genitales. Röntgenpraxis 10:403–406
3. Hötzinger H, Atzinger A, Ries G (1983) Transrektale Ultraschalltomographie des weiblichen Genitales: erste Ergebnisse. Röntgenpraxis 11:387–391
4. Hötzinger H (1984) Durch Intrauterinsonographie optimierte intrakavitäre Strahlentherapie bei Korpuskarzinomen. Strahlentherapie 160:600–604
5. Hötzinger H, Becker H, Becker V (1984) Intrauterine Ultraschalltomographie (IUT): Vergleich mit makroskopischen Präparatschnitten. Geburtshilfe Frauenheilkd 44:219–224
6. Requard CK, Wichs JD, Mettler FA (1981) Ultrasonography in the staging of endometrial adenocarcinoma. Radiology 140:781–785
7. Schwartz PE, Kohorn EJ, Knowlton AH (1975) Routine use of hysterography in endometrial carcinoma and postmenopausel bleeding. Obstet Gynecol 45:378–384
8. Wischnik A, Hötzinger H (1984) Intrauterine Ultraschalltomographie. Vorstellung eines neuen Verfahrens. Arch Gynecol 235:152–153

Interventional Radiology

GASTROINTESTINAL TRACT

Acute and Chronic Gastrointestinal Bleeding: Role of Angiographic Diagnosis and Management

S. L. Kaufman

Angiographic techniques have contributed significantly to the evaluation and management of patients with gastrointestinal bleeding. Acute gastrointestinal hemorrhage unresponsive to medical management can often be controlled nonoperatively using the techniques of transcatheter vasopressin infusion or embolization. Definitive diagnosis of previously occult sources of hemorrhage, such as those associated with colonic angiodysplasias, can now be made. This report summarizes our experience at the Johns Hopkins Hospital in the angiographic evaluation and management of patients with gastrointestinal hemorrhage.

Acute Gastrointestinal Bleeding

Diagnostic Approach

Careful clinical evaluation of the patient with acute gastrointestinal bleeding should always precede the decision to proceed with angiography. The initial diagnostic procedure should be the passage of a nasogastric tube. Even in the absence of hematemesis a positive aspirate from the nasogastric tube indicates an upper gastrointestinal site of hemorrhage (esophagus, stomach, or duodenum). Only 1% of patients with a negative nasogastric aspirate will have an upper gastrointestinal source of bleeding, usually due to duodenal ulcer with pyloric spasm or obstruction [1]. In patients with upper gastrointestinal hemorrhage, endoscopy should be performed next. A definitive etiology for the hemorrhage can usually be obtained with minimal morbidity using endoscopy [2]. If angiography is eventually necessary, the endoscopic diagnosis is helpful to the angiographer in determining which vessel to catheterize selectively and which therapeutic modality (vasopressin infusion or embolization) would be most effective. Sigmoidoscopy may be helpful in patients with lower gastrointestinal bleeding to localize a source of hemorrhage in the rectum or distal sigmoid colon. Barium studies should not be performed on patients with acute gastrointestinal bleeding. Endoscopy is more accurate than upper gastrointestinal barium examination in the diagnosis of acute upper gastrointestinal bleeding [3]. Hemorrhagic gastritis and Mallory-Weiss tears, for example, cannot be identified with barium. In addition, the presence of residual barium within the gastrointestinal tract makes angiography difficult or impossible. With the exception of those patients found to be bleeding from esophageal or gastric varices, patients with gastrointestinal hemorrhage should be given a trial of conservative medical management (bed rest, blood and fluid replacement, correction of clotting abnormalities) before angiography is considered. In the majority of patients, acute upper or lower gastrointestinal bleeding will stop spontaneously with these measures and angiography will not be required [4, 5]. Most patients with bleeding varices have been found to respond just as well to continuous low-dose intravenous infusion of vasopressin as to selective mesenteric artery infusions [6]. Intravenous vasopressin may be started immediately in these patients.

Angiography is indicated in those patients with massive acute gastrointestinal bleeding in whom the endoscopic diagnosis is equivocal and in those patients with upper or lower gastrointestinal bleeding who fail to respond to conservative management. Since evidence of extravasation is the only angiographic manifestation of most sources of acute upper and lower gastrointestinal bleeding, the patient must be actively bleeding at the time of angiography if the source of the hemorrhage is to be localized. In patients with upper gastrointestinal bleeding, an indwelling nasogastric tube is essential to ascertain whether active bleeding is occurring and to monitor the response to therapy following vasopressin infusion or embolization. With lower gastrointestinal bleeding, determination of the activity of the hemorrhage is more difficult. Most sources of lower gastrointestinal bleeding are intermittent [7]. Due to the intestinal transit time, the appearance of melena or even bright red rectal bleeding does not necessarily indicate that the bleeding is occurring at that moment. Serial falling hematocrits and the need for continued blood replacement are helpful in determining the activity of lower gastrointestinal hemorrhage but are not infallible. Imaging using labeled red blood cells [8, 9] or technetium-99m sulfur colloid [10] is a useful method for determining the activity of lower gastrointestinal hemorrhage. Radionuclide imaging may identify those patients who are actively bleeding and in whom emergency angiography should be performed. Angiography is generally not indicated in patients in whom no active bleeding is shown on nuclear medicine studies.

Angiographic Diagnosis of Bleeding

Upper Gastrointestinal Hemorrhage

Patients with massive active upper gastrointestinal bleeding unresponsive to conservative measures may frequently benefit from angiographic management. The endoscopic findings are helpful in determining which patients are most likely to benefit from angiography and in guiding the angiographer as to which vessel to selectively catheterize. In patients found endoscopically to be bleeding from hemorrhagic gastritis, Mallory-Weiss tears, or ulcers in the fundus of the stomach, angiographic management is effective and may eliminate the need for surgery [4, 11, 12]. The left gastric artery is usually the major source for bleeding from these lesions, and selective left gastric artery catheterization should be attempted first. Occasionally, bleeding in the fundus of the stomach may occur from branches of the phrenic arteries or from left gastric arteries which originate anomalously directly from the aorta (Fig. 1) [13]. If extravasation is not seen on selective left gastric artery arteriograms or on celiac arteriograms which demonstrate the left gastric artery, and if the patient is actively bleeding, the aorta should be searched for such anomalous vessels. Patients shown endoscopically to be bleeding from duodenal ulcers may be managed angiographically if they are poor surgical candidates. Patients who are good surgical risks are best managed by a definitive surgical procedure for both control of bleeding and ulcer management. Catheterization of the gastroduodenal or common hepatic artery should be attempted in patients with bleeding duodenal ulcers who come to angiography (Fig. 2). If subselective catheterization of the left gastric or gastroduodenal arteries is not possible in a reasonable amount of time in patients with upper gastrointestinal bleeding, a celiac arteriogram should be performed. Demonstration of extravasation of contrast material into the lumen of the stomach or duodenum is necessary to make an unequivocal diagnosis of the source of the bleeding. Extravasation, however, is nonspecific, and the determination of the etiology of the bleeding is dependent upon endoscopy.

In patients found to be bleeding from esophageal or gastric varices who have not responded to intravenous vasopressin, esophageal tamponade, or other conservative measures, and in whom some type of portosystemic shunting procedure is contemplated, diagnostic angiography should be performed to determine preoperatively the patency of the mesenteric and portal veins. High-dose superior mesenteric arteriography should be carried out immediately following injection of a vasodilator (tolazoline, 25 mg) into the superior mesenteric artery. If the patency of the splenic vein is in question or if a splenorenal shunt is contemplated, a selective splenic or celiac arteriogram should be performed to visualize the splenic vein.

Lower Gastrointestinal Bleeding

Angiography is indicated in patients with massive, acute, intractable lower gastrointestinal bleeding, both for diagnosis and for therapy. It is controversial as to which vessel, the superior or inferior mesenteric artery, should be selectively catheterized initially. Some angiographers feel that the inferior mesenteric artery should be studied first so that contrast material in the bladder from previous injections does not overlie arterial branches within the sigmoid colon or rectum. Since the superior mesenteric artery is the source of massive lower gastrointestinal bleeding in the majority of cases, we feel this should be the first vessel in which arteriography is performed. The most common cause of massive lower gastrointestinal hemorrhage is bleeding colonic diverticula [14]. Although colonic diverticula occur most frequently in the descending colon, approximately 75% of diverticula that bleed massively are in the right colon and are visualized by superior mesenteric arteriography [15]. Approximately

80% of bleeding colonic diverticula stop spontaneously, and of those that do stop, bleeding recurs in only one-third [16]. Angiography is only indicated, therefore, in those patients who do not stop bleeding spontaneously with conservative medical management or in whom recurrent massive bleeding occurs. When active bleeding is seen in the right colon without other angiographic abnormalities, bleeding colonic diverticula is statistically the most common etiology (Fig. 3). Since extravasation, however, is not specific, barium enema or endoscopy of the colon should be performed after control of bleeding is obtained to exclude the possibility of tumor or other abnormality. Other less common causes of massive lower gastrointestinal hemorrhage which can be diagnosed by superior mesenteric arteriography are bleeding Meckel's diverticula, ulcers of the small or large bowel, small bowel leiomyomas and leiomyosarcomas, and inflammatory bowel disease [17, 18]. Colonic angiodysplasia may occasionally be detected in patients with acute gastrointestinal hemorrhage, but is usually discovered in patients with chronic recurrent hemorrhage [19].

If superior mesenteric arteriography is negative, inferior mesenteric arteriography should then be performed. In most patients, evaluation of the entire inferior mesenteric artery circulation requires two separate contrast injections to visualize the area from the splenic flexure of the colon down to the rectum. Rarely, lower gastrointestinal bleed-

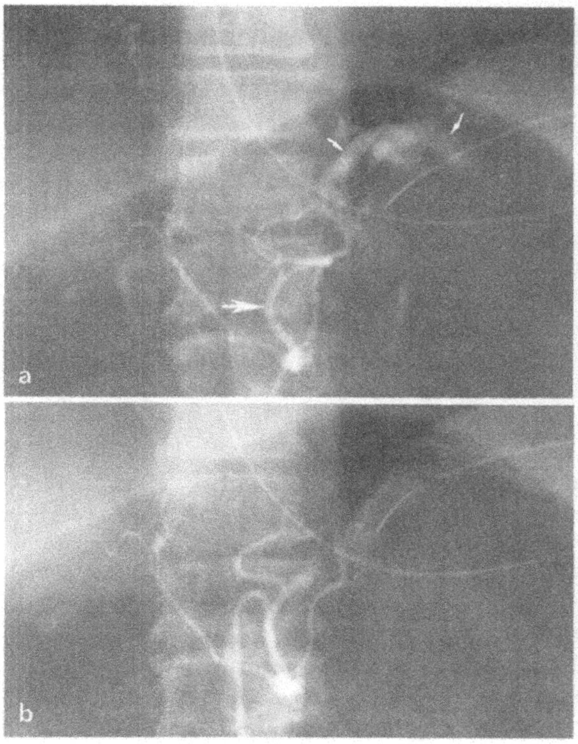

Fig. 1a, b. Bleeding Mallory-Weiss tear. **a** Left gastric arteriogram. The left gastric artery (*large arrow*) originates directly from the aorta in conjunction with the inferior phrenic arteries. There is contrast extravasation in the gastric fundus (*small arrows*). **b** Following gelfoam embolization of the left gastric artery hemorrhage was controlled

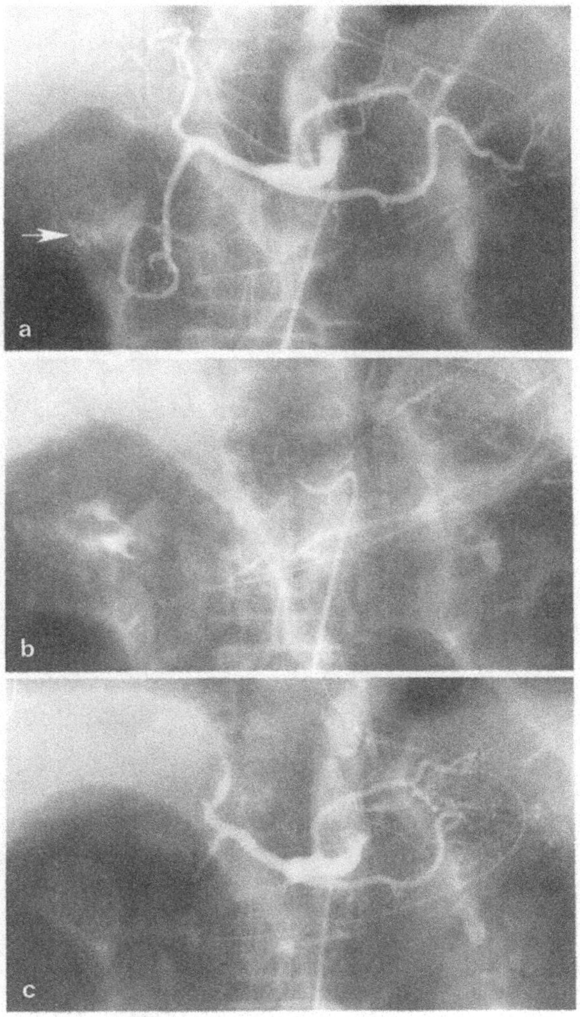

Fig. 2a–c. Bleeding duodenal ulcer. **a** Celiac arteriogram shows contrast extravasation (*arrow*) from a branch of the gastroduodenal artery. **b** Later phase of the arteriogram shows persistent extravasation in the duodenum. **c** Following gelfoam embolization of the gastroduodenal artery no extravasation is present. The gastroduodenal artery is occluded

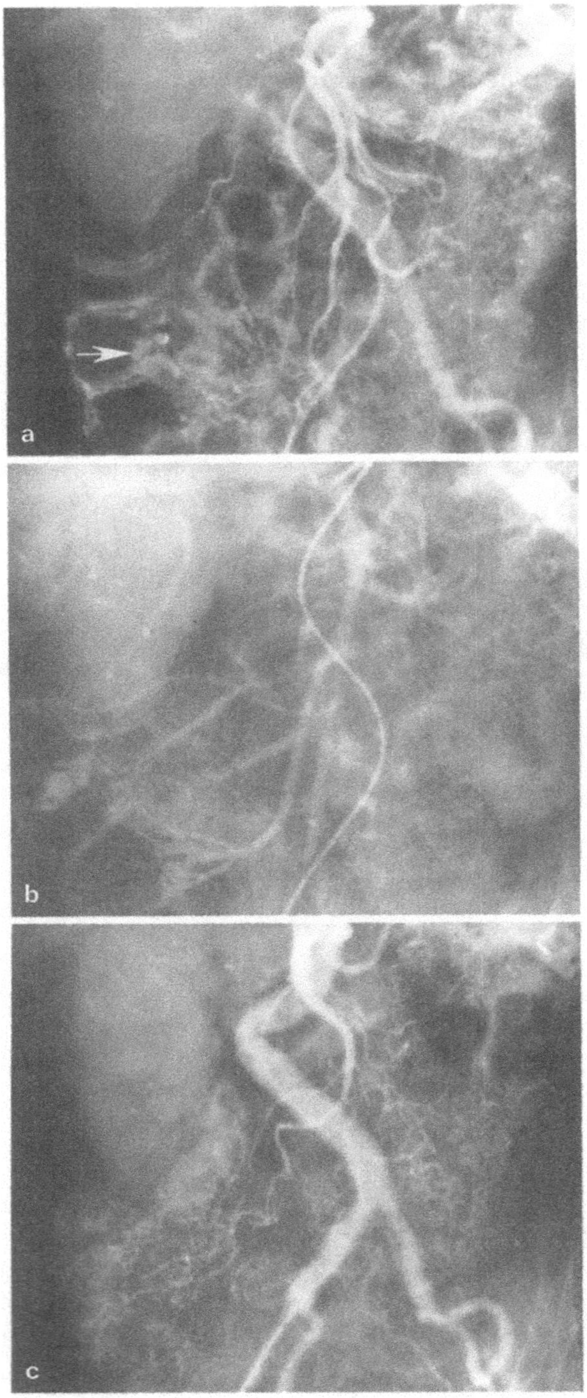

Fig. 3a–c. Bleeding colon diverticula. **a** Early arterial phase of superior mesenteric arteriogram shows contrast extravasation in the right colon (*arrow*). **b** Later phase of the arteriogram shows persistent contrast collection. **c** Superior mesenteric arteriogram after trial infusion of 0.2 U/min vasopressin for 30 min through the catheter shows no further extravasation

ing in a patient with negative gastric aspirate may have its source in the duodenum [1]. If superior and inferior mesenteric arteriography are negative and the patient is still felt to be actively bleeding, celiac arteriography should be performed. Since lower gastrointestinal bleeding is intermittent, patients may start and stop bleeding actively even on the angiography table. In selected cases, therefore, even after superior mesenteric, inferior mesenteric, and celiac arteriography are negative, a repeat superior mesenteric arteriogram may show active extravasation [7].

Angiographic Therapy

Acute gastrointestinal bleeding may be managed angiographically by vasopressin infusion or transcatheter embolization. Bleeding esophageal varices, hemorrhagic gastritis, and bleeding colonic diverticula may be controlled in over 80% of cases by vasopressin [4, 6, 15]. Intravenous vasopressin infusions are employed in the treatment of bleeding esophageal varices. Continuous intravenous infusions at an initial rate of 0.2–0.4 U/min should be started immediately after the diagnosis of bleeding esophageal varices has been made. Infusion at the lowest dose rate effective in stopping bleeding should be continued for 12 h. The infusion rate should be tapered at 0.1 U/min decrements every 12 h, provided bleeding remains controlled. Transhepatic portal venography and embolization of the coronary or short gastric veins have been used to sclerose or occlude bleeding varices. Successful results have been reported in several series [20, 21]. Other investigators have not achieved success with this method [11]. In addition, follow-up studies have showed recanalization of previously occluded veins and opening up of new collateral veins to fill the varices in a significant percentage of patients, with recurrent variceal bleeding in up to 55% [21, 22]. Complications of this procedure may include portal vein thrombosis and peritoneal bleeding. Because of the incidence of recurrence and portal thrombosis, which precludes subsequent shunt construction, we feel transhepatic embolization should only be used in patients who are not surgical candidates and in whom intravenous vasopressin and balloon tamponade of bleeding varices has failed.

Selective intra-arterial vasopressin infusions are more effective than intravenous infusions for bleeding not due to varices [23]. Bleeding hemorrhagic gastritis is best treated by selective left gastric artery vasopressin infusion [4]. If selective left gastric catheterization cannot be performed, celiac artery infusion may be effective [11]. Infusion of vasopressin into the superior or inferior mesenteric artery is required for treatment of bleeding colonic diverticula (Fig. 3c). Following angiographic localization of bleeding, a trial infusion of vasopressin at a rate of 0.2 U/min for 20–30 min is started, using a constant infusion pump. A repeat arteriogram is then performed to evaluate the therapeutic response. If bleeding is not controlled, the infusion rate may be increased to 0.4 U/min. The initial rate is maintained for 6–12 h. If bleeding remains controlled at 0.2 U/min the infusion rate is decreased at 0.1 U/min increments every 6–12 h. If bleeding still remains controlled, the catheter is left in place and physiologic saline is infused for another approximately 12 h, after which the catheter may be removed. If bleeding recurs, the vasopressin infusion may be restarted. Patients on continuous vasopressin infusions are best managed in the intensive care unit, where close monitoring of blood pressure, electrocardiogram, and urinary output can be performed. Vasopressin is a systemic and coronary arterial vasoconstrictor and may cause elevation of blood pressure and myocardial ischemia [24]. If severe hypertension or clinical or electrocardiographic manifestations of myocardial ischemia occur, the infusion should be stopped or the rate decreased.

Transcatheter embolization is most effective in bleeding due to large arterial sources. Although Mallory-Weiss tears have been treated successfully with left gastric artery vasopressin infusion, they may be controlled in over 90% of cases by transcatheter embolization (Fig. 1b) [12, 25]. If the left gastric artery can be entered, we feel embolization is the procedure of choice for control of bleeding due to Mallory-Weiss tears, as the need for an indwelling arterial catheter is eliminated. Bleeding ulcers do not respond well to vasopressin [26], and embolization is required for angiographic management (Fig. 2c). Selective catheterization is a required for transcatheter embolization in order to prevent inadvertent embolization of other circulations. Embolization of duodenal ulcers requires selective catheterization of the gastroduodenal artery, and embolization of gastric ulcers or Mallory-Weiss tears requires selective left gastric artery catheterization. Vigorous attempts at selective catheterization of the left gastric or gastroduodenal artery are justified for a reasonable period of time in attempts to control bleeding. If, because of difficult anatomy within the celiac axis, selective catheterization cannot be performed within 1–2 h and the patient is still actively bleeding, further attempts are usually ineffective and the best interests of the patient are served by discontinuing the procedure and resorting to surgery.

Gelatin sponge (Gelfoam, Upjohn, Kalamazoo) particles are the most commonly used embolic agent for control of gastrointestinal hemorrhage. Gelfoam is readily available, easy to inject through angiographic catheters, and provides arterial occlusion for periods of days to weeks [27]. This is adequate to control bleeding from most benign arterial sources. Particles of 1–2 mm in size suspended in dilute contrast material should be injected once selective catheter position has been achieved. Slow injection of small quantities of embolic material with continuous fluoroscopic monitoring is required to reduce the possibility of inadvertent embolization of neighboring vessels. Careful observation is especially important toward the end of the embolic procedure when flow in the vessel has slowed. For successful management of bleeding from duodenal ulcers, occlusion of the branch of the gastroduodenal artery to the site of hemorrhage is required, as well as of the gastroduodenal artery above and below the bleeding vessel. Since the duodenum has a dual supply from the celiac and superior mesenteric arteries, proximal occlusion of the gastroduodenal artery is inadequate, as bleeding will recur from inferior pancreaticoduodenal branches of the superior mesenteric artery. While embolization may control acute hemorrhage from bleeding ulcers, it does not treat the ulcer itself. Medical management of the peptic ulcer disease is required to assure that rebleeding does not occur.

The stomach and duodenum generally have extensive collateral circulation, and embolization with particulate materials such as Gelfoam rarely results in ischemic complications. Embolic agents which result in more distal arteriolar occlusion should be used with care in the gastrointestinal tract as they may preclude collateral circulation and result in ischemic ulceration or infarction [28]. Likewise, patients who have previously undergone gastric surgery with ligation of vessels should be embolized with care, as collaterals may be inadequate [29]. Patients who have undergone embolotherapy and in whom bleeding is not controlled should not undergo subsequent selective vasopressin infusion, as ischemia may result [30].

Embolization of branches of the superior or inferior mesenteric arteries has been described in patients with bleeding colonic diverticula in

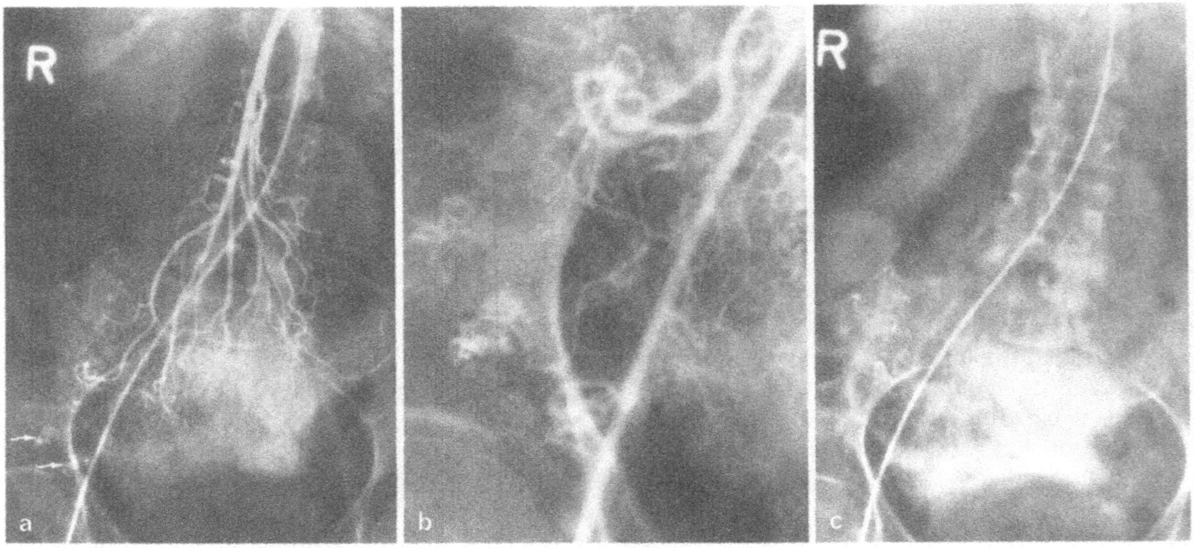

Fig. 4 a – c. Angiodysplasia of the colon. **a** Superior mesenteric arteriogram shows two vascular tufts (*arrows*) in the cecum. **b** Close-up view of the cecum shows the tufts in greater detail. **c** Late arterial phase shows early opacification of the ileocolic vein

whom vasopressin therapy has been unsuccessful [31]. Collateral flow in the small and large intestine is not as extensive as in the stomach and duodenum, however. Ischemic complications therefore occur more frequently with this form of therapy [32, 33]. Embolization in the superior or inferior mesenteric arteries should be performed with caution and only if the patient is a poor risk for surgical management.

Chronic Gastrointestinal Bleeding

Most causes of chronic, low-grade, recurrent gastrointestinal bleeding do not require angiography. Common causes of chronic gastrointestinal bleeding such as peptic ulcer disease, malignant neoplasms of the colon and stomach, colonic polyps, hemorrhoids, and inflammatory bowel disease are best diagnosed by barium studies and upper and lower gastrointestinal endoscopy. In general, a bleeding rate of approximately 1500 ml/day is required for visualization of contrast extravasation angiographically. Most sources of chronic gastrointestinal hemorrhage do not bleed at this rate and in most cases angiography is not indicated. In patients with continued chronic low-grade bleeding or multiple intermittent episodes of massive gastrointestinal bleeding in whom other diagnostic procedures are negative, angiography may reveal the source of bleeding even though extravasation may not be demonstrated. Colonic angiodysplasia is a cause of chronic gastrointestinal bleeding that is best diagnosed angiography [19, 34]. Most patients with colonic angiodysplasia are elderly and present with chronic low-grade bleeding or with repeated episodes of massive lower gastrointestinal bleeding often over the course of several years. The source of bleeding usually remains undiagnosed despite extensive evaluation, often including laparotomy. Colonic angiodysplasia occurs most frequently in the cecum and right colon. Although patients with colonic angiodysplasia may fortuitously be studied during an episode of acute hemorrhage, usually they are studied because of chronic recurrent bleeding. Characteristically, with angiodysplasia there is a small collection of abnormal vessels in the cecum or right colon associated with an early draining vein (Fig. 4). Often, this draining vein persists after the other mesenteric veins have emptied. Colonic angiodysplasia may be associated with calcific aortic stenosis in some patients [19], although there is probably no etiologic relationship. Since colonic angiodysplasia has been detected in up to 15% of nonbleeding patients [35], other etiologies for bleeding should be excluded before it is assumed that the angiodysplasia is responsible. Colonic tumors may also occasionally simulate the appearance of angiodysplasia [19]. The treatment of colonic angiodysplasia is surgical. Resection of the involved area of colon dem-

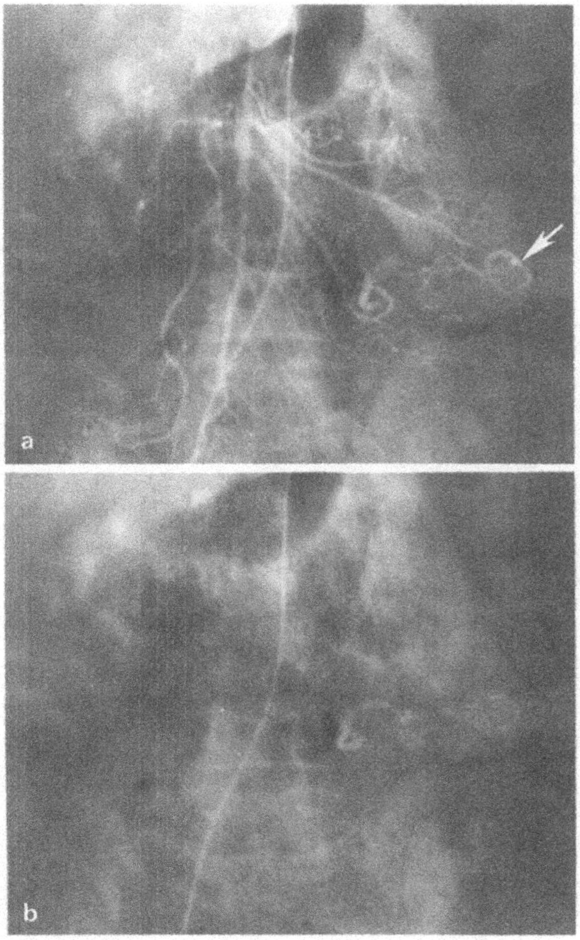

Fig. 5a, b. Small bowel arteriovenous malformation. **a** Early phase of superior mesenteric arteriogram shows the malformation (*arrow*) with a early appearance of draining vein. **b** Late arterial phase of arteriogram confirms early opacification of draining vein

onstrated on angiography should be performed. Frequently, the lesion cannot be detected even at surgery with the bowel opened. Injection of the pathologic specimen with silicone rubber preparations followed by specimen radiography has been helpful in documenting that the involved segment of colon has been removed [19]. Less frequently, arteriovenous malformations in the small bowel may be demonstrated as a source of chronic gastrointestinal bleeding (Fig. 5). The treatment for small bowel arteriovenous malformations is also surgical resection. As it may be difficult at surgery to determine the location of the arteriovenous malformation within the small bowel, selective catheterization of the branch of the superior mesenteric artery supplying the malformation immediately prior to surgery may be performed. Injection of a blue dye solution into the feeding vessel may aid the surgeon in localizing the segment of small bowel to be resected [36]. Small bowel leiomyomas or leiomyosarcomas not detected on small bowel barium examinations may occasionally be a source of chronic gastrointestinal hemorrhage. These tumors are frequently vascular, and may be detected angiographically without active extravasation.

References

1. Luk GD, Bynum TE, Hendrix TR (1979) Gastric aspiration in localizing of gastrointestinal hemorrhage. JAMA 241:576–578
2. Josen AS, Guiliani E, Voorhees AB et al. (1980) Immediate endoscopic diagnosis of upper gastrointestinal bleeding. Arch Surg 111:980–986
3. McGinn FP, Guyer PB, Wilken BJ et al. (1975) A prospective comparative trial between early endoscopy and radiology in acute upper gastrointestinal hemorrhage. Gut 16:707–713
4. Athanasoulis CA, Baum S, Waltman AC et al. (1974) Control of acute gastric mucosal hemorrhage. N Engl J Med 290:597–603
5. Eisenberg H, Laufer I, Skillman JJ (1973) Arteriographic diagnosis and management of suspected colonic diverticular hemorrhage. Gastroenterology 64:1091–1100
6. Johnson WC, Widrich WC, Ansel JE et al. (1977) Control of bleeding varices by vasopressin. Ann Surg 186:369–376
7. Sos TA, Lee JG, Wixson D et al. (1978) Intermittent bleeding from minute to minute in acute massive gastrointestinal hemorrhage: arteriographic demonstration. AJR 131:1015–1017
8. McKusick KA, Froelich J, Callahan RJ et al. (1981) ^{99m}Tc red blood cells for detection of gastrointestinal bleeding: experience with 80 patients. AJR 137:1113–1118
9. Ferrant A, Dehasque N, Leners N et al. (1980) Scintigraphy with ^{111}In-labelled red cells in intermittent gastrointestinal bleeding. J Nuclear Med 21:844–845
10. Alavi A, Dann RW, Baum S et al. (1977) Scintigraphic detection of acute gastrointestinal bleeding. Radiology 124:753–756
11. White RI JR, Harrington DP, Novak G et al. (1974) Pharmacologic control of hemorrhagic gastritis: clinical and experimental results. Radiology 111:549–557
12. Fisher RG, Schwartz JT, Graham DY (1980) Angiotherapy with Mallory-Weiss tear. AJR 134:679–684
13. Northrop CH, Studley MA, Smith GR (1975) Hemorrhage from the gastroesophageal junction. A cryptic angiographic diagnosis. Radiology 117:531–532

14. Dunphy JE, Mikkelson WP, Moody FG et al. (1973) Massive gastrointestinal bleeding: A panel by correspondence. Arch Surg 107:367–372
15. Athanasoulis CA, Baum S, Rösch J et al. (1975) Mesenteric arterial infusions of vasopressin for hemorrhage from colonic diverticulosis. Am J Surg 129:212–216
16. Athanasoulis CA, Waltman AC, Novelline RA et al. (1976) Angiography: its contribution to the emergency management of gastrointestinal hemorrhage. Radiol Clin North Am 14:265–280
17. Casarella WJ, Galloway SJ, Taxin RN et al. (1974) Lower gastrointestinal tract hemorrhage. New concepts based on arteriography. AJR 121:357–368
18. Cavaluzzi JA, Kaufman SL, White RI Jr (1976) Vasopressin control of massive hemorrhage in chronic ulcerative colitis. AJR 127:672–675
19. Athanasoulis CA, Galdabini JJ, Waltman AC et al. (1978) Angiodysplasia of the colon. A cause of rectal bleeding. Cardiovasc Radiol 1:3–13
20. Bengmark S, Borjesson B, Hoevels J et al. (1979) Obliteration of varices by PTP. A follow-up of 43 patients. Ann Surg 190:549–554
21. Widrich WC, Robbins AH, Nabseth DC (1980) Transhepatic embolization of varices. Cardiovasc Intervent Radiol 3:298–303
22. Athanasoulis CA (1980) Therapeutic applications of angiography. N Engl J Med 302:1117–1125
23. Davis GB, Bookstein JJ, Coel MN (1977) Advantage of intraarterial over intravenous vasopressin infusion in gastrointestinal hemorrhage. AJR 128:733–735
24. Corliss RJ, McKenna DH, Sialer S et al. (1968) Systemic and coronary hemodynamic effects of vasopressin. Am J Med Sci 256:293–299
25. Carsen GM, Casarella WJ, Spiegel RM (1978) Transcatheter embolization for treatment of Mallory-Weiss tears of the esophagogastric junction. Radiology 128:309–313
26. Waltman AC, Greenfield A, Novelline RT et al. (1979) Pyloroduodenal bleeding and intraarterial vasopressin: clinical results. AJR 133:643–646
27. Barth KH, Strandberg JD, White RI Jr (1977) Long-term follow-up of transcatheter embolization with autologous clot, oxycel and gelfoam in domestic swine. Invest Radiol 12:273–280
28. Kaufman SL, Strandberg JD, Barth KH, White RI Jr (1978) Transcatheter embolization with microfibrillar collagen in swine. Invest Radiol 13:200–204
29. Goldman ML, Land WC Jr, Bradley EL III et al. (1976) Transcatheter therapeutic embolization in the management of massive upper gastrointestinal bleeding. Radiology 120:513–521
30. Prochaska JM, Flye MW, Johnsrude IS (1973) Left gastric artery embolization for control of gastric bleeding: a complication. Radiology 107:521–522
31. Bookstein JJ, Naderi MJ, Walter JF (1978) Transcatheter embolization for lower gastrointestinal bleeding. Radiology 127:345–349
32. Mitty HA, Efremidis S, Keller RJ (1979) Colonic stricture after transcatheter embolization for diverticular bleeding. AJR 133:519–521
33. Walker WJ, Goldin AR, Shaff MI et al. (1980) Per catheter control of haemorrhage from the superior and inferior mesenteric arteries. Clin Radiol 31:71–80
34. Baum S, Athanasoulis CA, Waltman AC et al. (1977) Angiodysplasia of the right colon: a cause of gastrointestinal bleeding. AJR 129:789–794
35. Kadir S, Athanasoulis CA, Waltman AC et al. (1979) Angiodysplasia of the colon: incidence and coexistence with other bowel lesions in nonbleeding patients (abstract). American Roentgen Ray Society, march 27
36. Crawford ES, Roehm JOF Jr, McGavran MH (1980) Jejunoileal arteriovenous malformation. Localization for resection by segmental bowel staining techniques. Ann Surg 191:404–409

Hepatic Artery Infusion and Embolization in the Management of Hepatic Tumors

K. H. Barth

The interventional radiologist participates in the treatment of patients with primary or metastatic tumors of the liver by providing a route for regional chemotherapy infusion and also by occluding tumor blood supply through therapeutic embolization. While the former technique has been practiced for well over a decade [1, 2], the latter has still found only limited acceptance mainly due to its complexity and inherent risks [3].

Theoretically, direct chemotherapy infusion into the hepatic arteries has several advantages. The hepatic parenchyma receives most of its nutrients from the portal venous system, whereas an intrahepatic tumor is predominantly supplied by the hepatic arteries [4]. Drugs administered arterially will reach the tumor tissue in higher concentrations without the dilutional effect of systemic administration. If the drug has a high hepatic clearance, relatively large doses can be given arterially with very low systemic levels. For example, 5-fluorouracil has a hepatic clearance of 80%, floxuridine of 95% [5]. Clinical studies attesting to the advantage of regional chemotherapy infusion have usually not been comparative; however, failures of systemic infusion frequently respond to regional chemotherapy infusion. Recently, intermittent short-term infusions have been abandoned in favor of long-term infusions by implantable pumps. This extension of infusion periods seems to increase the therapeutic yield [6].

Infusion can be delivered by a percutaneously placed catheter [7] or by a surgically implanted catheter [8]; both can be connected entirely subcutaneously to an implanted infusion pump. Both techniques have their advantages and disadvantages. Surgical implantation requires a laparotomy but generally affords a more stable catheter position and effective diversion of gastric and duodenal blood supply away from the route of infusion. The percutaneous placement is less invasive, malpositioned catheters can be adjusted, and the infusion system can be placed at the time of the initial diagnostic arteriogram, which is necessary for adequate delineation of the hepatic artery blood supply for both the surgical and the percutaneous technique.

The angiographer or surgeon involved in infusion catheter placement has to consider anatomic variations of the hepatic arterial supply, since the typical anatomy will only be found in 55% of patients [9]. The most frequent variation is origin of the right hepatic artery (RHA) from the proximal superior mesenteric artery (SMA). Next in frequency is the "trifurcation" of the hepatic artery, whereby the gastroduodenal artery (GDA) arises directly opposite the left hepatic artery (LHA) origin. Less common are origin of the LHA from the left gastric artery (LGA), origin of the LHA from the LGA, and replacement of the common hepatic artery (CHA) from the SMA.

Percutaneous catheterization can be performed via the femoral artery (FA) or via the left brachial artery (LBA). The FA route is used primarily for the initial diagnostic study and can be combined with a trial chemotherapy infusion for 5–7 days. If this initial chemotherapy infusion is successful in terms of local response, long-term infusion via the LBA may follow.

Hepatic artery infusion is usually confined to a single catheter. For this reason, hepatic arterial flow may have to be rerouted in the presence of dual arteries and bilobar liver tumor. Also, runoff of infusate into the gastric circulation needs to be limited as much as possible. The following are some suggestions pertaining to angiographic catheter placement.

If the right hepatic artery is replaced from the SMA selective infusion of the RHA with embolization of the LHA origin might be considered. It is known that collaterals will develop soon after occlusion of a proximal hepatic artery [9]. Similarly, the RHA may be embolized if the LHA is better suited for infusion in a fashion similar to GDA embolization.

If a hepatic trifurcation is encountered, the origin of the GDA should be occluded by permanent

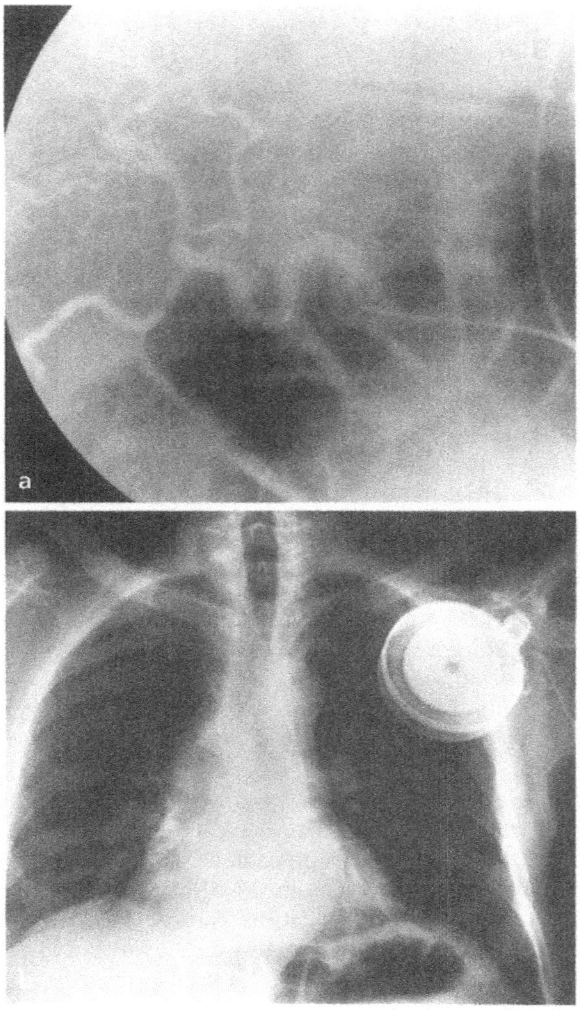

◂**Fig. 1.** **a** Percutaneously placed transbrachial catheter in proper hepatic artery for long-term chemotherapy infusion in a patient with bilobar metastastic carcinoma of colon. **b** Subcutaneous infusion pump superimposed over left lung field

◂**Fig. 2.** **a** Highly vascular metastases of gastrinoma with excessive gastrin production. **b** Selective hepatic artery infusion catheter (coaxial system). No significant response to chemotherapy. **c** Following embolization of right hepatic artery with Ivalon. Occlusion of entire right distribution with preservation of left hepatic blood flow

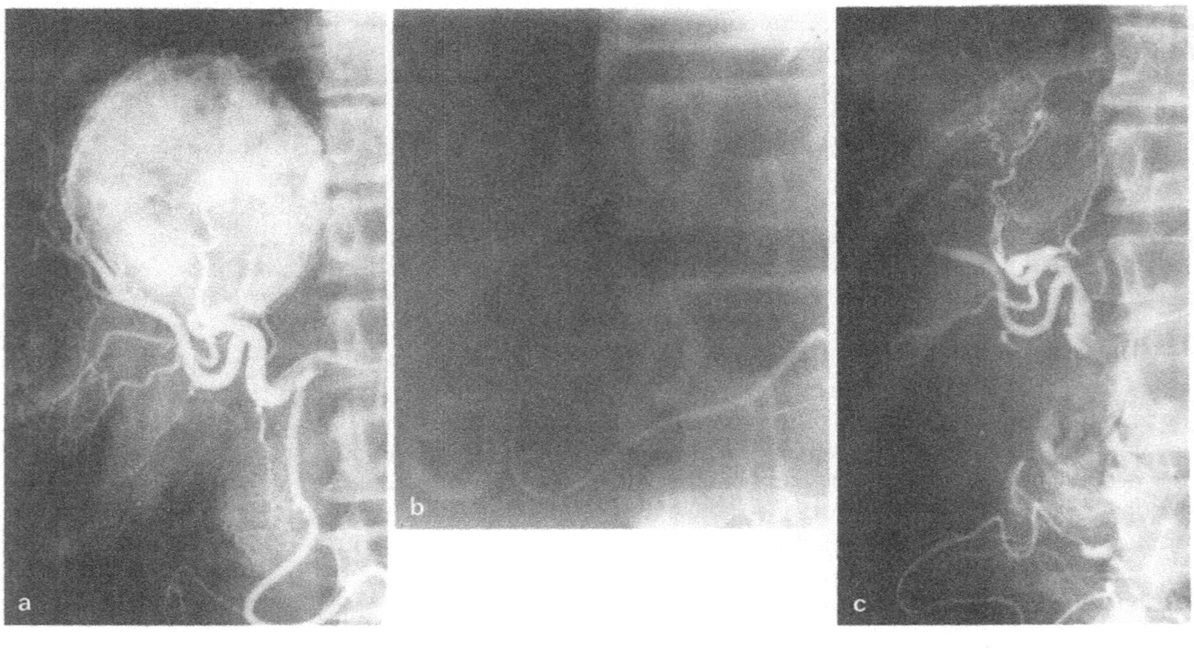

embolization. Gianturco coils are convenient for this purpose, but due to technical modifications they no longer occlude as effectively as the initial version, so that addition of a Gelfoam plug is advised.

Blocking GDA runoff from the CHA is justified by the high incidence (40%–50%) of chemical gastritis and duodenitis during hepatic artery infusion [10]. A problem for the angiographic approach is the right gastric artery (RGA), which usually arises from the proximal LHA. While this artery can be ligated during surgical catheter placement, selective catheterization and embolization is virtually impossible. During surgical catheter implantation, cholecystectomy may be performed to avoid 10% incidence of chemical cholecystitis. Recently, a 5% incidence of sclerosing cholangitis during long-term chemotherapy infusion has been reported [10]. The systemic toxicity from hepatic artery infusion is lower than from systemic chemotherapy.

When the femoral approach is used, retroflection of the catheter into the downward-directed celiac axis (CA), as well as the acute right turn of the CHA, frequently exhausts catheter directability at the mid or distal CHA. RHA origin from the SMA may pose similar problems, preventing stable catheter position, which is essential for safe infusion. In these instances we recommend placement of a coaxial 3-F catheter which can be advanced into either the RHA or the LHA. The 3-F catheter lumen is more than adequate for infusion. We have usually left the 6-F or 6.5-F outer catheter in place to preserve the CA or SMA entry. The LBA approach allows easier entry into the CA and CHA due to the obtuse downstream angles. The major limitation to the LBA approach is the caliber of this artery, limiting long-term catheters to 5F. Such catheters have little torque control; however, thin-walled 5-F catheters have a lumen large enough to perform embolizations as described above.

Before chemotherapeutic agents are infused through the catheter the definitive distribution of the infusate needs to be determined. This is best achieved by infusing ^{99m}Tc-macroaggregated albumin (MAA) or ^{99m}Tc-albumin microspheres (HAM) through the catheter, if possible, at the rate of the intended chemotherapy infusion. The distribution pattern on the flow scan should roughly correspond to the tumor [11]. The scan will also demonstrate potential flow to the gastric circulation, which requires redirection of the catheter. Scans should be repeated before each infusion; they also allow some means of evaluating the effect of chemotherapy when the extent of tumor activity is compared to previous scans [12].

Hepatic artery embolization is used to limit the growth of primary or metastatic liver tumors which are otherwise uncontrollable. The most significant benefits have been achieved with embolization of hepatomas and hormonally active hepatic metastases such as carcinoid tumors [4, 13, 14, 15]. It is essential to document patent portal blood supply prior to embolization if its occlusion represents a contraindication to embolotherapy [4, 13]. Embolization should be directed as selectively as possible to the tumor and only one lobe should be embolized at a time if the tumor blood supply cannot be interrupted exclusively. Permanent occluding agents are the choice. Ivalon particles appear to be very suitable [15]. Careful catheter position should avoid reflux of embolic material into the gastric and especially the mesenteric circulation [13–15]. Distal embolization reaching the liver sinisoids has to be avoided, since it would interrupt portal venous blood flow and result in liver infarction. For this reason liquid emboli are not considered safe. A "postembolization syndrome" can be expected consisting of abdominal pain, fever, nausea, vomiting, and elevated liver enzymes. Supportive treatment is required, as these symptoms persist for several days [13–15].

In summary, infusion of chemotherapeutic agents directly into the hepatic arteries exploits the predominance of tumor blood supply from the hepatic arteries, whereas normal parenchyma receives most of its nutrient flow from the portal venous system. Drugs with high hepatic clearance are preferred. Long-term infusion is presently the method of choice. Infusion catheters can be placed both percutaneously and surgically. With either method, catheters can be connected to subcutaneous infusion pumps. Effectiveness of catheter position should be assessed prior to each chemotherapy infusion by ^{99m}Tc-MAA or ^{99m}Tc-HAM scan. This test serves also as orientation for the distribution of tumor blood supply. The high incidence of chemical gastritis can be minimized by excluding gastric arteries from the route of chemotherapy infusion. Embolotherapy has its place as a palliative procedure in rapidly enlarging, highly vascular tumors, particularly in hormonally active hepatic metastases. Obstruction of the portal vein and presence of cirrhosis constitute contraindications to embolization.

References

1. Watkins E Jr et al. (1966) Surgical basis for arterial infusion chemotherapy of disseminated carcinoma of the liver. Surg Gynecol Obstet 130:581
2. Wirtanen GW (1973) Percutaneous transbrachial artery infusion catheter techniques. AJR 117: 696–700
3. Healey TE Jr (1965) Vascular patterns in human metastatic liver tumors. Surg Gynecol Obstet 120:1187
4. Furui S et al. (1984) Hepatocellular carcinoma treated by transcatheter arterial embolization: progress evaluated by computed tomography. Radiology 150:773–778
5. Ensminger WD et al. (1978) A clinical-pharmacological evaluation of hepatic arterial infusions of 5-fluoro-2-desoxyeridine and 5-fluorouracil. Cancer Res 38:3784–3792
6. Balch CM et al. (1983) A prospective phase II clinical trial of continuous FUDR regional chemotherapy for colorectal metastases to the liver using a totally implantable pump. Am Surg 198:567–573
7. Cohen AM et al. (1983) Treatment of hepatic metastases by transaxillary hepatic artery chemotherapy using an implanted drug pump. Cancer 51:2013–2019
8. Barone RM et al. (1982) Intraarterial chemotherapy using an implantable infusion pump and liver irradiation for treatment of hepatic metastases. Cancer 50:850–862
9. Chuang VP, Wallace S (1980) Hepatic arterial redistribution for intraarterial infusion of hepatic neoplasms. Radiology 135:295–299
10. Ensminger WD (1984) Intraarterial therapy of hepatic metastases. Symposium: intraarterial and intracavity chemotherapy 1984, San Diego, feb 24–25
11. Bledin AG et al. (1982) 99mTc-labeled macroaggregated albumin in intrahepatic arterial chemotherapy. AJR 139:711–715
12. Kaplan WD et al. (1982) Intraarterial hepatic infusion of Tc-99m-MAA: a predictive test of chemotherapeutic responses of liver tumors. J Nucleic Med 20:675 (abstract)
13. Yamada R et al. (1983) Hepatic artery embolization in 120 patients with unresectable hepatoma. Radiology 148:397–401
14. Allison DJ et al. (1977) Treatment of carcinoid liver metastases by hepatic artery embolization. Lancet 24:1323–1325
15. Chuang VP et al. (1981) Ivalon embolization in abdominal neoplasms. AJR 136:729–733

Update on Percutaneous Gallstone Extraction and Stricture Dilatation

H. J. Burhenne

General Considerations

Three access routes to the biliary tract are available for instrumentation: retrograde via gastrointestinal endoscopy, antegrade through the liver parenchyma, or through a postoperative drain tract. The latter two procedures involve interventional radiologic techniques in a transhepatic or subhepatic fashion.

The antegrade *transhepatic* approach was pioneered by radiologists as an offshoot of percutaneous needle cholangiography. It is primarily designed for bile drainage to palliate patients with a poor prognosis from carcinoma of the bile ducts or pancreas. The same approach can, however, be used for transhepatic removal of common duct stones and stricture dilatation. Recent reports, however, indicate that the transgression of the pleural space involves complications, including fatalities [12, 14]. The transhepatic approach for stone removal should be the last resort, as endoscopic sphincterotomy and stone removal carry less of a complication risk. Endoscopic removal of common duct stones is not possible if gastric surgery such as a gastrojejunostomy is present. The transhepatic approach may then be used for stone removal and can give satisfying results, particularly if the stones can be pushed into the duodenum.

The postoperative *subhepatic* approach is less time-consuming and less technically demanding. This interventional approach through postoperative sinus tracts has a lower complication rate, but cannot be used if no drainage tract from a T-tube or cholecystostomy or jejunostomy is available. The subhepatic approach also has advantages in biliary stricture dilatation if prolonged stenting is required. It permits use of larger stenting catheters [1]. Furthermore, sinus tract dilatation with coaxial catheters and angiographic dilatation balloons is more readily accomplished through postoperative drainage tracts and enterostomy sites than by the transhepatic technique.

Interventional radiologic procedures for stone extraction and stricture dilatation are usually carried out without anesthesia and in the ambulatory patient. Complicated cases require short-term hospitalization and coverage with antibiotics. Transhepatic procedures are often painful and are best performed after anesthesia with intercostal block.

Stone Extractions

Retention of stones in the biliary tract after surgery continues to be a problem, even with the routine use of operative cholangiography and choledochoscopy. Since nonoperative extraction has proven to be effective, reoperation for retained stones is no longer indicated. It carries a higher mortality and morbidity than the initial operative procedure.

Nonoperative extraction of retained stones from the biliary tract via postoperative drain tracts is a relatively easy radiologic procedure. The necessary equipment has undergone no essential change and has been described elsewhere [3]. Our experience now involves stone extractions in 1583 patients, with a success rate of 96%. This implies that even the last stone has been successfully removed in patients with multiple retained stones as seen on careful postinstrumentation cholangiography. The failures of retained stone removal continue to be patients with multiple impacted intrahepatic stones where mobilization of all retained concrements was impossible.

Percutaneous removal of large stones of more than 10 mm in diameter remains more difficult. The stone has to be engaged in the basket and then fragmented by strong traction (Fig. 1). The basket wires are sufficiently sharp to cut the bile duct stones. Larger fragments are extracted, and smaller fragments are usually passed spontaneously if the sphincteric portion of the distal common duct is not narrowed. It must be re-

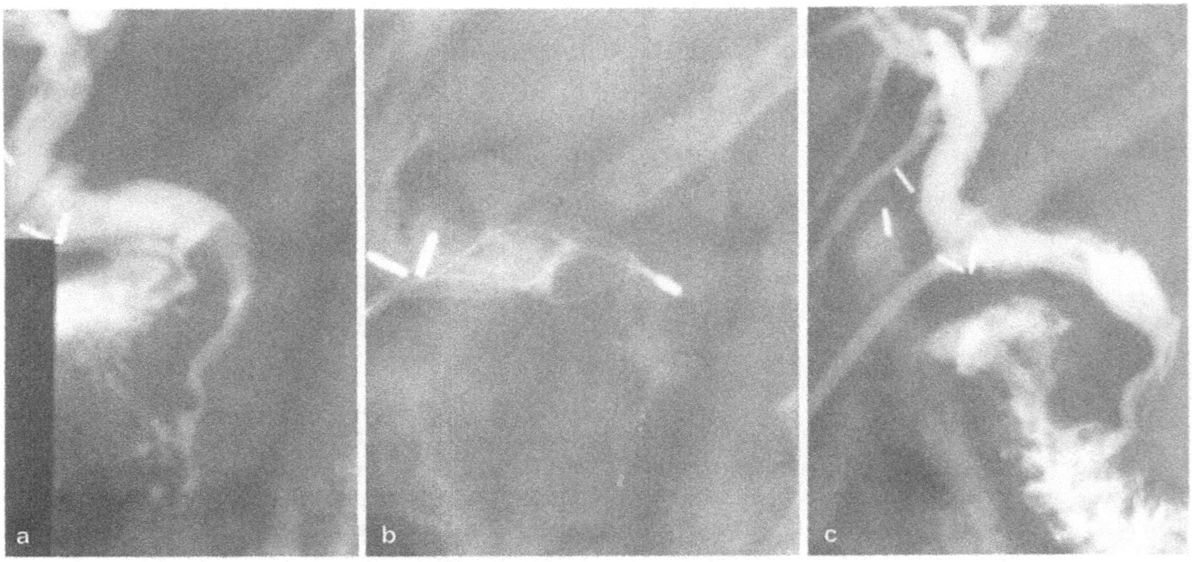

Fig. 1. **a** Large faceted stone retained in the common duct. **b** The stone has been engaged in the extraction basket. It is considerably larger than the sinus tract and it requires fragmentation by strong traction on the basket or by forcibly closing the basket in the bile duct. **c** The large fragments have been extracted, but the cholangiogram still shows multiple small fragments. Follow-up study 3 days later showed complete clearing of the bile ducts. Twenty-two percent of a series of 1583 patients with retained stones required stone fragmentation

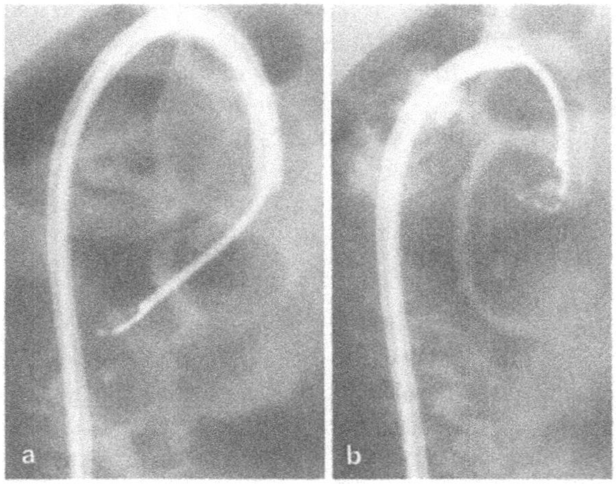

Fig. 2. **a** A stone dislodger (Cook Inc.) is maneuvered through the steerable catheter into the distal common duct just beyond an impacted stone. **b** The stone dislodger is opened and the stone is moved proximally for better engagement with the wire basket

membered that about a 40% magnification factor is involved when measuring retained stones on cholangiography. This means that a retained stone measuring 10 mm with magnification on cholangiography can just be extracted intact through the sinus tract of a 16-F T-tube [13].

Impacted stones at the distal end of the common duct may require a variety of maneuvers for successful extraction (Fig. 2) [3]. These bile duct stones often need mobilization with a Fogarty balloon catheter. The balloon is inflated with contrast for fluoroscopic visualization just distally to the stone. Gentle traction is then applied to move the stone more proximally for basket engagement (Fig. 3).

The percutaneous transhepatic approach has also been used for stone extraction [6]. This transhepatic stone removal technique, however, is only recommended if the subhepatic approach is not possible or if endoscopic papillotomy and stone removal are contraindicated or unsuccessful. The technique involves standard percutaneous transhepatic cholangiography followed by insertion of a guide wire and sheath, followed by a Dormia basket. The stones are then snared and the basket passed through the ampulla into the duodenum if possible. Mono-octanoin infusion through the catheter may be required in addition if stone fragmentation or passage of fragments is not possible [5].

More experience has been gained recently with stone extraction via cholecystostomy. If stones remain in the gallbladder after cholecystostomy, access with a steerable catheter is gained postopera-

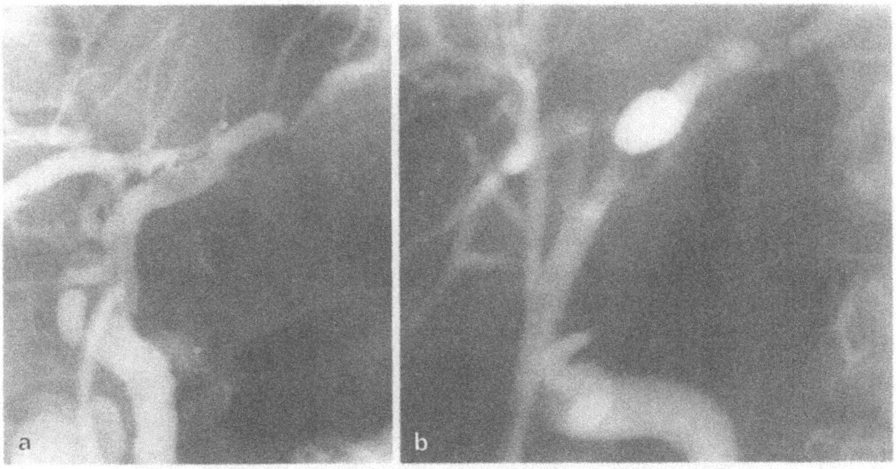

Fig. 3. **a** Stone retained in the left hepatic radicle. **b** A 4-F Fogarty balloon is maneuvered beyond the retained stone and the balloon is inflated with contrast. The stone is moved distally with gentle traction for subsequent engagement in the basket

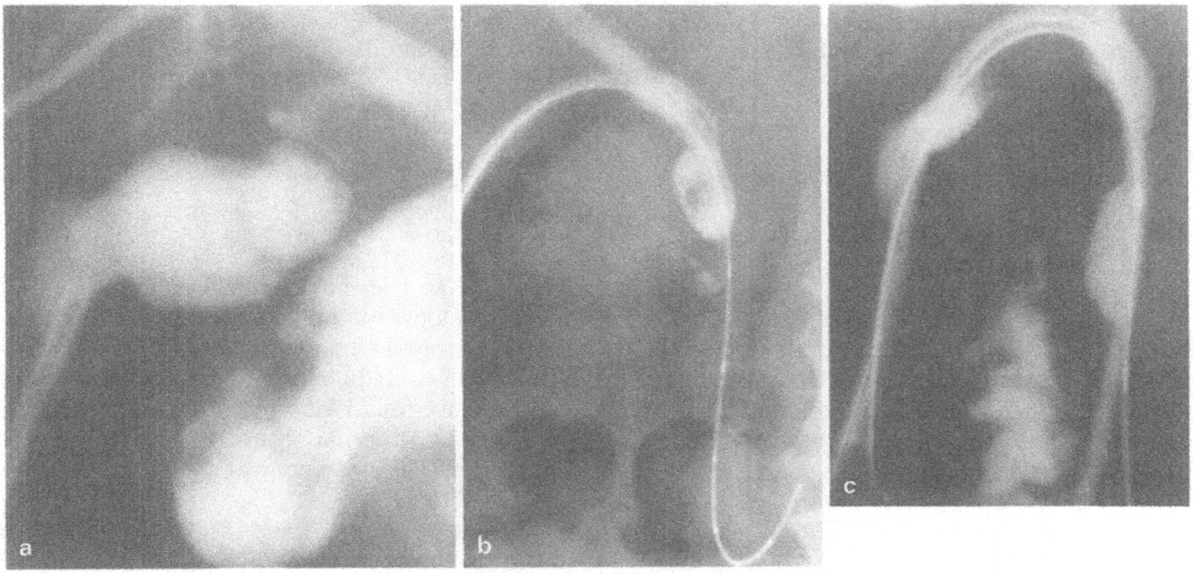

Fig. 4. **a** Using a cholecystostomy tract as access, one gallbladder stone was removed and the cystic duct was then negotiated with an 8-F. steerable catheter and a J-tipped guide wire. **b** A guide wire is placed through the 8-F steerable catheter alongside two retained stones in the common duct into the duodenum. **c** Closing cholangiogram after extraction of two common duct stones shows the duct system clear

tively through the drain tract. Stones may be removed with the use of a basket or by employing a stone forceps [1]. This procedure is indicated following drainage of acute cholecystitis if the patient's general condition does not indicate one-stage operative gallbladder removal. Gallbladder stones of any size may be crushed and removed through the cholecystostomy tract.

The same approach through the cholecystostomy tract can be used to gain access to the common duct for removal of biliary stones [10]. After cholecystocholangiography, J-tipped guide wires and a small 8-F steerable catheter are manipulated through the cystic duct into the major bile ducts. Cystic duct dilatation is then performed with the use of balloon catheters. The extraction of common duct stones is accomplished in the same manner as with percutaneous instrumentation through the postoperative T-tube tract (Fig. 4).

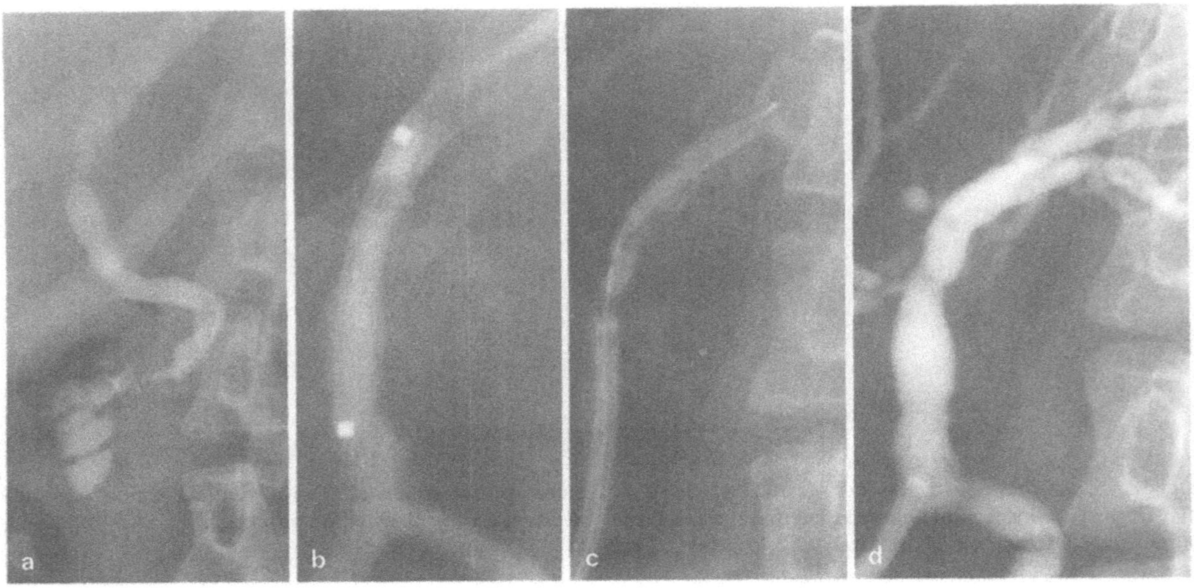

Fig. 5. **a** Operative cholangiogram demonstrates three small stones in the common duct and three stones in the left hepatic radicle above a bile duct stricture at the porta hepatis. The surgeon was unable to remove the stones in the left hepatic radicle. **b** Radiologic intervention 4 weeks after operation: Grüntzig balloon in place after stricture dilatation. **c** The retained stones in the left hepatic radicle were successfully extracted with the wire basket. **d** Closing cholangiogram shows the duct system clear. The dilated bile duct stricture was not stented, and recurred within 6 months. Note that the benign stricture also extends into the right hepatic radicles

Intrahepatic stones are often situated proximally to intrahepatic bile duct strictures. This made stone extraction more difficult until stricture dilatation was instituted as an interventional radiologic technique [2]. The use of the Grüntzig balloon catheter has greatly improved the success rate for stone extraction (Fig. 5) [4].

Stricture Dilatation

As in percutaneous stone extraction, the interventional radiologist can use either the transhepatic or subhepatic approach [1, 11]. The subhepatic approach through a postoperative drain tract or jejunostomy is preferred, as it is technically easier and larger retention catheters may be placed for maintenance of dilatation. Interventional dilatation of bile duct strictures is accomplished with Grüntzig balloon catheters using manual injection pressure (Fig. 5). It is indicated in postoperative iatrogenic strictures of the biliary tree, strictures at the hepatojejunostomy site, and inflammatory strictures. Dilatation and drainage has also been accomplished in patients with sclerosing cholangitis [9].

Percutaneous transhepatic balloon dilatation of benign postoperative biliary strictures usually requires repeated long-term high-pressure dilatations with subsequent stenting by large catheters [16]. We have found that stenting is often required for a prolonged period of time in order to prevent recurrence. It usually requires the placement of a 12-F, 14-F catheter.

Surgical injuries, occurring in most cases in the course of cholecystectomy, constitute 80% of all benign bile duct strictures [7]. Strictures caused by surgical injury show a marked tendency to progression and recurrence. Some are definitively cured by surgical repair. Hepatojejunostomy has been followed by good results in about two-thirds of the cases, although operative mortality rates from 5% to 8% have been reported [7]. Many authors use internal stents across a bile duct anastomosis to maintain the lumen while the fibrous tissue of the anastomosis matures in order to avoid recurrence of stenosis. Various stents have been placed, but many of them slip below the anastomosis, particularly if they have been placed from below. Surgical stenting in a transhepatic fashion from above, or placement of a U-tube, prevents tube displacement.

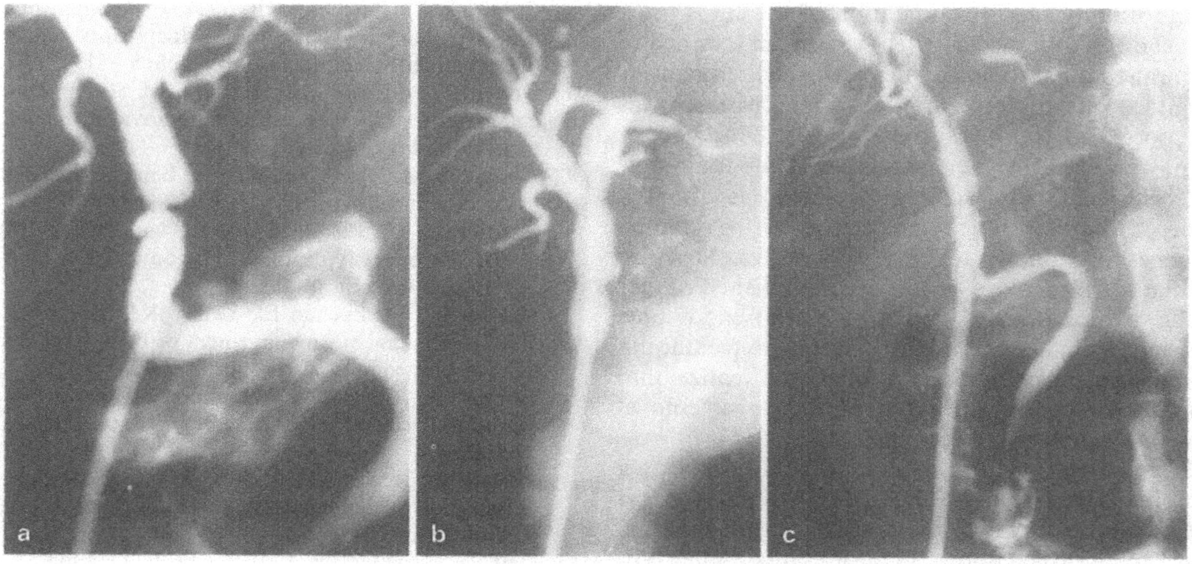

Fig. 6. a Cholangiogram 6 weeks after operation through a T-tube sinus tract demonstrates iatrogenic stricture in a jaundiced patient. **b** Balloon dilatation of the bile duct stricture using manual injection pressure. **c** Stenting catheter in place 3 months after stricture dilatation with decompression of intrahepatic bile ducts. Side-holes below the old stricture site and catheter closure at the skin provide for internal drainage. Four months after surgery, the stenting catheter was placed with its tip below the stricture site and the stricture recurred, requiring redilatation. After further stenting for 3 months, the old stricture site was stable and the stenting catheter was removed. The patient is asymptomatic on 2-year follow-up

If surgical stenting tubes become dislodged, the interventional radiologist can place a U-tube by adding a transhepatic approach, pulling the U-tube into position over a guide wire [4].

Some radiologists have reported good results with balloon dilatation of biliary strictures without subsequent stenting [15]. Our experience in 52 cases with balloon dilatation of biliary strictures is different: most strictures will recur without stent placement (Fig. 6).

After passage of a guide wire through the stricture, it is dilated with an angioplasty balloon catheter, and a catheter stent is placed to maintain the stricture dilatation. End- or side-holes are made in the stenting catheter above and below the stricture site for internal drainage. The catheter is closed at the skin. If the stenting catheter is placed from above in a transhepatic fashion, care must be taken that no side-holes are in the liver parenchyma. There should also be no side-holes in the stent in the sinus tract if the catheter is placed from below.

We prefer to leave the stenting catheter in place for 3 months, at which time the stent is withdrawn to a point outside the previous stricture but the catheter is left in place to maintain access. Control cholangiograms are obtained at 2-week intervals in order to assess possible stricture recurrence. If the stricture recurs, the stent is again inserted through the narrowed area. Slightly over half of the patients demonstrated stricture recurrence and needed such respositioning of the stent. These patients required an average stenting period of 8 months. The catheter was withdrawn in the remaining patients after 4 months. This is similar to the surgical experience, where indwelling splint catheters remained within previous stricture sites for a period of 8 – 14 months in order for the scar to mature and stabilize [18].

Patients tolerate indwelling catheters well. They return to work and are able to take showers without fear of losing the catheter. However, it remains controversial as to how long stents should remain in place [16].

Nonradiologic Techniques

Nonsurgical removal of retained biliary calculi has been recommended by means of choledochoscopy through the T-tube tract [19]. This technique, however, is more difficult, more expensive, and usually requires dilatation of the sinus tract. It shows a low success rate if stones are retained in intrahepatic ducts or in the cystic duct remnant. A failure rate of six extractions in 73 patients was reported in the best series [8]. Choledochoscopy may be used for stone extraction if the radiologic technique fails. Radiologic removal is also the procedure of choice in patients with retained stones proximally to biliary strictures. Stricture dilatation is more readily accomplished under fluoroscopic control. The high cost of endoscopic stone removal compared to radiologic techniques becomes more significant when we realize that multiple sessions are required for stone removal in over one-third of the patients.

Physical removal or fragmentation of biliary tract stones is preferable to chemical dissolution at this time since chemical dissolution of gallstones in the biliary ducts shows a considerably higher failure rate. Mono-octanoin and Capmul infusion also require hospitalization and are associated with a not inconsiderable complication rate.

In the treatment of benign strictures of the bile ducts, the technique of left hepatojejunostomy has been successful in the hands of experienced surgeons [7, 17]. Most of our patients undergoing interventional radiologic stricture dilatation in the biliary tract, however, had one or more stricture recurrences after surgical repair.

References

1. Burhenne HJ (1983) Biliary tract: radiology. In: Margulis AR, Burhenne HJ (eds) Alimentary tract radiology, 3rd ed. Mosby, St. Louis, pp 2318–2339
2. Burhenne HJ (1975) Dilatation of biliary tract strictures. Radiol Clin 44:153–159
3. Burhenne HJ (1980) Percutaneous extraction of retained biliary tract stones: 661 patients. AJR 134:888–898
4. Burhenne HJ, Morris DC (1980) Biliary stricture dilatation: use of the Grüntzig balloon catheter. J Can Assoc Radiol 31:196–197
5. Clouse ME, Falchuk KR (1983) Percutaneous transhepatic removal of common duct stones: report of ten patients. Gastroenterology 85:815–819
6. Dotter CT, Bilbao MK, Katon RM (1979) Percutaneous transhepatic gallstone removal by needle tract. Radiology 133:242
7. Fernandez M (1980) Treatment of benign strictures of the bile ducts. World J Surg 4:479–482
8. Jakimowicz JJ, Mak B, Carol EJ, van Baalen JM (1983) Postoperative choledochoscopy. A five-year experience. Arch Surg 118:810
9. Martin EC, Fankuchen EI, Laffey KJ, Sibley RE (1984) Percutaneous management of benign biliary disease. Gastrointest Radiol 9:207–212
10. Mazzariello RM (1974) Transcholecystic extraction of residual calculi in common bile duct. Surgery 75:338–347
11. Molnar W, Stockum AE (1978) Transhepatic dilatation of choledochoenterostomy strictures. Radiology 129:59
12. Neff CC, Mueller PR, Ferrucci JT Jr, Dawson SL, Wittenberg J, Simeone JF, Butch RJ, Papanicolaou N (1984) Serious complications following transgression of the pleural space in drainage procedures. Radiology 152:335–341
13. Nichols DM, Burhenne HJ (1984) Magnification in cholangiography. AJR 142:947
14. Nichols DM, Cooperberg PL, Golding RH, Burhenne HJ (1984) The safe intercostal approach? Pleural complications in abdominal interventional radiology. AJR 142:1013–1018
15. Ring EJ, McLean GK (1981) Interventional radiology: principles and techniques. Little, Brown, Boston
16. Salomonowitz E, Castaneda-Zuniga WR, Lund G, Cragg AH, Hunter DW, Coleman CC, Amplatz K (1984) Balloon dilatation of benign biliary strictures. Radiology 151:613–616
17. Warren KW, Jefferson MF (1973) Prevention and repair of strictures of the extrahepatic bile duct. Surg Clin North Am 53:1169
18. Warren KW, Whitcomb FF Jr (1971) Diagnosis and treatment of benign biliary tract stricture. Hosp Pract 6:62
19. Yamakawa T, Mieno K, Nogucki T, Shikata J (1976) An improved choledochofiberscope and non-surgical removal of retained biliary calculi under direct visual control. Gastrointest Endosc 22:160

Percutaneous Tissue Core Biopsy with the Tru-Cut Needle

N. Rupp, S. Feuerbach, M. Reiser, A. Schekatz, and K. Becker

Percutaneous aspiration biopsy for cytologic examination is a widely accepted and safe method of obtaining a correct diagnosis in many suspect masses in most anatomic sites with a high degree of reliability, when malignant cells are found [3, 10]. There are, however, certain drawbacks: for proper treatment oncologists often require histologic verification and differentiation of the malignant tumor. A cytologic report which is negative for malignant tumor does not exclude it, and histologic control is desirable. In certain parts of the body, CT-guided percutaneous large-core biopsy seems to yield material for histologic investigation just as good as that obtained by exploratory surgery with all its attendant risks.

Technique

The disposable Tru-Cut needle (Travenol GmbH, Munich) was used in all biopsies (Fig. 1). It has an outer diameter of 14 gauge and comes in three different lengths, 75, 114, and 152 mm. Virtually all structures of the body can be reached. The needle does not interfere with the CT gantry if the proper length is chosen and if the patient is placed in an excentric position. The needle is composed of two parts: an outer cannula with a cutting tip, and a removable stylet within which has a 2-cm-long excavation near its tip for acceptance of the specimen. The biopsy is performed in the following way (Fig. 2a, b): after larger vascular structures or hemangiomas are excluded, often by a preceding angio-CT, the mass for biopsy is located by thin-slice CT with a metallic marker on the skin at the presumed point of entry. Possible interposition of pleura or bowel is carefully excluded. After administration of local anesthesia in the skin and the deeper tissues, a new control CT is performed with the small anesthesia needle still in place, giving the direction of puncture, which is corrected if necessary. Using this guide needle the Tru-Cut needle is than advanced beside the anesthesia needle to a precalculated depth from the skin and a new control CT is performed, on which the distal 2.5 cm of the Tru-Cut needle should be exactly within the tumor mass. For biopsy, the inner stylet is held fixed while the outer cannula is pulled back to open the excavation of the stylet (Fig. 2a) and then pushed forward in order to cut the tissue (Fig. 2b). The stylet is then removed, the cannula remaining in place, and the tissue is placed into formalin solution for histologic examination. If necessary, biopsy is repeated, the outer cannula still being in place. If the complete needle is withdrawn, a new pass and control scan has to be done for the new specimen.

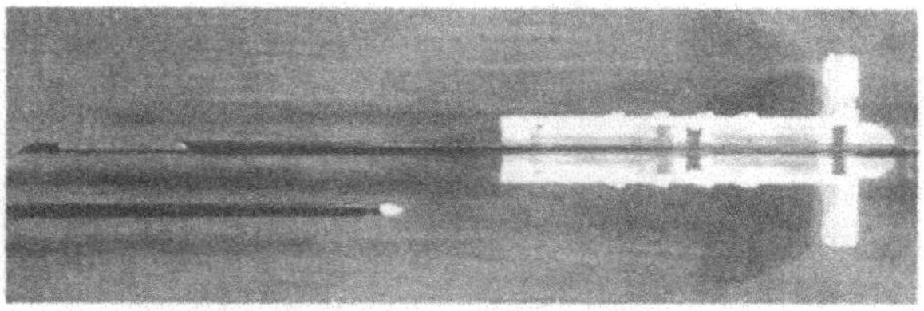

Fig. 1. Travenol Tru-Cut needle. *Below:* needle in closed position. *Above:* needle in open position; excavation in stylet can now be seen

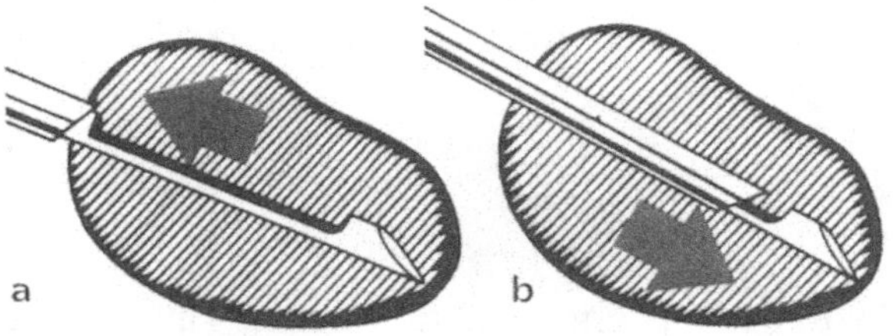

Fig. 2a, b. Biopsy technique. "Closed" needle is pushed into tumor mass, outer cannula is pulled back to open excavation (**a**), then cannula is pushed forward to cut tissue with its sharp edge (**b**)

Table 1. CT-guided biopsy with the Tru-Cut needle

Site	No. of patients
Liver	16
Pelvis	9
Retroperitoneal space	8
Abdominal wall	2
Thoracic wall	1
Lower limb	1
Total	37

Material

37 patients, 21 men and 16 women within an age range of 21 – 66 years, have been examined using the technique described. The different organs and structures examined are listed in Table 1. All patients were starved for at least 6 h prior to the intervention, and blood parameters like bleeding and clotting time were checked. Only inpatients were examined. The diameter of the masses was 2 cm and more. In all cases at least two specimens were obtained from slightly different sites. Further proof of malignancy, e.g. by operation, was only occasionally obtained, because percutaneous biopsy seemed to be reliable enough in most instances.

Results

All masses considered as suited for biopsy from a diagnostic point of view could be well examined technically. Neither CT artifacts from the metal needle nor the handling of the needle for biopsy were a problem. The procedure was described by most patients as annoying and sometimes slightly painful, but tolerable. As a rule, one single puncture was sufficient to obtain enough tissue material for examination, so we now rarely puncture more than once. Major complications needing further treatment were not encountered in any of our patients.

Liver

In 16 patients a total of 18 different tumors were examined by biopsy, 12 of them in the right and six in the left hepatic lobe. Twelve lesions were located near the liver surface, the rest more centrally but never near the hilum. In 15 of 16 patients the tissue core was sufficient for histologic examination, in two of them biopsies from two different masses both gave satisfactory results. In 12 patients metastases of an adenocarcinoma, and in three hepatocellular carcinomas, were found by histology. In the two patients with the double biopsy, each specimen revealed metastases of adenocarcinoma. In one patient with a large partially necrotic liver tumor only necrotic tissue was found on histology and the diagnosis could not be established. Histology of the operative specimen revealed hepatocellular carcinoma. Mainly the lateral or ventral approach was used, the patient lying supine or in left lateral decubitus. Masses in the apex of the liver or in its lower rim were punctured by angulation of the needle compared to the axis of the body in order to avoid penetration of pleura or bowel.

Pelvis

Nine patients with pelvic tumors, all in the perirectal and presacral spaces, were examined. In four patients, clinical and CT diagnosis was suspected recurrence of rectal carcinoma. In two of them histologic proof was obtained, whereas in the other two no malignancy was found in the specimen. CT control studies after 6 months confirmed this diagnosis. Biopsy of five patients with peri- and presacral mass with or without osteolysis revealed metastasis of an adenocarcinoma. In three of them the colorectal tumor was unknown before, in two the primary tumor was not found. The tissue specimen was sufficient for histologic examination in all nine cases, and histologic diagnosis was unequivocal. Two minor complications occurred, but did not need treatment: transient hematospermia 3 days after biopsy, and air penetration into the bladder, probably due to perforation. There were no further complaints in either patients. Only the dorsal approach was used in pelvic biopsy.

Retroperitoneal Space

Biopsy was performed in seven patients with retroperitoneal masses. Enlarged adrenal glands were examined in four patients: in two they were due to a squamous cell carcinoma (one known small bronchial carcinoma, the other unknown), one patient had adrenal lymphoma, and the fourth patient had a huge partly necrotic tumor,

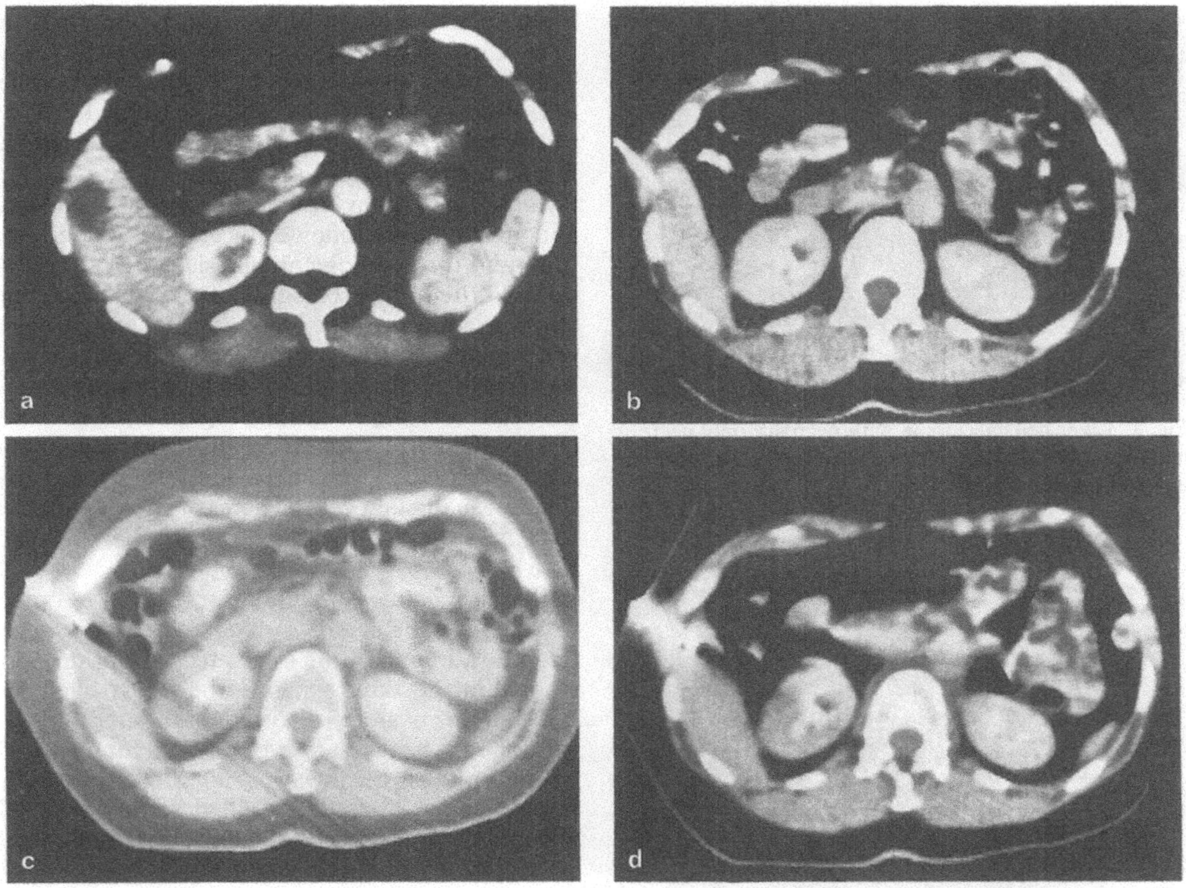

Fig. 3a–d. Biopsy of a liver metastasis. **a** Localization by CT; **b** biopsy direction given by small anesthesia needle; **c, d** CT slices with Tru-Cut in correct position

where the biopsy specimen was unsatisfactory for histologic examination. Retroperitoneal para-aortic and paracaval masses in one patient were due to lymphomas. In this patient a second tissue specimen was obtained for tissue typing, the cannula still being in place. In one patient a liposarcoma of the psoas muscle was diagnosed. All retroperitoneal masses were examined by dorsal approach.

Thoracic and Abdominal Walls, Limbs

In four patients rather superficial masses were examined by biopsy. In two patients masses of the abdominal wall were infiltrating into the peritoneum: biopsy showed in one of them granulomatous (Hodgkin) infiltration, and in the other a peritoneal metastasis with secondary infiltration into the subcutaneous tissue from a carcinoma of the ovary. In one patient, a tumor of the thoracic wall turned out to be a benign fibroma in histology. In another, a tumor of the thigh was found by histologic examination of the biopsy specimen and of the operatively removed tissue to be a benign lipoma. CT guidance seemed to be useful in restricting the biopsy to the tumor, preferably at the border, and avoiding necrotic tissue.

Discussion

Percutaneous tissue core biopsy with the Tru-Cut needle has definite *advantages* compared with fine-needle aspiration biopsy. Histologic examination of tissue from a suspected mass is usually more reliable than cytology and decreases the false-negative rate. The diagnostic decision whether a mass is malignant or not, is easier and more reliable. Besides this, histology leads to a specific tissue diagnosis and provides the cellular type or, in the case of metastasis, its possible

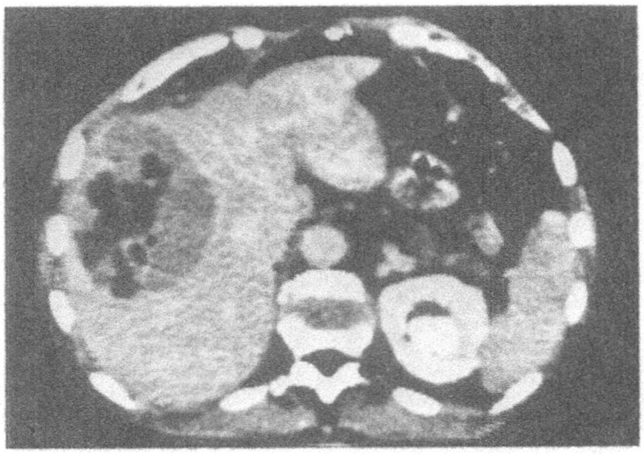

Fig. 4. Liver cell carcinoma with necrosis; only necrotic material obtained in biopsy specimen, therefore no histologic diagnosis possible

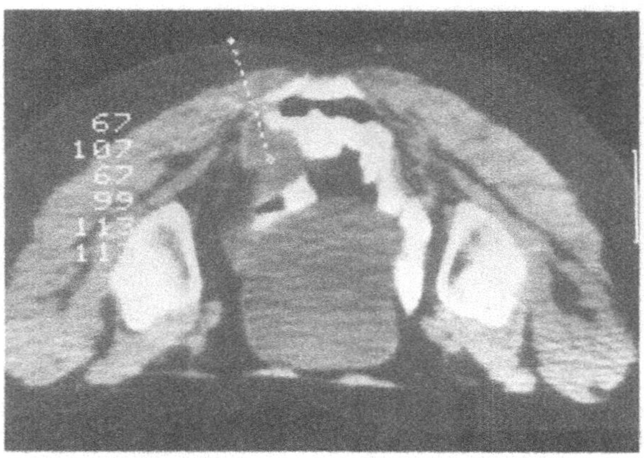

Fig. 5. Metastasis of sacrum from colon tumor: biopsy of soft tissue mass by posterior approach

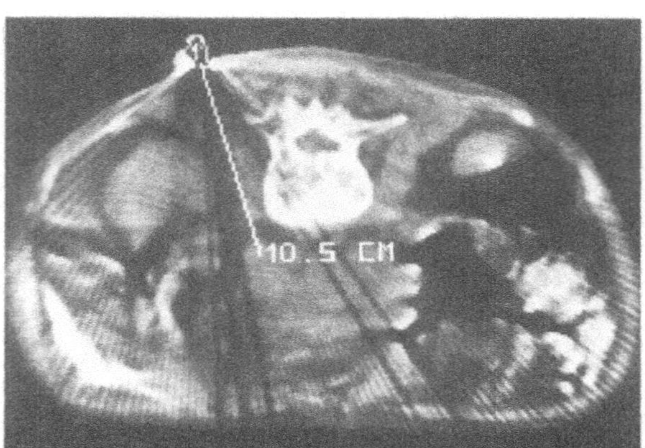

Fig. 6. Biopsy of paraaortal lymphoma, posterior approach. One needle pass was sufficient for two specimens, one for histologic diagnosis and one for additional tissue typing

origin. This seems to be especially important in liver metastasis when no primary tumor is known. Tissue core biopsy avoids purely explorative operations, and in some cases CT-guided biopsy can be more precise than laparatomy, for example in small intrahepatic masses.

Cytology is in many instances not reliable enough and must often be followed by explorative surgery to obtain the histologic diagnosis which is necessary in order that oncologists can decide upon the appropriate treatment. Here percutaneous biopsy can replace surgery. Furthermore, in certain tumors, such as lymphomas, core biopsy can furnish material for tissue typing, again in order to choose the correct treatment. In many benign tumors cytologic reports often simply show the absence of malignant cells, whereas histology is able to classify these tumors according to their cellular type [4, 5].

Different *requirements* must be observed in order to achieve satisfactory results from biopsy. The exact positioning of the excavated part of the stylet within the tumor mass is best controlled by CT, and this is more important in smaller tumors. Care should be taken to avoid the necrotic area of a tumor, the border always being preferable. Both failures in our material resulted from biopsy of necrotic tissue. For special sites, ultrasound-guided biopsy would be fine, but in fact there are as yet no biopsy devices available for the Tru-Cut needle.

In contrast to thin-needle biopsy, where virtually no precautions have to be observed [3, 6, 10] there are *limitations* in Tru-Cut needle biopsy. They are not yet proven, but they should be observed for safety reasons until there is more experience with the method. Large vessels of hypervascularized structures such as hemangiomas or hypervascularized tumors should be avoided in order to prevent peritoneal or retroperitoneal bleeding. This excludes certain anatomic sites from core biopsy, such as the hilum of the liver, the space near the aorta and the vena cava, the renal and the pelvic vessels. Often angio-CT becomes necessary prior to biopsy in order to exclude hypervascularity. No risk of bowel perforation and peritonitis should be taken. This excludes the ventral approach, as used in thin-needle biopsy for pancreas, spleen, bowel, and para-aortic lymph nodes, but masses in these organs are often just as accessible by the dorsal route. An alternative would be the use of smaller biopsy needles [5, 7, 8, 11]. Diaphragm, lungs, and pleural space should equally be avoided, to prevent pneumothorax or hematopneumothorax. This makes core biopsy of the dome of the liver rather difficult. If the biopsy needle is somewhat angulated in the cranial or ventral direction (Fig. 5) biopsy may be possible, but CT control is more difficult. The same is true for the lower border of the liver, where the bowel can be perforated.

The 14-gauge needle is relatively large, but tissue specimens are less damaged than with other needles, and it gives about 15 times as much tissue as a 22-gauge Chiba needle [1, 5, 9]. Our own experience with thinner-core biopsy needles is rather limited, because pathologists were too often unsatisfied with the tissue specimen obtained, despite several punctures. In contrast, one single biopsy with the Tru-Cut needle in smaller or moderately large tumors is usually enough for histologic diagnosis. A great advantage of this type of needle is the visual control of the specimen in the stylet without removal of the cannula, so that in case of failure on the first attempt, another tissue specimen can be obtained immediately without damage.

There have been two minor *complications* in our pelvic biopsy examinations, one transient hematospermia and one bladder wall perforation, neither of which required further treatment. There are, however, reports on bleeding after biopsy with larger needles [5], so it is wise to observe the patient for a certain time after biopsy until further experience with the method has been obtained. The same is true for malignant seeding within the puncture tract [2], although this has never yet been observed for the Tru-Cut needle.

Summary

Percutaneous tissue core biopsy has been performed in 37 patients using the Travenol Tru-Cut needle. Masses in the liver, retroperitoneal space, pelvis, thoracic and abdominal walls, and soft tissues of the limbs have been examined. Only two minor complications, not requiring treatment, were encountered. The advantage of this method is the possibility of histologic examination of tissue, leading to a specific tissue diagnosis. It often equals explorative surgery in accuracy, and may even be more accurate in smaller deeply located masses. In certain malignant tumors, especially in lymphoma, tissue for typing is obtained as well. However, the method is restricted to certain anatomic sites, where larger vessels, bowel, and the pleural space can avoided.

References

1. Andriole JG, Haaga JR, Adams RB, Nunez C (1983) Biopsy needle characteristics assessed in the laboratory. Radiology 148:659–662
2. Ferrucci JT, Wittenberg J, Margolies MN, Carey RW (1979) Malignant seeding of the tract after thin needle aspiration biopsy. Radiology 130:345–346
3. Göthlin JH, Rupp N, Rothenberger KH, MacIntosh PK (1981) Percutaneous biopsy of retroperitoneal lymph nodes. A multicentric study. Eur J Radiol 1:46–50
4. Haaga RH (1979) New technique for CT-guided biopsy. AJR 133:633–641
5. Haaga JR, LiPuma JP, Bryan PJ, Balsara VJ, Cohen AM (1983) Clinical comparison of small- and large-caliber cutting needles for biopsy. Radiology 146:665–667
6. Holm HH, Pedersen JF, Kristensen JK, Hanke S, Jensen F (1975) Ultrasonically guided percutaneous puncture. Radiol Clin North Am 13:493–503
7. Isler RJ, Ferrucci JT, Wittenberg J, Mueller PR, Simeone JF, van Sonnenberg E, Hall DA (1981) Tissue core biopsy of abdominal tumors with a 22 gauge cutting needle. AJR 136:725–728
8. Lieberman RP, Hafez GR, Crummy AB (1982) Histology from aspiration biopsy: Turner needle experience. AJR 138:561–564
9. Pagani JJ (1983) Biopsy and focal hepatic lesions. Comparison of 18 and 22 gauge needles. Radiology 147:673–675
10. Rupp N, Rothenberger KH, Bayer-Pietsch E, Feuerbach St, Esch U (1979) Die perkutane Feinnadelbiopsie von Lymphknoten. Fortschr Röntgenstr 130:328–331
11. Wittenberg J, Mueller PR, Ferrucci JT Jr, Simeone JF, van Sonnenberg E, Neff CC, Palermo RA, Isler RJ (1982) Percutaneous core biopsy of abdominal tumors using 22 gauge needles: further observations. AJR 139:75–80

New Developments in Caval Filters*

K. Amplatz

In patients with recurrent pulmonary emboli, placement of caval filters is a well-established beneficial procedure. This is particularly true in patients who cannot be anticoagulated. Among the various filters, the Greenfield and Mobin models are most widely used.

Because of the large size of the capsule, such filters are usually introduced by surgeons via jugular vein or, less commonly, femoral vein cutdowns. With the advent of the semirigid dilator the surgical approach is no longer necessary, and the filters can now be introduced by radiologists.

Technique

The jugular or femoral vein is punctured in routine fashion under local anesthesia. An angiographic catheter is introduced, and a cavogram is performed during the Valsalva maneuver. The level of the renal veins is thus identified. The vein is gradually dilated using semirigid dilators developed for renal stone removal (Cook Inc.). Dilatation to 24 F allows the introduction of a Teflon sheath which accepts the capsule of the Greenfield or Mobin filter. As soon as the capsule has been introduced the Teflon sheath is withdrawn.

For the introduction through the jugular vein it is of paramount importance that the patient is able to sustain breathing, in order to avoid air aspiration. At the University of Minnesota Hospitals, 27 such filters were introduced percutaneously by cardiovascular radiologists without complications [1]. In spite of the ease of introduction, the technique has not become popular because of the apparent large size of the capsule. It is therefore not surprising that different smaller devices have been developed in recent years. One such new development is the "bird-nest" filter, which can be introduced through an 8-F catheter. The filter is basically a wire mesh which is anchored to the wall of the cava. The new device is presently being tested in a few hospitals in the USA.

We have developed a different filter which can be introduced through a 14-F catheter and can be retrieved [2]. It is made from MP35N, an alloy of nickel, cobalt, chromium, and molybdenum which has proved to be very inert and is consequently used for the construction of pacemaker wires (Fig. 1). It has six prongs with wire loops limiting the penetration of the wires into the caval wall. Additional wires are placed between the six prongs in order to improve the filtering action. The filter is screwed to an introducing wire and delivered through a Teflon catheter introduced into the jugular vein. A small wire hook allows the withdrawal of the filter from below, using the standard cardiovascular snare introduced from the femoral vein (Fig. 1).

The filter has been successfully placed into the cava of dogs, and patency for several months has been proven. The filter has also been successfully removed up to 2 weeks after insertion (Fig. 2).

Discussion

Surgical ligation or plication can be used to interrupt flow in the inferior vena cava. Due to the decreased morbidity and mortality, the surgical technique has been replaced by the less invasive placement of filters. The Hunter balloon and the Greenfield and Mobin filter are the only commercially available devices at present.

The Mobin filter is the most effective, but it partially obstructs caval flow, which may result in early thrombosis of the cava and subsequent swelling of the lower extremities. The Greenfield filter is a compromise, but thrombosis of the cava is usually avoided. On the other hand, the filtering action is less effective than that of the Mobin filter. With our design, the filtering capacity is greater than with the Greenfield filter because the distance between the legs of the filter is much

* Addendum: Since the preparation of this report the filter has been percutaneously introduced into four patients

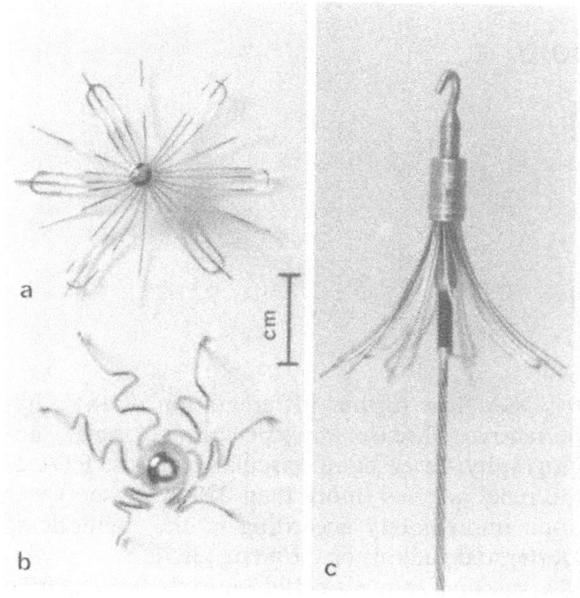

Fig. 1. a The new removable filter seen from above. **b** Greenfield filter for comparison. The spaces between the legs of the new filter are only half as big, improving the filtering efficiency. **c** Side view of filter attached to introducing cable

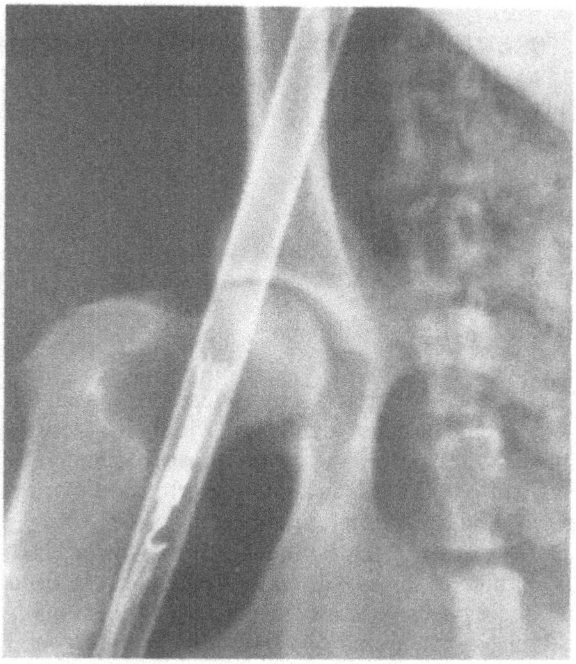

Fig. 2. Removal of the caval filter through a Teflon sheath introduced percutaneously into the femoral vein

smaller. Apparently our filter does not cause partial obstruction of caval flow, since thrombosis occurred in only one animal. Obviously, human tests will be necessary to determine the thrombogenicity in man.

The biocompatibility of the material MP35N has been well proven and a vast body of literature has accumulated on this alloy. MP35N does not contain iron, and since solder joints are avoided the filter very probably represents a corrosion-free long-term implant.

Patients undergoing major abdominal, pelvic, or hip surgery are in danger of developing pulmonary emboli, which may even be fatal. Although the incidence of this complication can be decreased by anticoagulation, some patients cannot be anticoagulated and are therefore at high risk of developing such emboli. In these patients prophylactic placement of a caval filter may be considered, provided it can be easily removed percutaneously. With the present design this requirement has been fulfilled, but removal is only feasible up to 10 days after insertion. After this period of time tissue ingrowth into the wire loops occurs, making removal difficult.

In a separate study, the filtering actions of the bird-nest, Mobin, Greenfield, and new filters were studied in a model. The filters were inserted into vinyl tubing which was connected to a pump delivering saline at a flow rate corresponding to human inferior vena cava flow. Coagula were then injected and the filtering action was observed. The Mobin filter was the best, followed by the newly described retrievable filter. The Greenfield and bird-nest filters were the less effective.

Summary and Conclusion

A new retrievable filter is described that can be percutaneously introduced through the jugular vein. The filter has been tested in animals and its filtering capability has proved to be superior to that of the Greenfield filter. The new filter can be removed via percutaneous puncture of the femoral vein and therefore its prophylactic use is feasible.

References

1. Formanek A, Castaneda-Zuniga W, Knight L, Amplatz K (1977) Three-year experience with percutaneous introduction of inferior vena cava filter. Rev Interam Radiol 2:171–175
2. Lund G, Rysavy JA, Salomonowitz E, Cragg AH, Kotula F, Castaneda-Zuniga W, Hunter DW, Coleman CC, Amplatz K (1984) A new vena caval filter for percutaneous placement and retrieval: experimental study. Radiology 152[2]:369–372

Present Workup of Renal Hypertension

E. Löhr

The causes of arterial hypertension associated with renal diseases can vary widely. Infections and vascular processes are the most frequent. The classical pathways leading to hypertension involve extra- and intrarenal vascular processes, mostly arteriosclerotic, releasing the renin-hypertensin mechanism. Chronic infections and noninfectious nephritic processes must be discussed; hormonally influenced extrarenal diseases must be excluded.

Renal hypertension can develop as a consequence of trauma, by means of an organized renal or perirenal hematoma narrowing the capsule and main renal artery. Systemic and metabolic diseases, especially diabetes, are also accompanied by hypertension. Renal transplants in different phases of rejection can develop hypertension of different origins.

Arterial hypertension of unknown origin, if the above mentioned diseases can be excluded, are commonly named "essential". Not a small percentage of these hypertensions are due to vascular malformations of the segmental and cortical renal vessels classified as nephrosclerotic. These regional, mostly cortical processes can be overlooked in conventional and even in selective renal angiography. In the course of the last 5 years we have diagnosed a series of cases of infantile and juvenile nephrosclerosis, some of which were primarily suspected to be caused by stenosis of the renal artery. In approximately half the patients, recurrent microhematuria was the reason for carrying out further diagnostic examination.

Patients and Methods

We are currently following up more than 500 patients examined by us in the last 5 years with hypertension induced by renal inflammatory or vascular disease.

In most of these patients hypertension had been known for many years. All of them were pre-examined by IVU and nuclear studies, some also by DSA. For further differentation of their hypertensive disease we performed renal angiography. In cases of vascular stenosis, PTA of the renal arteries (more than 220 at present) was done immediately according to the methods of Dotter and Judkins or Grüntzig [3, 5].

If a vascular stenosis could be excluded – which effectively can only be done be intravascular pressure measurements [8, 9] – we examined our images thoroughly with the EMH apparatus (Electronic Magnification and Harmonization unit, Siemens), which is really a precursor of digital imaging in radiology and possesses high spatial resolution [8]. The pictures were projected onto the monitor screen, photographed with the Leitz system, and thoroughly evaluated. Special attention was paid to the configuration, size, and formation of the interlobar, arcuate, and interlobar-cortical vessels.

Results

The EMH system was used routinely in evaluating vascular disease, and was also employed when vascular deformations or stenosis had already been observed without it. The findings are presented below according to the diseases listed in Table 1.

Arteriosclerotic Disease

Changes of caliber in all larger and segmental, even cortical, vessels are obvious. Renal hypertension is due to generalized vascular illness, whereas arteriosclerosis of the kidneys finally leads to vascular obstruction and renal insufficiency.

Stenosis of the Renal Arteries

In renal artery stenosis combined with arteriosclerosis, the same observations can be made as in

Table 1. Causes of renal hypertension

a) "Essential" hypertension		Congenital
		Nephrosclerotic
b) Hpertension in nephritic disease	Extrarenal	Fibrodysplastic
		Arteriosclerotic
c) Hypertension caused by vascular disease	Intrarenal	Systemic
		Embolic
		Diabetic
		Vascular malformation
d) After trauma	Incompatiḇility caused by:	
e) Hormonally induced	Immunologic reaction	
f) Metabolic	Vascular disorders	
g) After renal transplant	Infection	
	Original kidneys producing renin	

arteriosclerosis alone, with one difference: the vasculature of the ipsilateral kidney does not show such severe arteriosclerotic lesions of the segmental and corticomedullary vessels (in the range of 49%) as in the nonaffected kidney, where those severe vascular processes exceed than 80.9% [7].

These findings probably influence the results of PTA of renal arteries: although the PTA could be done completely (we are currently following up 225 cases), in about 40% the renal hypertension could be cured [1]. In hypertension due to fibrodysplastic disease, the corticomedullary vascular lesions are less severe.

Hypertension with Nephritis

Hypertension in patients with nephritic processes (interstitial bacterial and nonbacterial) releasing renin can be differentiated by means of EMH, as previously described by Friedenberg et al. [4].

The kidneys of patients with interstitial bacterial nephritis mostly have extended or localized cortical scars, with irregular-shaped vessels in the cortical zone, sometimes obstructed. Within the scarred region there is localized edema.

In kidneys with a suspected nonbacterial interstitial nephritis these problems are absent. The stretching of the corticomedullary arteries is not marked. The localized edema can be detected too, but not to such an extent as in bacterial nephritis.

Interstitial nephritis due to chronic phenacetin consumption (always bilateral) demonstrates extended destruction of those vessels, accompanied by a generalized edema.

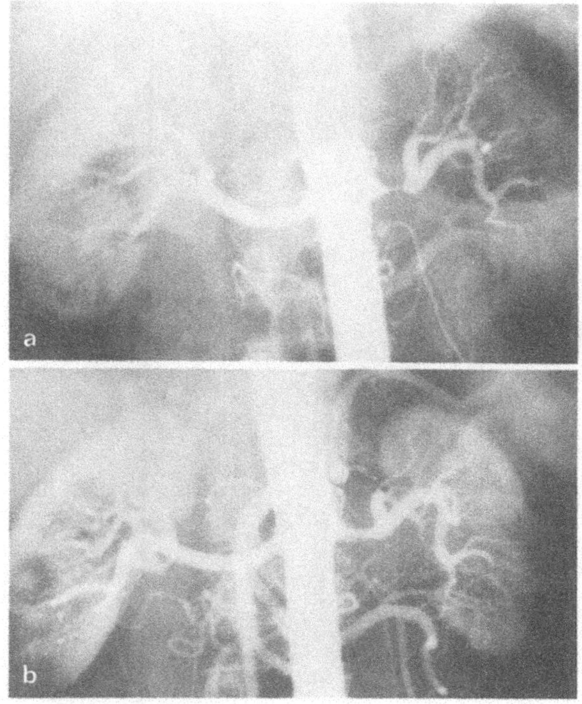

Fig. 1a, b. Stenosis in a 46-year-old patient suffering for more than 6 years from hypertension. The stenosis of about 90% could be treated successfully with PTA, blood pressure values now normal for last 15 months

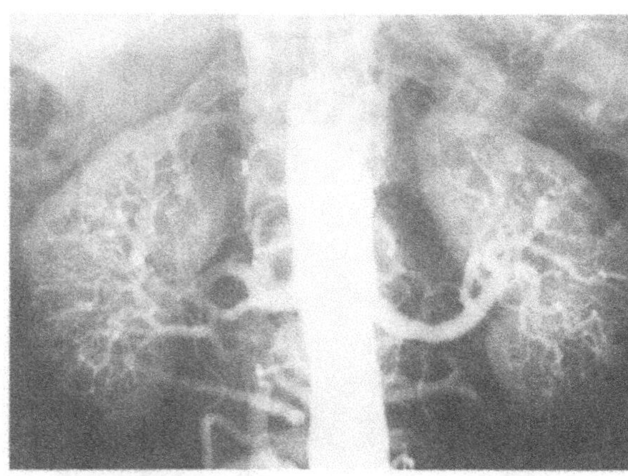

Fig. 2. Renal arteriogram of a 41-year-old patient with hypertension for several years. Typical torqued vessels and rarefication of the cortical zone: malignant nephrosclerosis

Congenital Vascular Lesions

Patients with congenital vascular lesions leading to hypertension often have combined defects such as bilateral stenoses of the renal artery and/or coarction of the abdominal aorta (we observed

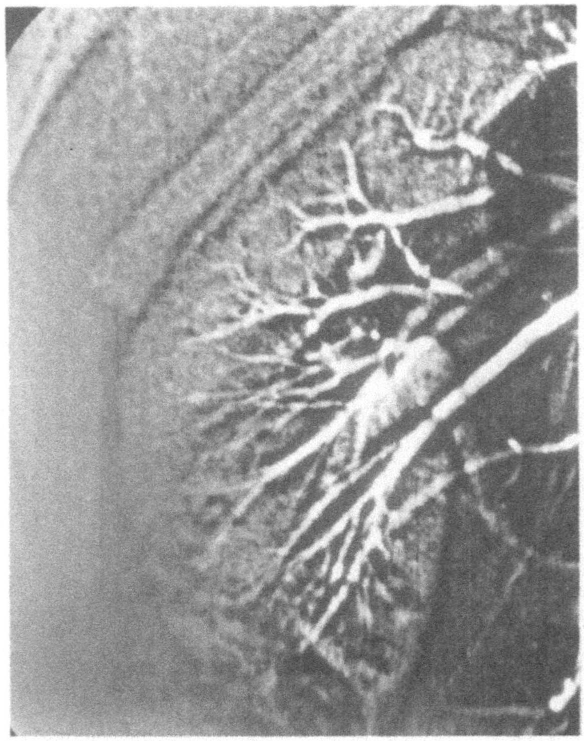

Fig. 3. EMH image of a 7-year-old boy with hypertension. The stretching of the interlobar vessels and the rarification of the corticomedullary vessels is typical for juvenile malignant nephrosclerosis

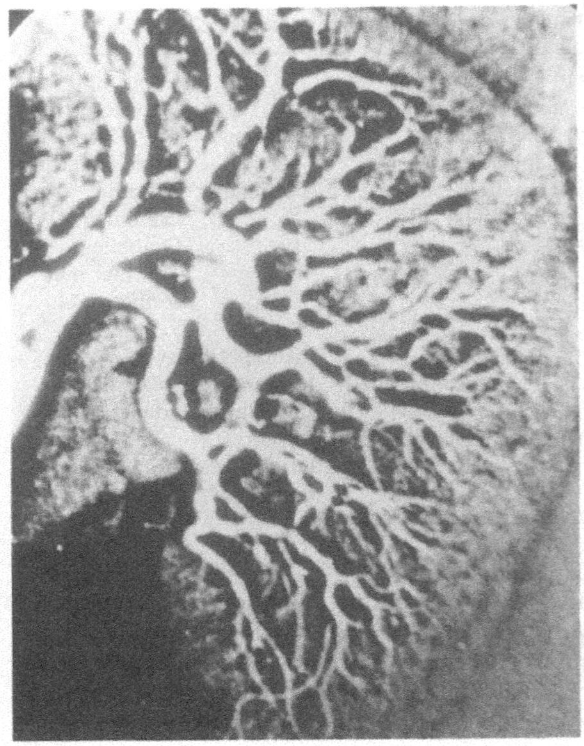

Fig. 4. Section (EMH) of an angiogram of a patient with nonbacterial interstitial nephritis: rarefication of the cortical zone and circumscript cortical edema

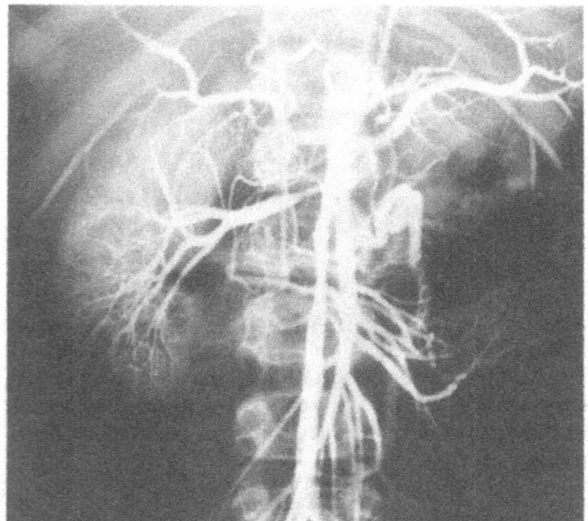

Fig. 5. Abdominal angiogram of a 6-year-old boy with hypertension: stenosis of the right renal artery and coarctation of the abdominal aorta. (The patient had already been operated on: in the postoperative period there was also obstruction of the left renal artery, which had a high graded fibrodysplastic stenosis.)

two such cases). If the angiographic examination is carried out early there could be still a chance of surgical correction.

Essential Hypertension

Patients with essential hypertension must be examined with special care, regardless of their age. The true diagnosis can in the majority of the cases be established as nephrosclerosis.

By means of EMH we were able to detect, even in very young individuals (6 and 7 years respectively), typical lesions of the cortical, medullary, and even lobular arteries which could be identified as nephrosclerotic. By means of EMH it is possible to analyze vessels as small as approximately 15 µm in diameter.

There are hints of congenital factors causing nephrosclerosis: we detected identical vascular lesions in the kidneys of a 41-year-old father and his 8-year-old son, both suffering from severe essential hypertension.

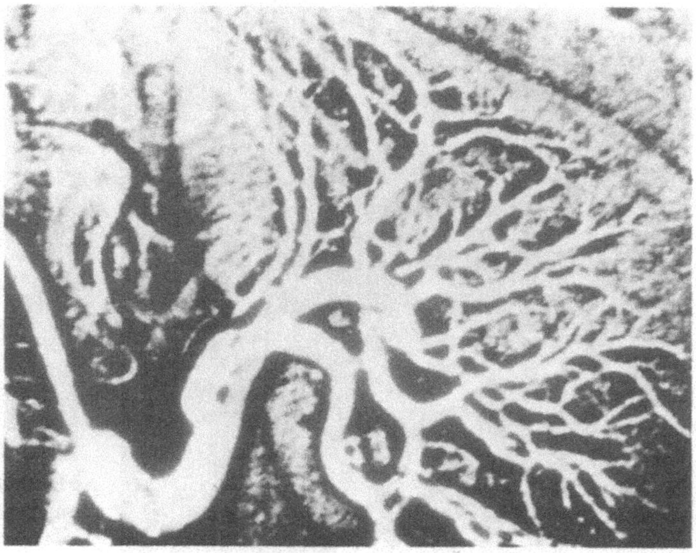

Fig. 6. Section (EMH) of the left kidney in a 35-year-old patient suffering from essential hypertension. The irregular shape and caliber of the vessels and the stretching of even the arcuate and interlobular arteries are typical for nephrosclerosis

Diabetic Angiopathy

Patients suffering from diabetes (examined because of microhematuria and hypertension) generally showed advanced vascular lesions of all sizes in the renal arteries, demonstrating the fact that diabetic angiopathy, as a generalized disease, occupies all vascular regions of the body. Moreover, EMH reveals localized cortical hemorrhages causing microhematuria.

Systemic Diseases

A number of systemic diseases, e.g., lupus erythematosus, sclerodermia, and periarteriitis nodosa, affect the kidneys in the course of visceral spread. The images of the kidneys present different pathologic vasculature patterns: sometimes microaneurysms, always advanced rarification of the cortical vasculature which is responsible for the maintenance of renally induced hypertension.

Hypertension After Renal Transplants

Hypertension in transplanted kidneys has been known for several years. It is due to vascular obstruction or kinking of the newly anastomized renal artery, sometimes by infection, usually due to immunologic incompatibility between donor and host.

In such cases cortical edema is prevalent, leading to stretching and obstruction of the corticomedullary vessels, which is similar to acute interstitial nephritis of infarction e.g. nonspecific. Of course, rejection of a transplanted kidney can be investigated by ultrasound, which should be the first step of examination.

Discussion

The onset of the renally induced hypertension is caused by different factors, all of them originating in a reduced supply of arterial blood. The site of reduction of arterial flow can be localized both in the larger and in the smaller vessels. The obstruction may be of inflammatory, vascular, or immunologic origin.

In cases of localized stenosis of the renal artery based on arteriosclerotic of fibrodysplastic origin, PTA may be successful [6, 8, 9, 12, 13, 14, 15]. Hypertension may only be classified as essential if congenital, generalized, and inflammatory disease can be excluded. This vascular disease, probably developing in the arterioles [2] starts very early in life. EHM enables the radiologist to ascertain the diagnosis at a very early stage. Differential diagnostic statements are possible.

In the detection of suspected renal hypertension the first examination should be IVU. Ultrasound and nuclear studies can be helpful, but are not specific.

DSA is of particular use. Except for stenoses of the renal arteries, which can be detected by intravenous bolus injection, only arterial administration of contrast media leads to optimal spatial resolution of the renal vasculature. In our opinion and experience, EHM combined with renal arteriography possesses the highest validity in the

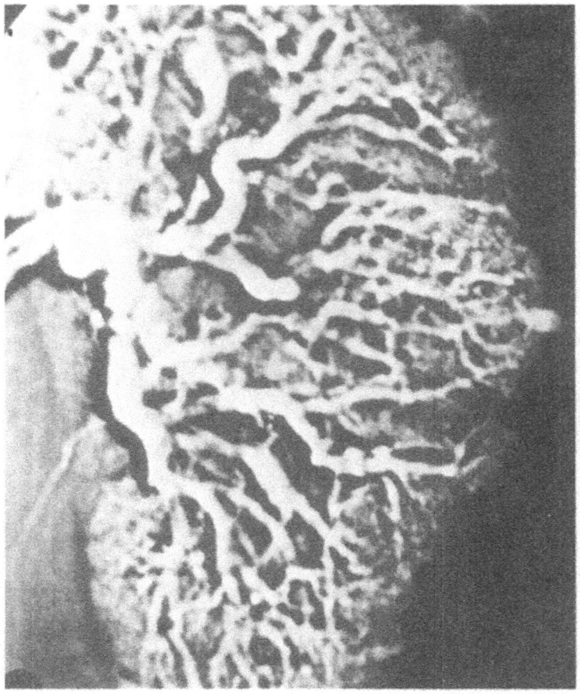

Fig. 7. Section of the left kidney (abdominal angiography in a 54-year-old patient with hypertension, diabetes, and microhematuria). The EMH image reveals multilocular vascular disorders in all parts of the kidney, demonstrating that diabetic angiopathy is a generalized disease. Moreover, the tiny lacuna observed in the cortex would correspond with subcortical hemorrhages leading to microhematuria

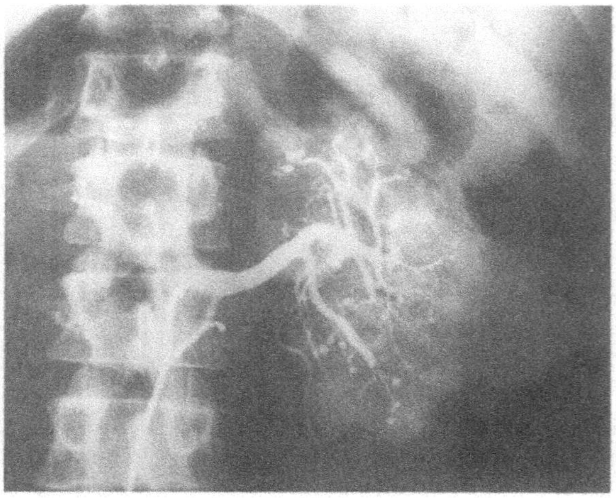

Fig. 8. Renal angiogram of a patient suffering from lupus erythematosus. Several aneurysms can be detected in all parts of the renal vasculature, which shows signs of rarefications

differentiation of renal vascular processes, as it did previously in the detection of poorly vascularized renal tumors [11].

References

1. Birkner P, Löhr E (1984) PTA bei Patienten mit Nierenarterienstenosen: Ergebnisse und Verläufe. Dtsch Med Wochenschr (in press)
2. Bohle A (1982) The compensated and decompensated form of benign nephrosclerosis. Pathol Res Pract 174:357–367
3. Dotter CT, Judkins MP (1984) Transluminal treatment of arteriosclerotic obstruction. Description of a new technique and a preliminary report of its application. Circulation 30:654–670
4. Friedenberg MJS et al. (1965) Renal angiography in pyelonephritis, glomerulonephritis and articular nephrosclerosis. AJR 95:349–363
5. Grüntzig A et al. (1978) Treatment of renovascular hypertension with percutaneous transluminal dilatation of renal artery stenosis. Lancet I:801
6. Ingrisch H et al. (1982) Röntgenologische und nuklearmedizinische Diagnostik von Nierenarterienstenosen im Hinblick auf deren perkutane transluminale Angioplastie (PTA), Vasa 11[44]:347–352
7. Löhr E, Langmack B (to be published) The detection of early nephrosclerosis by means of EMH technique in renovasography.
8. Löhr E et al. (1980) Nicht-operative Gefäßdilatation von Nierenarterien. Verh Dtsch Röntgenkongress, Köln
9. Löhr E et al. (1983) Percutaneous transluminal angioplasty of renal arteries – therapeutic principle. Case report of 128 patients with renovascular hypertension. In: Dotter CT, Grüntzig AR, Schoop W, Zeitler E (eds) Percutaneous transluminal angioplasty. Springer, Berlin Heidelberg New York Tokyo, pp 281–285
10. Löhr E, Mellin P (1973) Zur Diagnose und Differentialdiagnose entzündlicher Nierenveränderungen im Röntgenbild. Internist Praxis 13–73
11. Löhr E, Mellin P (1968) Angiographische Diagnose von gefäßarmen Nierentumoren unter besonderer Berücksichtigung des elektronischen Subtraktions- und Harmonisierungsverfahrens. Electromedica 4:121–124
12. Mahler F et al. (1982) Percutaneous transluminal dilatation of renal artery stenoses: methods and results. Vasa 11(4):353–357
13. Schwarten DE (1980) Percutaneous transluminal angioplasty of renal artery. Cardiovasc Intervent Radiol 34:197–206
14. Sos TA, Pickering TG, Suiderman K et al. (1984) Percutaneous transluminal renal angioplasty in renovascular hypertension due to atheroma or fibromuscular dysplasia. Radiology 151:547
15. Tegtmeyer CJ et al. (1982) Percutaneous transluminal angioplasty: the treatment of choice for renovascular hypertension due to fibromuscular dysplasia. Radiology 143:631–637

Percutaneous Transluminal Angioplasty in Renal Arteries

F. Olbert, N. Muzika, and A. Schlegl

In hypertensives, transluminal dilatation of renal artery stenoses is performed both to reduce hypertension and to improve renal function.

This method of treating arterial hypertension was first rendered possible by the balloon catheter developed by A. Grüntzig [1]. The interventions reported in this paper were carried out with the catheter system developed by the author [2, 4].

The Olbert balloon catheter differs from other catheter systems in that only a minimal puncture of the vascular wall is required to permit insertion of the balloon into the vessel, since the balloon itself and the rest of the catheter are identical in diameter at the time of insertion and the balloon is inflated only at the actual site of the stenosis or occlusion. The balloon, at the distal end of the slender catheter, is designed in such a way as to ensure that its cylindrical shape is maintained even under maximum pressure and that its lumen is reduced to that of the catheter as soon as the pressure is released. This is ensured by a telescopic coaxial catheter system shortening the balloon under pressure and elongating it upon pressure release. Accordingly, the distal end of the catheter moves slightly forward when stenoses are dilated or occlusions recanalized. This phenomenon does not affect the vascular wall, however, since the diameter of the extended balloon is the same as that of the rest of the catheter, so that there is no contact with the wall. At the same time the balloon reaches its minimum length before being inflated to its maximum diameter, so that vascular wall damage by this process is also avoided. In addition, the catheter may be advanced or retracted in the vascular lumen only with the guide wire in place, so that even during the intervention the extended, uninflated catheter may be advanced without giving rise to plaque detachment.

The catheter may also be inserted via a system of commercially available guide tubes permitting the painless exchange of catheters when different balloon diameters or balloon or catheter lengths are required.

The balloon is designed to withstand pressures of up to 12 atm without losing its predetermined diameter. Thus, no annular impressions will occur at the site of the stenosis.

Patients eligible for dilatation of a renal artery are hypertensives with diastolic pressures in excess of 100 mm Hg (Table 1). Prior to the intervention the following examinations have to be performed (Table 1):

1. Determination of peripheral renin.
2. Determination of central renin from selective blood samples taken from the left and right renal veins after insertion of a catheter by the Seldinger technique. Blood samples for renin determination are taken before and after stimulation with Lasix.
3. Isotope examination with indication of the perfusion rate.
4. Renal clearance for the differential diagnosis of renovascular or renoparenchymatous hypertension.
5. Digital subtraction angiography (DSA) following selective central renin determination.

In the presence of significantly increased renin levels, and if the isotope examination of the kidneys yields results compatible with DSA findings,

Table 1. Indications and preliminary investigations

Clinical indications

1. Arterial hypertension (especially high diastolic pressure)
2. Reduced renal function

Investigations performed before dilation

1. Peripheral renin levels + furosemide stimulation
2. Isotopes: a) clearance
   b) nephrography
3. Venous blood sampling + furosemide stimulation
4. DSA
5. Aortography

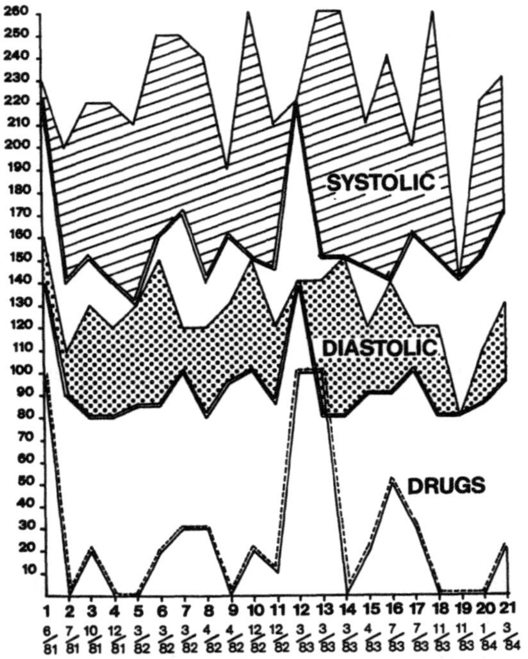

Fig. 1. Blood pressure in relation to antihypertensive medication needed after dilation. *Abscissa,* patients in chronological order

Table 2. Sex, age, and disease of patients

$n = 21$		
Male:	12	Average age: 48.5 years
Female:	9	Average age: 43.8 years
Fibromuscular stenoses	3	
Arteriosclerotic stenoses	18	

Table 3. Results

Improvement of	*n*
Renal parameters	15
Renin level	17
Angiographic results	
Ad integrum	10
⅓ remaining stenosis	7
⅔ remaining stenosis	3
No effect	1

PTA should be recommended after consultation with the surgeon.

Prior to PTA, survey aortography is performed by means of a pigtail catheter. A sidewinder or cobra catheter is used to probe the renal artery ostium. The stenosis is penetrated by a sidewinder catheter with or without guide wire (0.35) serving as a "splint" for the dilatation catheter.

During the intervention the guide wire remains in place or is advanced far beyond the stenosis. After dilatation, control angiography is performed by means of a pigtail catheter inserted via the contralateral route. In this way, successful dilatation can be immediately verified. If necessary, the dilatation catheter is reinserted along the guide wire, still in place in the renal artery, and the dilatation procedure is repeated.

Before angioplasty is performed the patient is given half a tablet of aspirin each day for 3 days. Immediately before insertion of the angiography catheter, i.e., immediately before survey aortography, 5000 units heparin are administered intra-arterially. Immediately before dilatation another 5000 units heparin are selectively administered intra-arterially. Four times 5000 units heparin per day are administered subcutaneously for 3 days following the intervention. Administration of half a tablet of aspirin per day is recommended for the next 3 months. Lidocaine has proved successful in the treatment of any spasms that may occur.

From June 1981 to March 1984, 21 patients with a stenosis of the renal artery were treated at our department by PTA. The distribution of age and sex can be seen in Table 2. In most cases blood pressure could be reduced significantly. Antihypertensive therapy was not necessary in some cases and could be reduced in many other cases of renal artery dilatation (Fig. 1). Figure 2 shows the trend with time and experience of percentage of total clearance before and after dilatation. Figure 3 illustrates one difficult case. The functional and angiographic results of renal artery angioplasty are summarized in Table 3. So far, no complications have been observed.

Summary

The literature available so far [3, 5, 6] suggests that transluminal dilatation of the renal artery is preferable to surgery, while purely conservative treatment of arterial hypertension due to renal artery stenosis has proved unsuccessful, since the underlying disease promotes progressive arteriosclerosis in the rest of the arterial system and thus accelerates coronary sclerosis and/or sclerosis of the carotid, the renal arteries, and the aorta. Dilatation resulted in an average increase in longitudinal and transverse kidney diameters by 1.5 ± 0.5 cm.

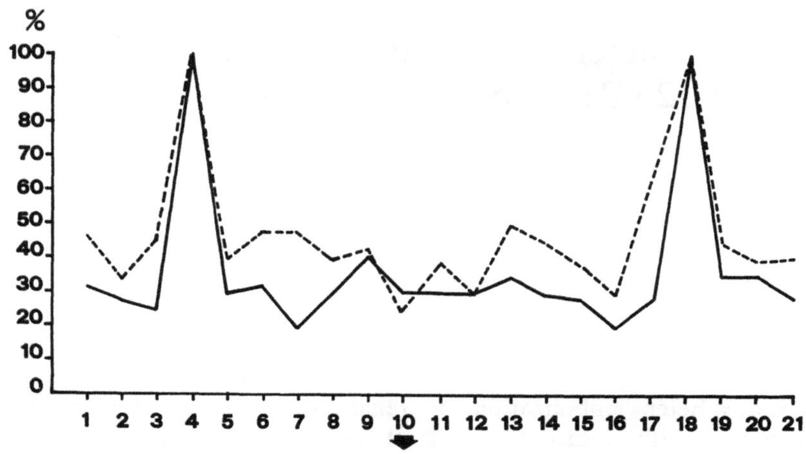

Fig. 2. Total clearance (%) before (*solid line*) and after (*broken line*) dilation. In patient 10 there was a decrease

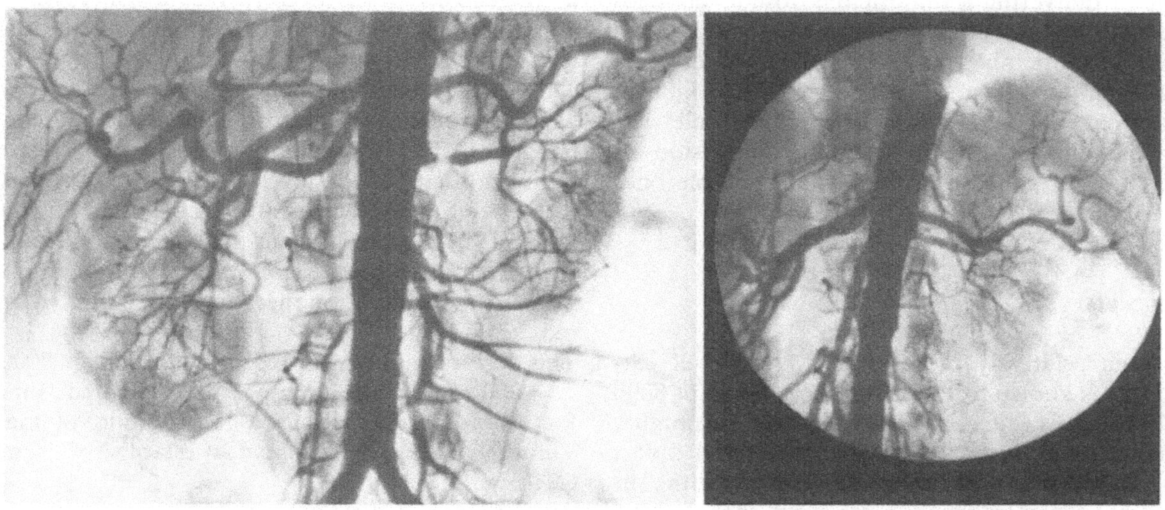

Fig. 3. Case 17, July 1983. The severe stenosis of the left renal artery could be removed by dilation. The blood pressure improved from RR 230/120 to RR 140/90

References

1. Grüntzig A, Hopff H (1974) Perkutane Rekanalisation chronischer arterieller Verschlüsse mit einem neuen Dilatationskatheter. Modifikation der Dotter-Technik. Dtsch Med Wochenschr 99:2502
2. Hanecka L, Olbert F (1977) Ballonkatheter. OE Patentschrift, 17. 2. 1977. Patent number 348.094
3. Mahler F, Probst P, Haertel M, Weidmann P (1982) Lasting improvement of renovascular hypertension by transluminal dilatation of atherosclerotic and nonatherosclerotic renal artery stenoses: a follow-up study. Circulation 65:611–617
4. Olbert F, Kasprzak P, Muzika N, Schlegl A (1984) Percutaneous transluminal dilatation and recanalization: long-term results and report on experience with a new catheter system. Ann Radiol 27, 4:349–356
5. Puijaert CBAJ, Boomsma JHB, Ruijs JHJ et al. (1981) Transluminal renal artery dilatation in hypertension: technique, results and complications in 60 cases. Urol Radiol 2:201–210
6. Sos TA, Pickering TG, Sniderman K et al. (1983) Percutaneous transluminal renal angioplasty in renovascular hypertension due to atheroma or fibromuscular dysplasia. N Engl J Med 309:274–279

Transcatheter Embolization of Renal Cell Carcinoma with I-125 Particles

E. K. Lang

Transcatheter embolization of renal cell carcinomas with radioactive infarct particles is undertaken to create an interstitial implant capable of delivering a tumoricidal dose to the neoplasm. This modality is advocated for the treatment of inoperable renal cell carcinoma or renal cell carcinoma in a solitary or remaining kidney, management of metastases of renal cell carcinoma, and downstaging of inoperable lesions in the hope of converting them into operable ones [1–4].

Concepts

Though relatively radioresistant, renal cell carcinoma is known to respond to dose levels of 8000 – 16 000 rads (80 – 160 Gy). Moreover, this highly immunogenic tumor is known to respond favorably to an improved host immune status if the tumor burden is reduced. Care must therefore be exercised as not to adversely influence host immune response (such as with suppression attendant on radiation) while attempting to ablate the primary neoplasm [5].

Interstitial radiation therapy is ideally suited to reduce the tumor burden while keeping the integral dose to the host to a minimum. Appropriate choice of the radionuclide can limit effective radiation for practical purposes to the tumor.

I-125 is a radiopharmaceutical ideally suited to this purpose. The low energy levels (27 and 35 KEV) and long half-life (59.6 days) ensure that the radiant energy, for practical purposes, is totally absorbed in the tumor [1, 2]. A rapid fall-off of dose in adjacent tissues can be documented, and the integral dose to the host is kept to a minimum.

The long half-life of the radionuclide exposes the tumor to prolonged irradiation, hopefully during phases of mitotic activity, at which time the cells tend to be most sensitive to radiation damage.

Transcatheter embolization is used to seat the I-125 particles and to create an interstitial implant capable of delivering 8000 – 16 000 rads to the tumor-bearing area. In order to achieve more or less homogeneous irradiation of the tumor volume, particles must be distributed throughout the tumor at even intervals [1, 2, 3].

This can be accomplished by superselective engagement of many tumor branch vessels and embolization of the muscular branches (Fig. 1). Seating of particles at the level of muscular branches insures retrograde perfusion of the affected tissue volume via collaterals. Thus there is no significant reduction in oxygen tension in the tumor, and effectiveness of radiation therapy is not curtailed or reduced.

The dose in millicuries necessary to deliver 8000 – 16 000 rads to the tumor is precalculated from Patterson-Parker tables for a given tumor volume. Tumor volume itself is readily established from CT (Fig. 2).

An acceptable distribution of infarct particles throughout the tumor can be accomplished not only by using a relatively large number of infarct particles and distributing them by superselective catheterization of many tumor branch vessels, but also by seeding infarct particles according to prevailing flow characteristics within the tumor [1–3]. Release of approximately one-third of the infarct particles into the main tumor vessel at the first session will distribute particles throughout those areas of the tumor manifesting the most prominent flow characteristics.

The effect of radiation therapy on the exposed tumor components is a sharp reduction in flow attendant on the resulting fibrosis [1–3]. Therefore, release of a second generation of infarct particles into the main tumor arteries some 6 weeks later will result in an entirely different distribution, usually to areas hitherto spared radiation therapy. An identical procedure followed for a third transcatheter embolization series will finally distribute infarct particles into those areas of the tumor spared until this point in time (Fig. 3).

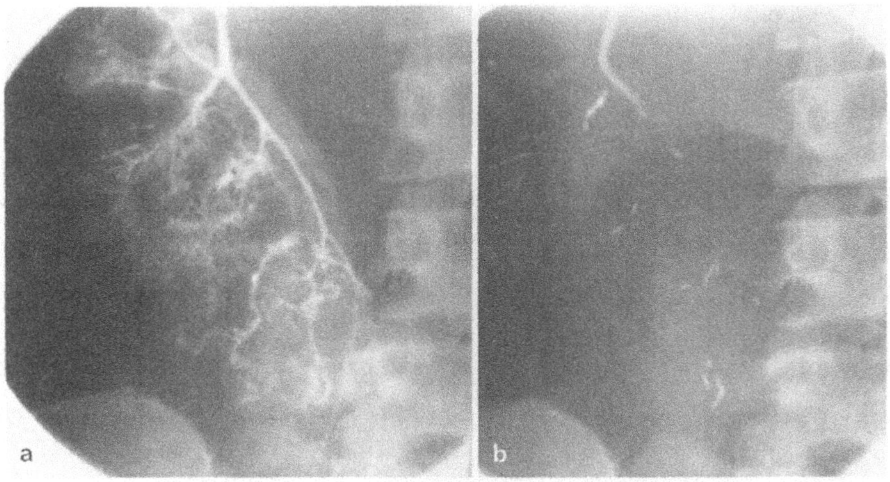

Fig. 1. **a** A branch supplying the anterior component of a large tumor involving the lower pole of the right kidney has been engaged and is injected superselectively. **b** Following release of I-125 particles midstream in this tumor branch vessel, the particles are seated in muscular branches and distributed according to flow characteristics existing in the tumor at the time of release

An infarct implant with acceptable distribution, can thus be seated with minimum effort relying solely on the flow characteristics existing in the tumor at a given point in time to determine the distribution of the released infarct particles.

I-125 particles manufactured for needle implantation into the prostate fortuitously fit through a 6.3 and 7.2 angiographic catheter, and are thus readily available for creating such infarct implants. The particles are loaded into the end of the catheter with a straight guide wire and ejaculated into the tumor vessel. From there transport into the peripheral muscular branch arteries is determined by the flow characteristics existing within the tumor.

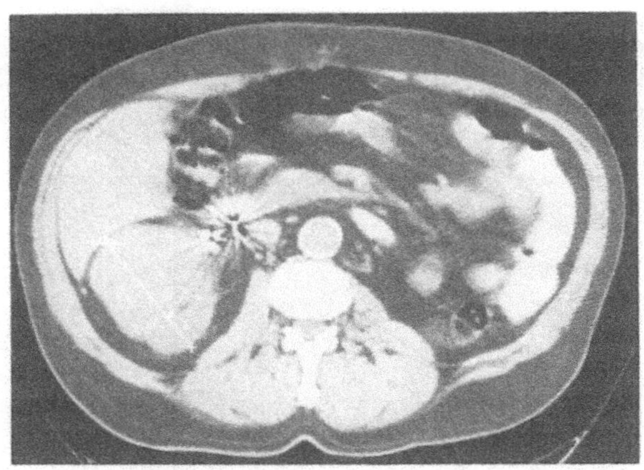

Fig. 2. The volume of the tumor is easily computed by CT. Moreover, the location of the radioactive seeds can be identified on the various slices obtained through the tumor

Dose Calculation

The location of each radioactive infarct particle is determined by CT (Fig. 4). Computers can then calculate the dose delivered to the tumor or any of its segments and to adjacent tissues [6]. Progressive shrinkage of the tumor in response to interstitial radiation therapy causes a change in the geometric relationship of the implanted radioactive sources. This necessitates reassessment of tumor volume and location of radioactive sources at fixed intervals and renewed computation of dose rate. The final tumor dose is established from the mean of fractional dose rates [3].

The deep location of a renal cell carcinoma results in an almost complete absorption of radiant energy and such implants therefore do not constitute a radiation hazard to nursing personnel and attendants. Even the integral dose to the patient is extremely low since almost complete absorption of the low gamma energy radiation (27.3 and 35.4 KEV) occurs within the tumor [1, 2].

Efficacy of I-125 Infarct Implants

Eradication of the neoplasm is the ultimate aim, but available therapeutic modalities often permit only palliation. Radical surgery, feasible in pa-

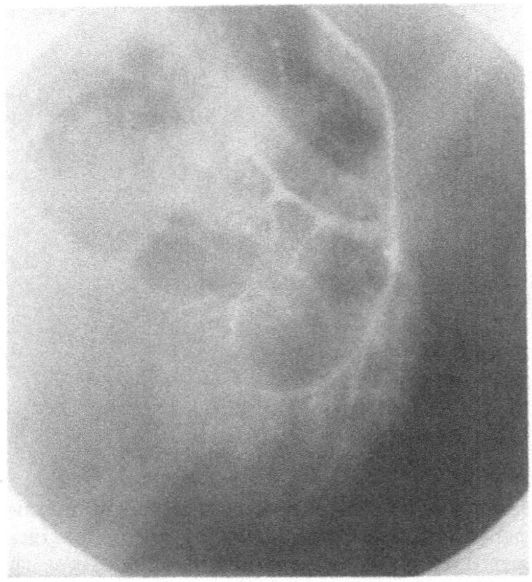

Fig. 3. An arteriogram performed after two prior transcatheter embolizations with I-125 particles shows predominant flow to segments of the tumor hitherto spared interstitial radiation therapy. Release of infarct particles midstream at this point in time will therefore tend to seat them in segments of the tumor not yet adequately seeded

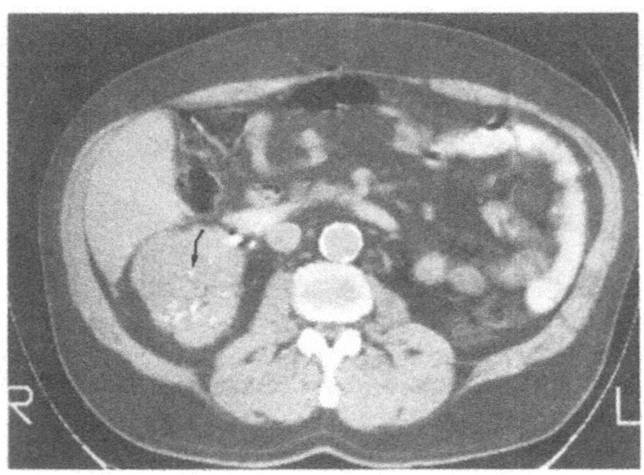

Fig. 4. The location of each radioactive seed is readily determinable by CT (*arrow*)

Table 1. Survival of patients treated for renal cell carcinoma with known metastases by interstitial radioactive infarct implant (at risk/surviving)

Stage	2 Years	5 Years	10 Years
$T_4(N_{4-3})M_1$	4/2	4/2.	3/0
$T_4N_xM_1$	9/3	4/1	1/0
$T_3(N_{3-0})M_1$	3/3	3/2	1/0
$T_3N_xM_1$	16/7	6/2	2/0
$T_2N_2M_1$	1/1	1/0	–

tients with localized renal cell carcinoma, has been credited with a 5-year survival rate of 57% and a 10-year survival rate of 44%. Conversely, survival of patients presenting with metastases has been dismal, regardless of therapy [7, 8].

However, there appears to be a relationship between tumor volume and potential for survival in patients with metastatic disease [5]. Spontaneous regression of metastases has been reported in occasional cases after removal of the primary lesion [9, 10]. It has been suggested that debulking of the tumor may make the host immune defense mechanisms more effective and perhaps initiate remissions and regression of known metastases.

The series of patients treated by interstitial radiation therapy by an infarct implant demonstrates remarkably improved survival (Table 1). A 2-year survival rate of 48% and a 5-year rate of 38% represent an four-fold improvement over the rates achieved by surgical management of similarly advanced lesions. Admittedly, there is a significant difference in the survival potential depending on whether there is known lymph node involvement at the time of discovery and also depending on the site of metastatic disease. Patients presenting with bone metastases fared better than those presenting with other soft tissue metastases, particularly to the spleen, brain, or skin [1–3]. The latter group seemed to follow an inexorable course and most patients were dead within 6 months, irrespective of any interstitial radiation or other adjuvant therapy (Table 2). The grade of the tumor also greatly influences survival. However, the more undifferentiated tumors also tend to present at a more advanced stage and with metastatic disease to nodes [7].

The gratifying response of our patients with known skeletal metastases to interstitial radiation therapy by radioactive infarct implant supports our concept that we may have induced and altered immune response (Fig. 5). The proven ability of such patients to survive despite extensive primary and metastatic tumors implies the presence and action of a host immune mechanism. Thus, if the tumor burden is substantially reduced (by interstitial radiation therapy), the host immune mechanism may retard or even control tumor growth for a period of time and thus initiate a remission [1 – 3, 5].

Such remissions were heralded in our patients by improved well-being, weight gain, and cessation of any pain and hematuria present. Normalization of abnormal erythrocyte sedimentation rates was observed almost uniformly in patients in clinical remission [1–3]. If tumor markers, such as

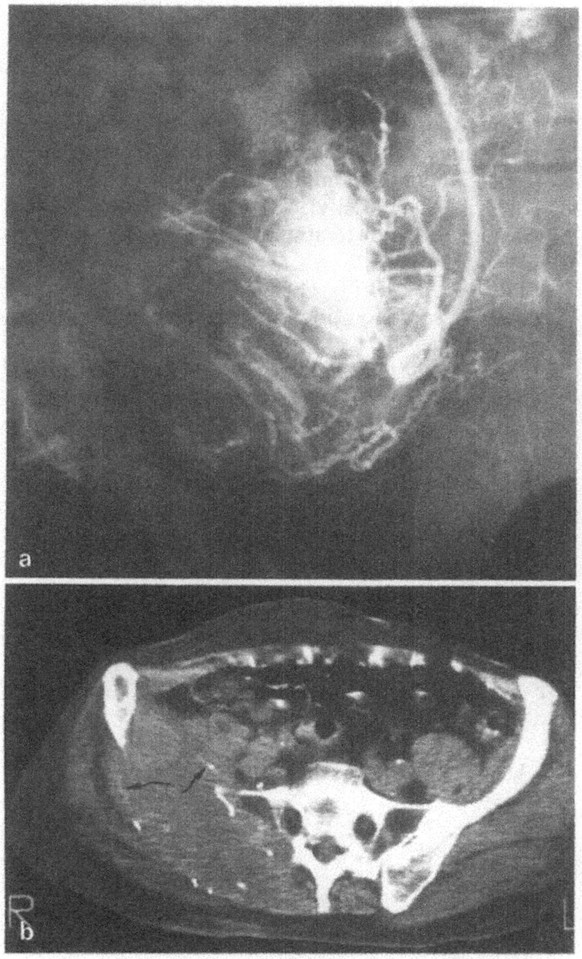

Fig. 5. **a** A selective arteriogram of the right superior gluteal artery demonstrates abundant tumor neovascularity and destruction of the sacroiliac joint area. **b** A CT scan obtained some 3 months after radioactive infarct implant was seeded demonstrates incipient redeposition of calcium in the remaining osseous matrix (*arrows*)

Table 2. Survival of patients treated for advanced renal cell carcinoma by interstitial radioactive infarct implant, arterial chemotherapy, surgery, and sometimes adjuvant external therapy (at risk/surviving)

Stage	2 Years	5 Years	10 Years
$T_{3-2}N_{2-x}M_{1-0}$	9/5	9/3	9/1

elevated erythropoetin, renin, or serum chorionic gonadotropin, were present prior to therapy, they disappeared or occurred at a much reduced level. It was of interest to note that even in several patients who died of unrelated causes during a period of apparent remission, viable tumor was found at autopsy. Often, however, such tumor appeared incarcerated within fibrotic pseudocapsules.

Eventually the tumor resumed an active growth pattern in most of our patients, and repeat interstitial radiation therapy proved unable to induce another remission.

Bony metastases of renal cell carcinoma treated by interstitial radiation therapy (by radioactive infarct implant) not only demonstrated a spectacular regression of neovascularity, but also eventually showed redeposition of calcium in the remaining bone matrix (Fig. 5). Thus, osseous structures seemingly destroyed by renal cell carcinoma metastases sometimes demonstrated repair to such a degree that they could assume weight bearing function again (Fig. 5) [1, 2].

In an earlier series, radioactive infarct implants were seated with the intent of converting inoperable lesions into operable ones [4]. The results in this group exceeded expectations, since the survival rate was clearly better than one would expect in virgin, locally advanced renal cell carcinoma handled by radical surgery. Host immune response is once again suspected of creating this favorable milieu [2, 3].

The survival statistics of patients with renal cell carcinoma presenting with metastatic disease and treated by interstitial radiation therapy (by transcatheter radioactive infarct implant) only almost match those of radical nephrectomy in early renal cell carcinoma [7]. Since there is abundant evidence that the neoplasm is not totally eradicated, it must be assumed that the reduction of the tumor burden creates a favorable setting in patients with existing host immune response to their tumors [10, 11].

In our experience, interstitial radioactive infarct implants are useful for

(1) treatment of advanced primary renal cell carcinomas and their metastases nonamenable to surgical intervention, and (2) reducing the size of advanced primary neoplasms and thus rendering them amenable to surgical resection.

References

1. Lang EK, Sullivan J, DeKernion JB (1983) Work in progress: transcatheter embolization of renal cell carcinoma with radioactive infarct particles. Radiology 147:413–418
2. Lang EK, DeKernion JB (1981) Transcatheter embolization of advanced renal cell carcinoma with radioactive seeds. J U 126:581–586
3. Lang EK (1984) Transcatheter embolization of renal cell carcinoma with radioactive infarct particles. In: Libertino JA (ed) Current concepts of uro- radiology. Williams and Wilkins, Baltimore, pp 226–236
4. Lang EK (1971) Superselective arterial catheterization as vehicle for delivering radioactive infarct particles to tumors. Radiology 98:391–399
5. Droller MJ, Levy HJ (1984) Immuno therapy of metastatic renal cell carcinoma with poly IC LC. 79th annual meeting of the American urologic association, paper # 301, may 6–10
6. Ling CC, Yorke ED, Spiro IG et al. (1978) Physical dosimetry of I-125 seeds of a new design for interstitial implant. NCRP publication CA 30378
7. Skinner DJ, DeKernion JB (1978) Clinical manifestations and treatment of renal parenchymal tumors. In: Skinner DJ, DeKernion JB (eds) Genitourinary Cancer. Saunders, Philadelphia, pp 107–133
8. Katz SA, Davis JE (1977) Renal adenocarcinoma: prognostics and treatment reflected by survival. Urology 10:10–19
9. Bloom HJG (1973) Hormone induced and spontaneous regression of metastatic renal cancer. Cancer 32:1066–1071
10. Bloom HJG (1973) Adjuvant therapy for adenocarcinoma of the kidney, present position and prospects. Br J Urol 45:237–245
11. DeKernion JB, Katsuoka Y, Ramming KP (1980) Immunology of human renal adenocarcinoma. In: Sufrin G, Beckley SA (eds) Renal adenocarcinoma: a series of workshops on the biology of human cancer. International Union Against Cancer, Geneva, pp 96–113 (report 10)

Noninvasive Renal Stone Therapy with Extracorporal Shock-Wave Lithotripsy

F. Eisenberger, G. Fuchs, K. Miller, and J. Rassweiler

Removal of calculi from the upper urinary tract is, by and large, mandatory when they cause symptoms and when their size prevents spontaneous passage.

Chemically dissolution has been effective only in uric acid calculi, by means of alkalinization. Similar attempts at dissolution with other types of stones have not yet yielded any promising results within a reasonable period of treatment.

Stone removal via the exposed renal pelvis constitutes the surgical ideal, obviating direct parenchymal damage. However, in a quarter of such operations, the need arises for additional parenchymal incisions. In these cases, either single or multiple radial nephrotomies are indicated.

The operative techniques have become widely standardized. They encompass (a) operations on the ischemic kidney, with either surface cooling, or in situ hypothermic perfusion as developed by us, and (b) ex situ renal surgery with autotransplantation and the development of microscurgical techniques. Intraoperative stone localization by ultrasonography and mapping of intrarenal vessels by a Doppler probe has enabled the surgeon to cut down onto these stones without resorting to renal ischemia and still preserve the vascular integrity of the parenchyma. Stone recurrence – ranging in the literature between 20% and 70% – requires repeated operations, in many cases leading to progressive loss of renal function. Finally, about 8% of dialysis cases are linked with urinary stone disease. Furthermore, it has to be noted that although morbidity from conventional renal surgery has decreased considerably, a number of patients still suffer harmful consequences from such an open operation.

In recent years, percutaneous nephrolithotomy (PCN) has been shown to be a safe procedure for removal of stones from the renal pelvis, calices, and upper ureter. As more information is gained and with increasing experience, even partial staghorn calculi can be successfully treated. Compared to standard operative procedures, the main advantages of PCN are the feasibility of access to the renal pelvis with minimal trauma and the fact that it can be performed under regional or local anesthesia.

A new and revolutionary method for the treatment of urinary stones became available once it was clinically proved that high-energy, focused shock waves, applied externally, could lead to contact-free disintegration of kidney stones without the need to resort to any kind of operation [14].

A nonphysicist confronted with the term "shock wave" might think of devastating pressure waves such as those resulting from explosions. Any attempt to convince him that such waves could be applied to the body in order to destroy calculi without causing serious injuries would probably be met with skepticism or amazement. Our experiments using shock waves aiming at contact-free destruction of urinary stones began in 1972. These studies on the effect of high-energy shock waves on biological systems have been carried out at the Urological Clinic and the Institute for Surgical Research in Munich and have led to the development of a noninvasive, contact-free method for disintegrating renal calculi in laboratory animals [1–3, 7–10, 16, 17].

Experimental Phase and Method

Extracorporally generated shock waves are focused at the renal stone, or target (Fig. 1) [16, 17]. The shock waves are generated by an underwater, high-voltage condensor spark discharge lasting 1 ms. The spark electrodes are placed in the geometric focus of an ellipsoidal reflector (Fig. 1). The high-voltage discharge of the condenser causes explosive evaporation of the water between the tips of the electrode, which in turn generates a shock wave because of the sudden expansion.

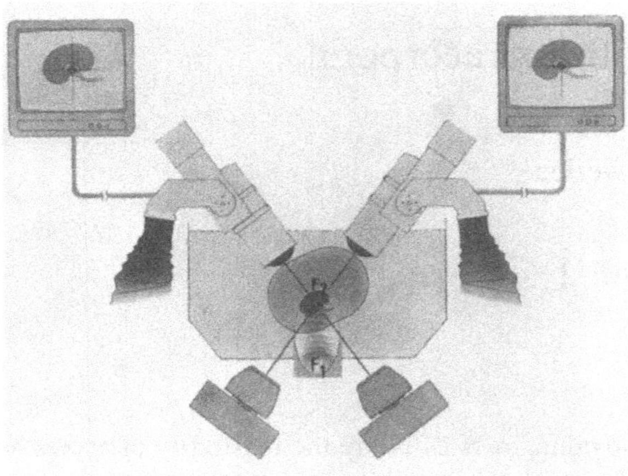

Fig. 1. The layout of the lithotripter, with the ellipsoid, the focal points F1 and F2 and the X-ray systems

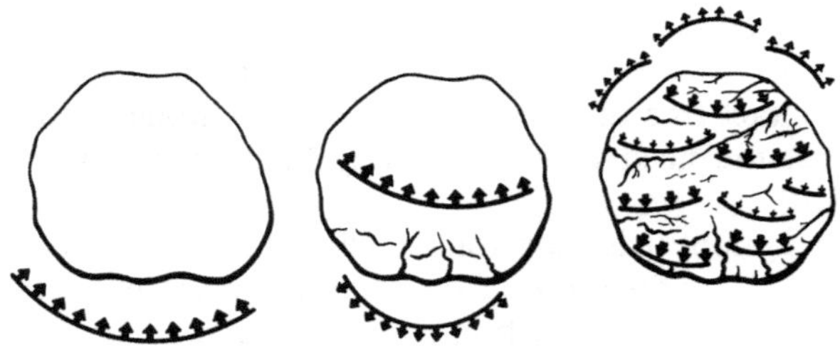

Fig. 2. Stone disintegration by shockwaves

As the shock waves' source is at one focal point of a half-ellipsoid, all the energy produced is reflected from the surrounding wall and collected again at the second focal point (Fig. 1) [16, 17]. The target must be situated at this point of highest energy density (Fig. 1) [16].

Shock waves spread through the body evenly, since the acoustic impedance of most body tissues is close to that of water. The shock wave is partially reflected when it reaches the stone, but the remainder enters the stone, being absorbed because of the abrupt change in acoustic impedance (Fig. 2). This leads to the build-up of a high pressure gradient and the formation of tear and shear forces, which eventually disintegrate the brittle material when the limit of the stone's comprehensive strength is exceeded. The portion of the penetrating shock wave reflected at the opposite, i.e., inner surface of the stone has the same effect, and finally the stone is reduced into smaller and smaller particles (Fig. 2).

After technical prerequisites had been met by the development of adequate equipment, the next step, before moving on to more complex experiments with animals, was to clarify two fundamental questions using simple parameter-free tests in vitro:

1. Is the amplitude of energy sufficient to disintegrate kidney stones?
2. To what degree could traction waves of this kind produce undesirable effects on other organs?

By 1976 we could answer these questions, and the results of our fundamental work were awarded with the C. E. Alken prize [7]. After stones, irrespective of their chemical composition, had been destroyed by means of shock waves we concentrated on the effect of shock waves on cell cultures, tissues, and organs of live animals [1, 7]. In our first trials, we demonstrated that the stimulation ability and proliferative potential of human lymphocytes showed no alteration after repeated exposure to shock waves. Secondly, we found that serum concentration of hemoglobin increased slightly with the number of treatments when directly exposed to the shock waves. When live bone or bone marrow was subjected to shock waves no damage besides small petechial bleedings occurred, whereas bone of dead animals was broken by the impact of the shock wave energy.

Exposure of eventrated intestine and parenchymal organs of rats also caused no damage besides small petechial bleedings. Shock wave exposure of the lungs, however, resulted in alveolar rupture and hemorrhage because of the abrupt change of the acoustic impedance between the parenchyma and the air filled alveoli.

As the results of in vitro and in vivo investigations were promising, an experimental series in animals was started [1, 7, 8].

For this purpose a prototype apparatus has been constructed for the experiments on animals, consisting of a control and an energy unit, as well as the half-ellipsoid attached to the floor of the exerimental tub [7, 8]. With the aid of an adjusting device, samples, and later larger animals, such as dogs with implanted human kidney stones, were placed at the second focal point. This experimental apparatus made it possible to concentrate high-energy shock waves at an area of approximately 1.5 cm^2 [1, 7, 8]. With this apparatus 64 mongrel dogs were successfully treated; in all cases the stone fragments passed spontaneously. Thereafter the animals were killed and checked for morphologic and histologic alterations. In no case we have found any alterations other than the above-mentioned petechial bleedings, which have no overall significance [8].

After our series had ruled out any possible damage to biological systems and the experiments with animals had demonstrated the feasibility of contact-free destruction of kidney stones, the method was ready for clinical application in humans. A prototype for the treatment of humans was therefore constructed and technically improved for clinical use [4, 5].

Indications

In February 1980, this method was applied on the first patient at the University of Munich by our former co-worker Christian Chaussy [4, 5], and since then more than 2800 patients have been successfully treated at 11 centers in the Federal Republic of Germany and the United States. The center in Stuttgart was inaugurated in October 1983, and so far more than 500 patients have been treated [22]. At the onset, indications were limited, and only patients with pelvic stones smaller than 1 cm and single caliceal stones were eligible [4, 5]. Since then the range of indications has been cautiously extended and encompassed about 70% – 80% of all stone-bearers by the end of 1983, including stones larger than 1 cm up to incomplete staghorn calculi, ureteral stones above the iliac crest, multiple stones, high-risk patients, and infective stones [5, 6, 12].

Patients with complete staghorn stones and patients with obstruction distal to the stones are still excluded from treatment by extracorporal shock-wave lithotripsy (ESWL). As stone treatment by PCN was already a well-established method in our department when our ESWL unit was opened, the question was how the range of indications could be extended with the combination of PCN and ESWL [18].

Especially in large stones, the rationale for this treatment concept is based on the observation that the period of stone passage after ESWL mainly depends on the size of the intact stone or the number and size of stone fragments [6, 11, 18–21, 25, 26]. With larger stones, usually more than one sitting is required to reduce the stone to a size where the particles can pass spontaneously. As the fragments have to pass spontaneously, no ureteric obstruction should be present when the next session is performed. This leads to a prolonged treatment time, and during this period obstruction due to the large number and volume of fragments may occur at any time, leading to hydronephrosis with the possible hazards of superinfection and urosepsis [15, 20, 25, 27].

Being aware of the pitfalls of each of the methods applied alone, we developed the combination of both techniques and now use it routinely for the treatment of large incomplete or complete staghorn stones [20, 25].

This procedure has major advantages when compared to each of the methods alone. The number of sittings, and accordingly the duration of hospital stay, can be considerably reduced.

Only one percutaneous track is necessary, and no urinary obstruction can occur, as the stone fragments can easily pass through the nephrostomy tube [20, 25].

We have now successfully treated 45 patients, including 17 with complete staghorns and three with bilateral staghorns. Due to the good results we could forgo open surgery for all of these patients.

Results

The ages of the 540 patients treated from October 1983 to May 1984 ranged from 6 to 79 years, with a mean of 49.1 years. Sixty percent of the stones were located in the renal pelvis, 30% in the calix (nine upper, six middle, 15 lower), and in the ureter above the iliac crest 10%. Multiple stones were treated in 16%, incomplete and complete staghorns in 14%, and 35% of the patients had had to undergo one or more operations for renal stones.

All stones in our series could be treated with our device regardless of their composition. A typical case is illustrated in Fig. 3. Epidural catheter anesthesia is the method of choice for eliminating pain; general anesthesia is performed only in patients where epidural anesthesia is not possible or if requested by the patient. In no case have we encountered any problems from the anesthesia or thereafter from the epidural catheter, which has usually been left in place until treatment is definitely finished.

The duration of treatment is between 10 and 60 min, with an average of 40 min. The number of shock-wave applications ranges from 300 to 1800, with an average of 1100. X-ray exposure for stone localization and for the monitoring of disintegration during the treatment is between 2 and 80 s, with an average of 35 s.

In 28% of patients pain or colic occurred during the period of stone passage. In about 50% of these cases this could be managed with antispasmodics by mouth or as suppositories; in the rest it was necessary to resort to infusions and antispasmodics or narcotics given intravenously. Fever was

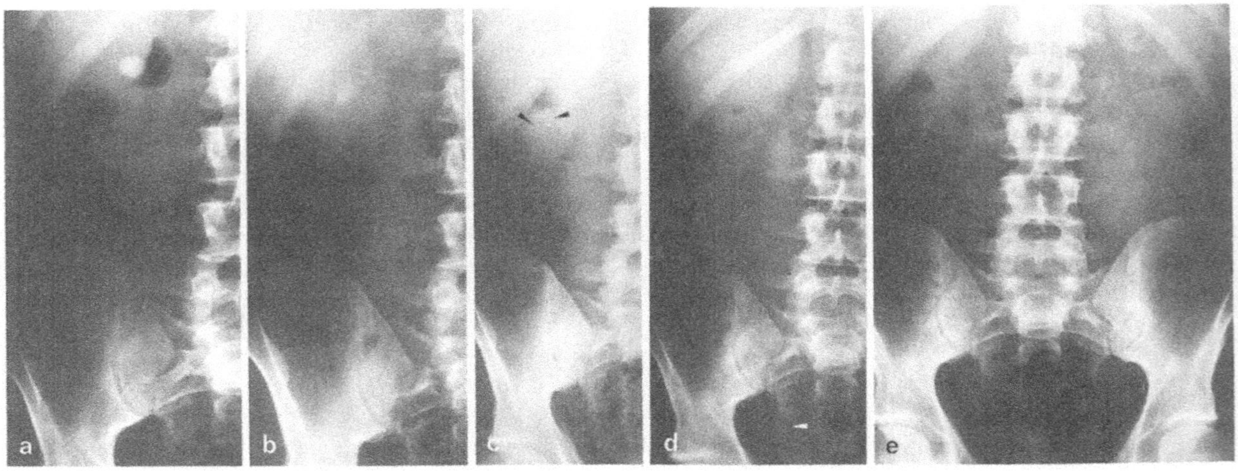

Fig. 3 a – e. Typical course after ESWL: 30-year-old patient with a pelvic stone on the right side. **a** Plain X-ray before treatment. **b** Control X-ray after treatment: disintegrated stone fragments in the renal pelvis and lower calix. **c** Control X-ray 3 days after treatment: fewer fragments in the collecting system (*arrowheads*), incipient prevesical *Steinstraße*. **d** Control X-ray 5 days after treatment: stone-free kidney, more pronounced prevesical *Steinstraße* (day of discharge). **e** Control X-ray 14 days after treatment: stone-free

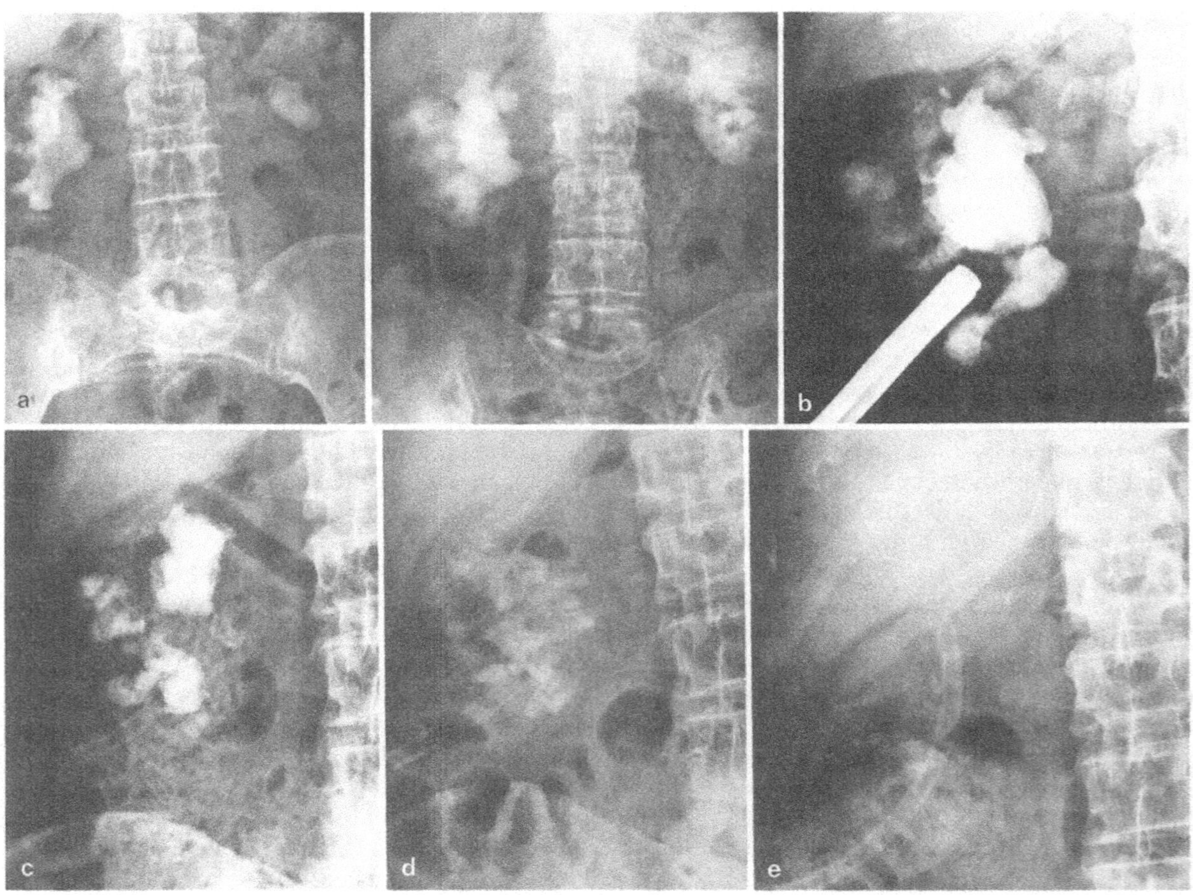

Fig. 4 a – e. Combination of PCN and ESWL in a 60-year-old female patient with a large pelvic stone in the left renal pelvis and a complete staghorn stone in the right kidney. **a** Plain abdominal Y-ray and IVP. **b** In a first sitting a percutaneous track to a lower posterio calix and onto the stone is established and most of the stone mass in the lower calix and the renal pelvis is removed with an ultrasound probe. **c** Result after percutaneous treatment. **d** In a second session – usually after 2 days – the remaining saliceal parts of the stone are treated with ESWL. **e** Stonefree kidney 1 week after ESWL seen in 2% of patients, but never led to urosepsis when ureteral obstruction was immediately relieved.

Though in 60% of cases various degrees of distension of the collecting system have been noticed in routine ultrasound examinations, the overall necessity for auxiliary measures was not higher than 20% [20, 23]. Auxiliary measures are necessary if complete reduction of the stone cannot be achieved in the first sitting and for relief from colicky pain or from a longer persisting obstruction [20, 23]. In our series, they were required in 8.6% of cases because of insufficient reduction of the stone. In 7% of cases a second session was necessary, and was mainly performed as a planned procedure in larger stones [20].

Open surgery for this reason has been performed on five patients – three with ureteral stones and two with pelvic stones – all of whom were amongst our first 100 patients. Since then we have not had to operate on any patient because of incomplete stone disintegration.

PCN secondary to ESWL has been performed on 0.8% of patients, mainly in cystine stones (Fig. 4). PCN was indicated because these stones had broken into fragments too large to be passed spontaneously. During stone passage auxiliary measures to relieve from ureteral obstruction have been necessary in 60% of cases. Insertion of a percutaneous nephrostomy because of obstructing stone fragments has been required in 1% of cases, loosening of a so-called ureteral *Steinstraße* with a ureteral catheter or stone extracting using a Zeiss sling has been performed on 2% of patients, and in 3% of the cases this could only be accomplished under direct view using a ureteroscope [20].

Overall, 98.4% of urinary stones subjected to our ESWL treatment could be efficiently reduced into spontaneously passable fragments. Ultrasonic follow-up studies have given no evidence of damage to the kidney, and in no case has any damage to adjacent organs been noticed. On reevaluation after 3 months, split renal function has been found unchanged or improved after successful treatment of obstructive stone disease [20, 23].

On reevaluation after 3 months we found 85% of patients to be stone-free. Residual stones which were considered spontaneously passable remained in 11%, and in 3% fragments larger than 4 mm remained [20]. It has to be noted that all these patients with residual fragments are symptom-free and that no infection persisted after successful treatment. During the period of stone passage, extraction of prevesical stone particles using a Zeiss sling or a ureteroscope was undertaken in 1% of patients whom we had to readmit to hospital because of longer persisting obstruction [23]. In no case has an open operation been necessary for longer persisting obstruction or for any other complication.

Change of Indications in Urinary Stone Management

Due to the introduction and development of PCN, ureterorenoscopy, and particularly ESWL, the treatment of urinary stone disease has undergone a fundamental change in the past 2 years [13, 15].

Until July 1983 we had no problems in deciding how to treat stone patients: open surgery was mandatory for all but spontaneously passable stones, except prevesical ureteral stones which could be initially treated with the Zeiss sling. In that month, PCN and ureterorenoscopy were introduced in our department. We began to remove kidney stones – at the beginning lower caliceal and pelvic concrements – via a percutaneous track, and ureteral stones via the transurethral route. When the second kidney lithotriptor was installed in October 1983, indications for stone treatment had to be changed again. Meanwhile, increasing experience with the different techniques has led to clearly defined indications and finally to a new concept of stone treatment. Before July 1983, for example, all ureteral calculi had to be operated on, but from that time on the number of open operations decreased steadily as PCN, ureterorenoscopy, and ESWL were more frequently used. In the last 2 months before writing, open surgery for removal of ureteral stone was only necessary in 24% of all cases [20, 28].

This trend gives an idea of our present policy concerning stone treatment: whenever possible, stones are initially treated with the least invasive technique. In cases of failure, progressively more invasive methods are used until success is achieved. Usually, high ureteral stones with a history not longer than 6–8 weeks are primarily treated with the noninvasive ESWL, with success in about 70% of the cases [26, 28]. If this treatment is not successful and the calculus shows no sign of disintegration 2 days after ESWL, then the stone can be mobilized and pushed up into the renal pelvis using an ureteral catheter. In the renal pelvis, the stone can more easily be treated with ESWL. Whenever mobilization with an ureteral catheter is not possible, we use the ureterorenoscope, either to remove the stone directly or to push it up into the renal pelvis for consecutive ESWL treatment. Open operation, the most invasive technique, is required if all other methods have failed. The same policy is applied to kidney stones: pelvic and caliceal calculi up to incomplete staghorns are primarily treated using ESWL.

Slightly opaque or nonopaque concrements can be disintegrated by shock waves using a contrast medium for stone localization. However, as it is difficult to assess size and localization of the stone fragments during and after treatment, we prefer PCN in these cases.

In our experience, relative obstruction distal to the stone does not handicap the passage of fragments after ESWL, assuming the fragments are sufficiently reduced in size. When spontaneous passage does not occur after 2–3 days, the fragments are removed by PCN. In cases of kidney stones and hydronephrosis caused by stenosis of the ureteropelvic junction (UPJ), an open operation is indicated and we usually perform a dismembered pyeloplasty.

The distribution of kidney stone treatment in our hospital from October 1983 to June 1984 confirms the new indications: 98% of all patients could be treated using ESWL, PCN or the combination of these two methods, and only 2% of the patients had to undergo open surgery [20, 26].

So what place is left for open surgery in the treatment of urinary stone disease? We have already mentioned that when obstruction at the UPJ causes severe hydronephrosis and resultant kidney stone disease, the obstruction has to be relieved [13, 15, 26].

Children smaller then 120 cm are still excluded from ESWL treatment for two reasons: first, they will not fit on to the patient support, and second, due to the close anatomic relationship between kidney and lung in smaller children, the shock waves may damage alveolar tissue [19].

Finally, about 25% of ureteral stones cannot be managed with one of the new techniques and still need open surgery [13, 26, 27].

Summary

ESWL has been proved to be a safe and easily reproducible method to reduce kidney stones to a size where they can pass spontaneously with the urine. As our experience has shown, approximately 80% of nonselected stone patients can be treated with ESWL alone, and by combining ESWL with endourological methods, open operation can be avoided in more than 90% of stone patients [13, 15, 20, 25, 26]. We anticipate that in the not too distant future many stone patients will be able to benefit from urological centers where all facilities – ureterorenoscopy, PCN, ESWL, and open operation – are available. Problems still may occur during the period of stone passage, requiring auxiliary measures in about 16% of patients [20, 23]. For this reasons the patients need to be closely followed by their urologist to prevent the possible hazards of longer persisting hydronephrosis and ensuing infection with the threatening hazard of urosepsis [23].

References

1. Chaussy C, Eisenberger F, Wanner K, Forssmann B, Hepp W (1976) In vitro-Untersuchungen und erste in vivo-Untersuchungen mit fokussierten Stoßwellen. Wissenschaftliche Berichte, Meersburg, Juni
2. Chaussy C, Schmiedt E, Forssmann B, Brendel W (1979) Contact free renal stone destruction by means of shock waves. Eur Surg Res 11:36
3. Chaussy C, Brendel W, Schmiedt E (1980) Extracorporeally induced destruction of kidney stones by shock waves. Lancet 13:1265–1268
4. Chaussy C, Schmiedt E, Jocham D, Brendel W, Forssmann B, Moser E (1981) Berührungsfreie Nierensteinzertrümmerung durch Stoßwellen. Deutsches Ärzteblatt 18:881–886
5. Chaussy C, Schmiedt E, Jocham D, Brendel W, Forssmann B, Walther W (1982) First clinical experience with extracorporeally induced destruction of kidney stones by shock waves. J Urol 127:417–420
6. Chaussy C, Schmiedt E, Jocham D, Walther V, Brendel W (1983) Stoßwellentherapie zur Behandlung von Nierensteinen. Münch Med Wochenschr 125:151–155
7. Eisenberger F, Chaussy C, Wanner K (1976) Extrakorporale Anwendung von hochenergetischen Stoßwellen – Ein neuer Aspekt in der Behandlung des Harnsteinleidens. C. E. Alken-Preis
8. Eisenberger F, Chaussy C, Wanner K (1976) Entwicklung eines steintragenden Hundemodells zur in vivo-Untersuchung der Wirkung fokussierter Stoßwellen auf Nierensteine. Biophysikalische Verfahren zur Diagnose und Therapie von Steinleiden der Harnwege. Wissenschaftliche Berichte, Meersburg, Juni
9. Eisenberger F, Schmiedt E, Chaussy C, Wanner K, Forssmann B, Hepp W, Pielsticker W, Brendel W (1977) Berührungsfreie Harnsteinzertrümmerung (Stand der Forschung). Deutsches Ärzteblatt 74:1145
10. Eisenberger F, Chaussy C, Wanner K (1977) Extracorporale Anwendung von hochenergetischen

Stoßwellen. Ein neuer Aspekt in der Behandlung des Harnsteinleidens. Akt Urol 8:3

11. Eisenberger F, Fuchs G, Miller K, Rassweiler J (1983) Alternatives to open surgery for renal calculi. XI Conferencia Urologica, Rio de Janeiro, November
12. Eisenberger F, Fuchs G, Miller K (1983) Nierensteintherapie: erste klinische Erfahrungen mit der berührungsfreien Nierensteintherapie (ESWL) am Katharinenhospital Stuttgart. Ärzteblatt Baden-Württemberg 12:504
13. Eisenberger F, Fuchs G, Miller K (1984) Endourology and stone-machine – the end of open surgery for renal calculi? Symposium of Japanese Urological Association, Osaka, April
14. Eisenberger F, Fuchs G, Miller K (1984) History and theory of extracorporeal shockwave lithotripsy. Symposium, Keio University, Tokio, April
15. Eisenberger F, Fuchs G, Miller K (1984) Stone-machine and endourology: competitive or combined methods in the treatment of urinary stone disease? First international Course on Urological Surgery and Endoscopy, Milan, May
16. Forßmann B, Hepp W, Hoff G, Chaussy C, Eisenberger F, Wanner K (1976) Entwicklung eines Verfahrens zur berührungsfreien Zerkleinerung von Nierensteinen durch Stoßwellen. Symposion, Biophysikalische Verfahren zur Diagnose und Therapie von Steinleiden der Harnwege, Meersburg, Juni
17. Forßmann B, Hepp W, Chaussy C, Eisenberger F, Wanner K (1977) Eine Methode zur berührungsfreien Zertrümmerung von Nierensteinen durch Stoßwellen. Biomed Tech 22:164
18. Fuchs G, Miller K, Rassweiler J, Eisenberger F (1984) Alternatives to open surgery for renal calculi. In: Schilling A (ed) Acute ischaemic renal failure and intrarenal surgery. Zuckschwerdt, München (klinische und experimentelle Urologie, vol 8)
19. Fuchs G, Miller K (1984) ESWL – a revolutionary new therapy for urinary stones. Second Charles D. Branch Symposium (Spectrum of Urinary Stone Therapy), Peoria, May 12th
20. Fuchs G, Miller K, Bub P, Eisenberger F (1984) Extracorporeal shockwave lithotripsy (ESWL): clinical experience and results. Second World Congress on Percutaneous Renal Surgery, Mainz, 14–15 June
21. Fuchs G, Miller K, Eisenberger F (1984) Extracorporeal shockwave lithotripsy (ESWL) – clinical experiences and results. Symposium, Japanese Urological Association, Osaka, April
22. Fuchs G, Miller K, Eisenberger F (1984) Extracorporeal shockwave lithotripsy – indications. Symposium Keio University, Tokio, April
23. Fuchs G, Miller K, Eisenberger F (1984) Ultrasound before, during and after ESWL. Reduction of X-Ray exposure. Second World Congress on Percutaneous Renal Surgery, Mainz, June
24. Miller K, Fuchs G, Rassweiler J, Eisenberger F (1984) Financial analysis, personnel planning and organizational requirements for the installation of a kidney lithotripter at an urological department. Eur Urol (in press)
25. Miller K, Fuchs G (1984) Combination percutaneous nephrolithotomy (PCN) – extracorporeal shockwave lithotripsy (ESWL). Symposium, Keio University, Tokio, April
26. Miller K, Fuchs G (1984) New treatment modalities – ureterorenoscopy (URS) and percutaneous nephrolithotomy (PCN) as adjunct to extracorporeally induced shockwave lithotripsy (ESWL). Second Charles D. Branch Symposium (Spectrum of Urinary Stone Therapy), Peoria, May 12th
27. Miller K, Fuchs G, Eisenberger F (1984) New endoscopic methods for the treatment of urinary calculi. Ureterorenoscopy (URS) and percutaneous nephrolithotomy (PCN). Symposium, Japanese Urological Association, Osaka, April
28. Rassweiler JJ, Miller K, Fuchs G, Eisenberger F (1984) Ureterorenoscopy (URS) – its role in the management of ureteral stones. Second World Congress on Percutaneous Renal Surgery, Mainz, June

Percutaneous Stone Removal

K. Amplatz

Shortly after Fernstrom [1, 2] described the first percutaneous stone removal, a urologist, Dr. Arthur Smith, and a radiologist, Dr. Robert Miller, started the systematic percutaneous removal of renal calculi at the University of Minnesota. Due to the close cooperation between cardiovascular radiologists and urologists, numerous new techniques were developed.

With the advent of the ultrasonic lithotriptor [3–5], the percutaneous approach has gained wide popularity, and at the present time surgery is considered obsolete for most renal calculi. Renal calculi can be removed under fluoroscopic guidance or under direct vision. In recent years the endoscopic techniques have largely replaced the fluoroscopic approach, but both techniques are still applicable.

Technique

There is great controversy about the type of anesthesia [6, 7]. In our opinion, general anesthesia is only indicated in very apprehensive patients. The stone extraction can be carried out under local or epidural anesthesia without significant discomfort to the patient in one single sitting.

The renal pelvis has to be opacified prior to puncture. This can be accomplished by the intravenous injection of contrast medium intravenously by skinny needle puncture, or preferably through a retrograde catheter.

All patients undergoing percutaneous stone removal have a retrograde catheter placed prior to the procedure, preventing stone fragments from entering the ureter. Furthermore, contrast medium can be injected and the pelvis can be opacified and distended, facilitating punctures.

Prior to puncture of the kidney, the radiologist and urologist have to agree on the approach and instrumentation to be used. This consultation between the two specialists is of paramount importance. An error in approach strategy may result in failure.

The kidney should be entered at its lateral aspect, which is relatively avascular. This can be accomplished using a C-arm, but it is preferable to place the patient in a $30° - 35°$ oblique position. If the kidney is punctured too medially in the prone position, large arteries and veins may be intersected, resulting in a higher level of bleeding, which is the most common complication of percutaneous stone removal. On the other hand, the lateral approach may, on very rare occasions, result in a transcolonic perforation, which is treated conservatively.

The radiologist has to have a clear concept of the anatomy of the renal calices. Almost invariably, the posterior calices project medially to the anterior calices because of the oblique position of the kidney along the psoas muscle (Fig. 1).

Preferably, a posterior renal calix is punctured. Sometimes the differentiation between anterior and posterior renal calices may be difficult. The injection of air or carbon dioxide is most useful to identify the posterior calices. The alternative technique is identification of the posterior calices by their paralactic shift during fluoroscopic observation.

Since the calix is a relatively small target for percutaneous puncture, punctures have to be made in the direction of the central X-ray beam. Some investigators advocate oblique punctures, but they cannot equal the accuracy of central beam punctures.

If a handle is used for puncture, the respiratory motion of the kidney is no longer important. The patient can be instructed to stop breathing in any phase of respiration. The puncture can even be performed during respiration under fluoroscopic observation. Many patients who are heavily sedated may not be able to stop respiration.

The operator's hands are not exposed to radiation (Fig. 2).

The Minnesota experience was that ultrasound was an unnecessary complication of the procedure, since the renal pelvis can be well opaci-

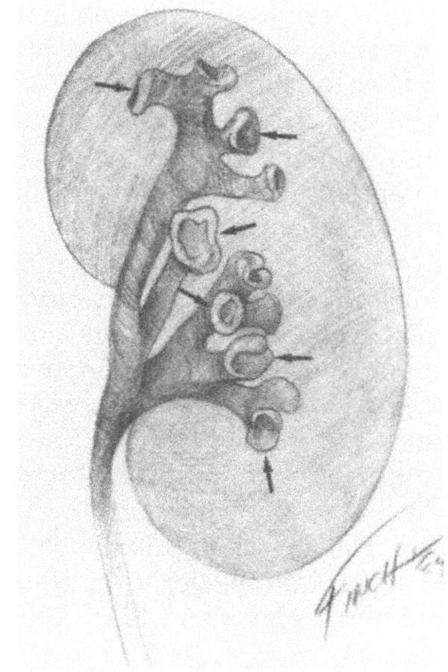

Fig. 1. Artist's drawing of a normal kidney demonstrating the posterior calices (*arrows*)

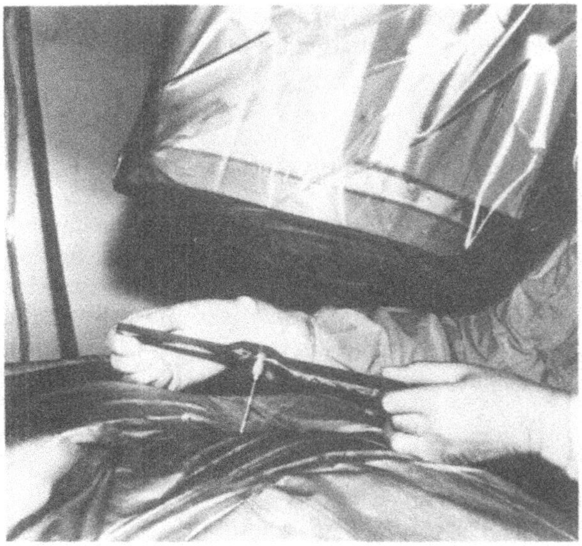

Fig. 2. Puncture of the kidney with an 18-gauge needle exactly in the direction of the central beam using a C-arm. The hands of the operator are kept outside the fluoroscopic field by means of a radiolucent plastic handle

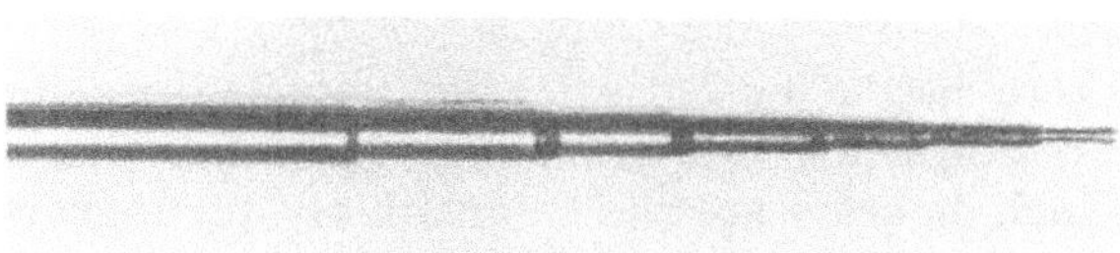

Fig. 3. Rigid coaxial dilator system for dilatation of the tract. This instrument, designed by Alken, is mostly used in Europe

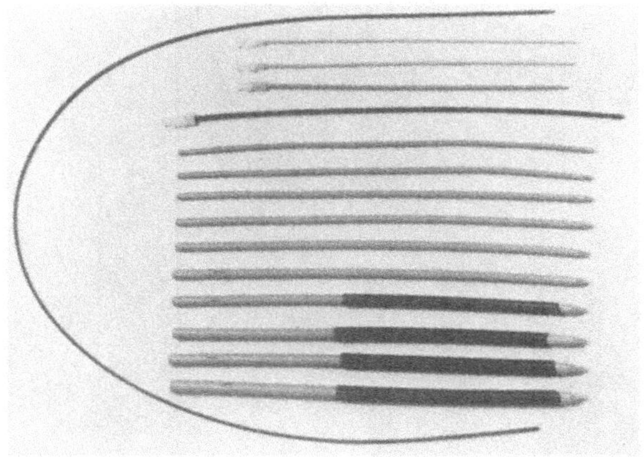

Fig. 4. Semirigid dilator set which is passed coaxially over an 8-F Teflon catheter. The Teflon catheter is passed into the ureter. The larger dilators, French 24, 26, 28, and 30 F, have snugly fitting Teflon sleeves which facilitate the manipulation of instruments and scopes. This system is one of the most popular in the United States

fied by injection of contrast medium through the retrograde catheter. The European investigators, on the other hand, found ultrasonic guidance very useful.

Dilatation of the Nephrostomy Tract

Dilatation is an important step in the sequence of percutaneous stone removal. The nephrostomy tract has to be dilated to 26 F or even 34 F in order to admit the passage of instruments or scopes. Dilatation of the tract can be accomplished by the use of metal telescopic bougie sets, as designed by Alken, or by semirigid plastic dilators (Figs. 3, 4). The dilatation of the tract by the semirigid dilators requires the passage of sequentially larger dilators, which is somewhat time-consuming. The more expedient way to dilate the tract is to use a balloon catheter. Only balloon catheters with high pressures, such as the Olbert, Cook reinforcer, or USCI catheters, can be used (Fig. 5). However, not all tracts can be dilated with balloon catheters.

Stone Removal Under Fluoroscopic Control

Many stones can be removed under fluoroscopic guidance without endoscopy. Baskets and rigid stone extraction can be employed for stones in the renal pelvis, and the Randall forceps (Fig. 6) is particularly useful. However, the use of rigid for-

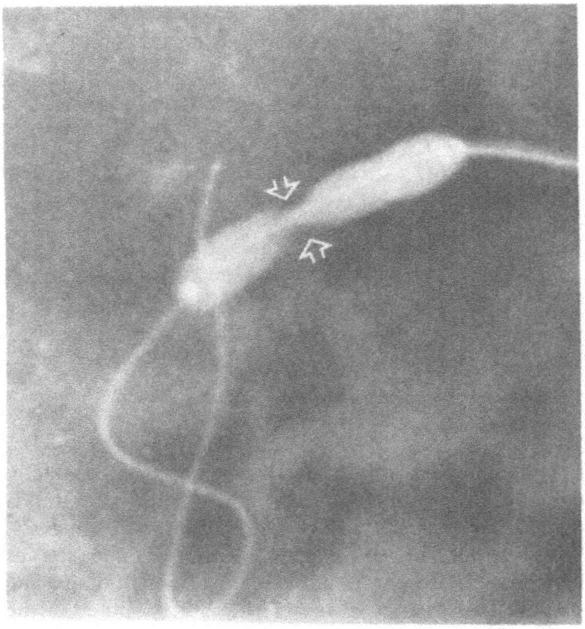

Fig. 5. Dilatation of the nephrostomy tract using a high-pressure balloon catheter. The waste (*arrowheads*) at the level of the renal capsule is well demonstrated. Balloon catheter dilatation works in most cases, but has the disadvantage that the catheter has to be discarded, at least in the United States. Consequently, it adds significantly to cost

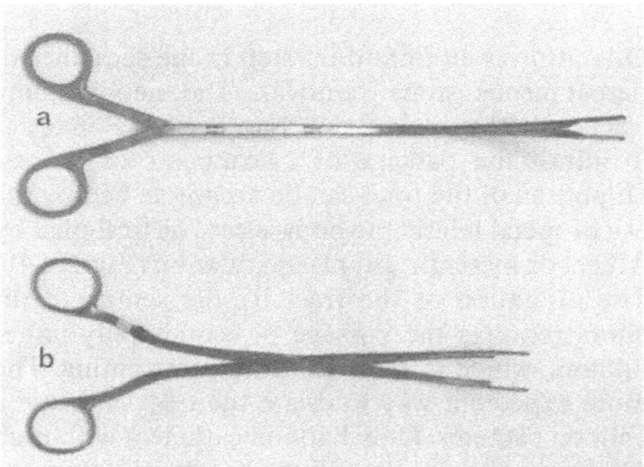

Fig. 6. The Caprini forceps (*A*) and the Randall forceps (*B*). Both instruments are used for stone removal under fluoroscopic control. The Caprini forceps has the advantage that it can be passed through smaller nephrostomy tracts than the Randall forceps

ceps tends to be more traumatic than manipulation under direct vision, and baskets are less useful in the renal pelvis than in the upper ureter.
Balloon catheters are useful for delivering stones from the renal calix into the renal pelvis. The catheter (Fogarty) is passed behind the stone and pulled from the calix into the pelvis.
Large stones have to be fragmented. This can be accomplished by an electrohydraulic lithotriptor.
An electrode is introduced and placed in close proximity to the stone, and the lithotriptor then generates a spark which propagates a shock wave, shattering the stone.
The advantage of the electrohydraulic lithotriptor is its power, which allows the fragmentation of even oxalate stones. The major disadvantage is the impossibility of aspirating the fragments, which remain in the renal pelvis and have to be removed by other techniques.
For larger stones, the preferred instrument is the ultrasonic lithotriptor, which creates very small fragments that are simultaneously aspirated. This device, designed by Alken [3–5], has largely replaced the electrohydraulic lithotriptor and represents the greatest advance in the history of renal stone removal.

Care Following the Procedure

A 24-F or 26-F catheter is introduced to tamponade the tract for 2–4 days. If there are no free stone fragments as determined by laminography, and free urinary flow as determined by nephrostography, the tube is removed and the patient can be discharged.

Results

At the University of Minnesota, 500 stones have been removed percutaneously. In the last 100 patients, the success rate was 99%. It is our feeling that all stones can be removed percutaneously with an almost 100% success rate, and surgery is no longer indicated. The successful removal of 45 staghorn calculi proves the obsolescence of surgery.
There has to be close cooperation between the radiologist and the urologist, since the failures which do occur are almost invariably due to inappropriate puncture of the kidney in relation to the position of the renal stone.

References

1. Fernstrom L (1983) Percutaneous pyelolithotomy. A new extraction technique. Scand J Urol Nephrol 10:257–259
2. Fernstrom L (1983) Percutaneous extraction of renal calculi: technique and results. Br J Urol [Suppl] 25–36
3. Alken P, Altwein JE (1980) Die perkutane Nephrolitholapaxie. Verh Dtsch Ges Urol 31:109–112
4. Alken P et al. (1982) Percutaneous kidney stone removal. Eur Urol 8:304–311
5. Alken P (1984) Percutaneous nephrolithotomy. Eleventh World Congress on Percutaneous Renal Surgery, Mainz, 14–16 June
6. Günther R et al. (1979) Percutaneous nephropyelostomy using a fine-needle puncture set. Radiology 132:228–230
7. Clayman RV et al. (1983) Nephrostolithotomy: percutaneous removal of renal and ureteric calculi. Br J Urol [Suppl] 6–10

Percutaneous Stone Litholapaxy and Extraction

R. Günther and P. Alken

Percutaneous stone manipulation has gained increasing popularity in the past 5 years. Following initial experience with stone dissolution as the least invasive form of percutaneous stone manipulation, litholapaxy and extraction emerged as a more efficient method of treatment which is independent of the composition of the calculi. With an average of 4–6 days of hospital stay and a low complication rate, percutaneous litholapaxy has now become an attractive alternative to operation.

Technique

The combination of both litholapaxy and extraction is advisable for larger stones. The following steps are essential: (1) puncture of the kidney, (2) dilatation of the track, (3) endoscopy, (4) litholapaxy, and (5) extraction. It should be noted that contrary to our initial concept, all these steps are now performed in one session.
Several variations concerning positioning of the patient, access to the renal collecting system, and dilatation of the needle track have been added to the initial technique [1–3, 6, 7, 12–14, 16, 18].

Anesthesia

Percutaneous stone manipulation can be done under local anesthesia; peridural anesthesia, however seems to be more convenient for the patient. General anesthesia is only applied if the patient desires it.

Positioning of the Patient

We prefer the patient to be in prone position, some authors have found the prone oblique position to be more favourable for the puncture of the collecting system.

Puncture

Failure to take individual topographic and renal anatomy into consideration may cause unnecessary complications [10]. In order to avoid a major arterial lesion, peripheral puncture of the renal parenchyma aiming at the lower posterior calix is most appropriate. This provides access to the renal pelvis and upper calices, whereas the middle calix serves as access to the renal pelvis and the ureter. A posterolateral approach is preferred to a direct posterior one.
Three-dimensional orientation is a prerequisite for successful puncture. For this reason, real-time ultrasound is very helpful, and is optimally combined with fluroscopy. Puncture of a nondilated collecting system may occasionally be found very frustrating. Other definite aids include i.v. urogram, fine-needle puncture [8], and retrograde ureteral blockage using a balloon catheter.
The instruments required for puncture and initial catheter insertion comprise a 5-F Longdwell needle, a 1.0-mm J guide wire, and a 9-F introducer sheath. The sheath is used for insertion of the guide rod of the telescopic bougies.

Dilatation

In contrast to stone dissolution, litholapaxy and stone extraction require dilatation of the nephrostomy track up to 26 F or even 34 F. Despite this, there is only minimal scarring along the track, as shown in animal experiments [17]. Dilatation of the track may be performed using a metal telescopic bougie set, as designed by Alken [19], fascial Teflon dilators, or balloon catheters (Grüntzig or Olbert type).

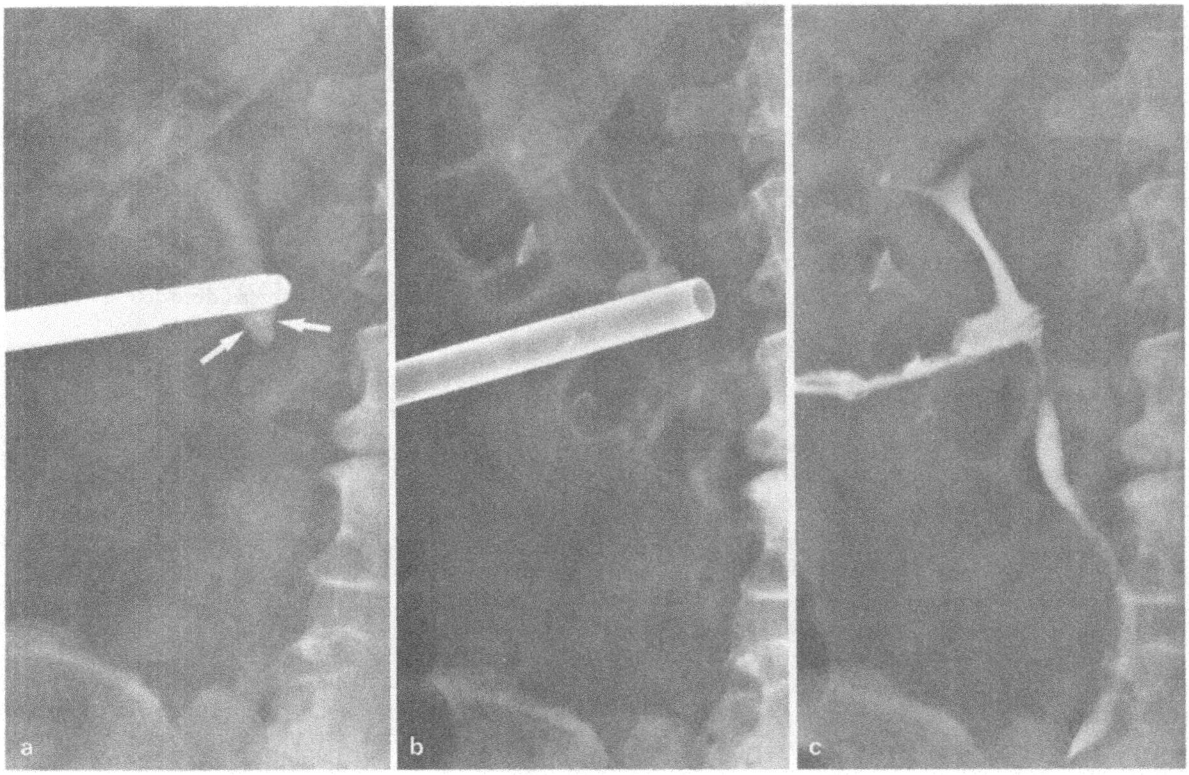

Fig. 1 a–c. Percutaneous stone extraction. **a** Percutaneous nephrostomy and dilatation up to 24 F using a telescopic bougie set. **b** Sheath of the set through which the stone is extracted. **c** Reinsertion of a nephrostomy tube (12 F) following successful stone removal

Instruments

Stone manipulation is done under direct vision using a rigid endoscope. The flexible endoscope is a useful addition for removal of caliceal stones.

The most important instruments for breaking stones are (1) the ultrasound lithotriptor, (2) the electrohydraulic lithotriptor, (3) the stone punch, and (4) forceps.

Simple mechanical fragmentation of small stones is done by forceps. Only in a capacious collecting system may a stone punch be used. Larger stones can be fragmented by the rigid ultrasound lithotriptor (10 F), which is preferred by most authors because of its safety. The electrohydraulic lithotriptor is less frequently used, but has the advantages of smaller caliber (5 F) and flexibility.

Extraction of ureteral stones can be accomplished using a snare or a Dormia stone basket. To ensure that the track can be re-entered following the procedure, insertion of a spare guide wire is recommended during manipulation.

Care Following Procedure

Following the procedure a 14- to 26-F nephrostomy tube is reinserted and left in place for 2–4 days to enable control of bleeding or obstruction. If nephrostography demonstrates complete stone clearance and free urinary flow, the tube is then removed.

Results

From 1977 to 1983, 200 renal units were treated in the Urological Department of Mainz University. Percutaneous nephrostomy was feasible in 98%, although the majority of patients had a nondilated renal collecting system. Complete stone removal was achieved in 168 of 181 patients with percutaneous nephrostomy. Failures were due to inability to gain access, unsuitable access, inadequate track, limited intrarenal access, or unfavorable stone position. No stones were resistant to ultrasound litholapaxy.

In the literature, the removal rate of renal stones varies from 71% to 89% [5–7, 13, 14, 18]. Segura reports a success rate of 98% with renal stones. The success rate in ureteral stones may be up to 86%. Operation time ranges from 45–70 min, and hospital stay 4–6 days.
As demonstrated by functional studies [11, 17] and CT [9], alterations of the kidney are minimal following percutaneous stone manipulation.

Complications

Complications such as bleeding, pneumothorax, hydrothorax, septicemia, extravasation, and ureteral obstruction are rare, but may arise during puncture, dilatation, and endoscopic manipulation. The complication rate in 1571 cases compiled by Alken [3] from the literature was 1.7%. The majority of them, however, were managed conservatively. In our series, three major complications were encountered, including bleeding, perforation of the colon and development of a subpelvic stenosis. Only the last-mentioned had to be corrected operatively, and there was no mortality.
According to Segura et al. [16], the most significant complication remains the development of an arteriovenous fistula in 0.5%–0.6% of cases.

Conclusion

Percutaneous manipulation has proved to be a safe and efficient method of stone treatment. However, with the advent of [4] extracorporal shock-wave lithotripsy (ESWL) its clinical application has been considerably reduced, since the majority of patients can be treated by this technique. However, percutaneous litholapaxy has not been completely rendered obsolete by this. First, there are only a small number of units currently available. Second, there are some calculi not suitable for ESWL, such as nonradiopaque stones, staghorn calculi, or stones proximal to a stenosis. For the treatment of staghorn calculi, the combination of initial percutaneous litholapaxy and subsequent ESWL offers a complete nonoperative approach. The need for surgery will be restricted to approximately 10%–15% of stone patients in future.

References

1. Alken P, Altwein JE (1980) Die perkutane Nephrolitholapaxie. Verh Dtsch Ges Urol 31:109–112
2. Alken P et al. (1982) Percutaneous kidney stone removal. Eur Urol 8:304–311
3. Alken P (1984) Percutaneous nephrolithotomy. Second World Congress on Percutaneous Renal Surgery, Mainz, 14–16 June
4. Chaussy C et al. (1982) First clinical experience with extracorporeally induced destruction of kidney stones by shock waves. J Urol 127:417–420
5. Clayman RV et al. (1983) Nephrostolithotomy: percutaneous removal of renal and ureteric calculi. Br J Urol [Suppl] 6–10
6. Fernström I, Johansson B (1976) Percutaneous pyelolithotomy. A new extraction technique. Scand J Urol Nephrol 10:257–259
7. Fernström I (1983): Percutaneous extraction of renal calculi: technique and results. Br J Urol [Suppl] 25–36
8. Günther R et al. (1979) Percutaneous nephropyelostomy using a fine-needle puncture set. Radiology 132:228–230
9. Hruby W, Marberger M (1984) Morphological alterations of the kidney and perirenal structures after PCN. Second World Congress on Percutaneous Renal Surgery, Mainz, 14–16 June
10. Kaye KW, Goldberg ME (1982) Applied anatomy of the kidney and ureter. Urol Clin Am 9:3–13
11. Le Duc A et al. (1984) Assessment of cortical function of the kidney by 99mTc DMSA scintigraphy pre and post percutaneous procedure. Second World Congress on Percutaneous Renal Surgery, Mainz, 14–16 June
12. Newhouse JR, Pfister RC (1981) Therapy for renal calculi via percutaneous nephrostomy: dissolution and extraction. Urol Radiol 2:157–164
13. Marberger M (1983) Ultrasonic lithotripsy of renal calculi: a 3-year experience. Br J Urol [Suppl] 41–50
14. Miller RA et al. (1983) Percutaneous destruction of renal calculi: clinical and laboratory experience. Br J Urol [Suppl] 51–54
15. Raney AM, Handler J (1975) Electrohydraulic nephrolithotomy. Urology 6:439–446
16. Segura JW et al. (1984) Results of percutaneous removal of ureteral and renal stones. Second World Congress on Percutaneous Renal Surgery, Mainz, 14–16 June
17. Webb DR, Fitzpatrick JM (1984) Percutaneous nephrolithotomy; structural and functional effects. Second World Congress on Percutaneous Renal Surgery, Mainz, 14–16 June
18. Wickham JEA et al. (1981) Elective percutaneous, nephrolithotomy in 50 patients: an analysis of the technique, results and complications. Br J Urol 53:297–299
19. Alken P (1981) Teleskopbougieset. Zur perkutanen Nephrostomie. Akt Urol 12:216–219

The Effects of Digitization and Processing on Diagnostic Images

K. N. Vizy

The recent proliferation of digital signal-processing systems, particularly as they apply to medical diagnostic images, has brought with it a new set of effects on these images. These effects are sometimes benign, sometimes tolerable, and at times very objectionable. The degree to which a diagnostician accepts these effects in his daily interaction with the images will no doubt be a very personal affair – for our tolerances and visual capabilities are quite personal in nature – but description of the effects for proper communication with fellow professionals will require a new lexicon to describe the pictorial results.

The medical diagnostic information will in most instances be digital in nature, meaning that the pictorial content will exist as a long sequence of numbers, each defining the gray level of the picture elements (pixels) for which they stand. This was thoroughly explained in an earlier publication [1].

Now image processing in general refers to the individual or collective manipulation of these numbers so as to yield a more easily interpretable diagnostic image. The manipulation usually takes place in a computer through the use of special programs or algorithms which are part of the system's software package. Ample literature exists on the processing methods [2–5]. The journal *Image and Vision Computing* [6] provides periodic updates on what is being done in the field.

The processed data sets representing images collected in various ways [7, 8] are then exhibited either as soft images on CRT monitors or other such display devices, or as hard copies on film or paper for human use. Jensen [9] and Sherr [10] provide good technical support for display designs and evaluations. It is on the output medium of these displays where one will come in visual contact with the potential effects of digitization, processing, or both.

The Effects of Digitization

There are five main digitization effects, which have been addressed by a number of speakers at recent conferences on electronic imaging in medicine.

Aliasing Effects

When an information-rich field is under-sampled with too coarse a scan spot, or when in a scan con-

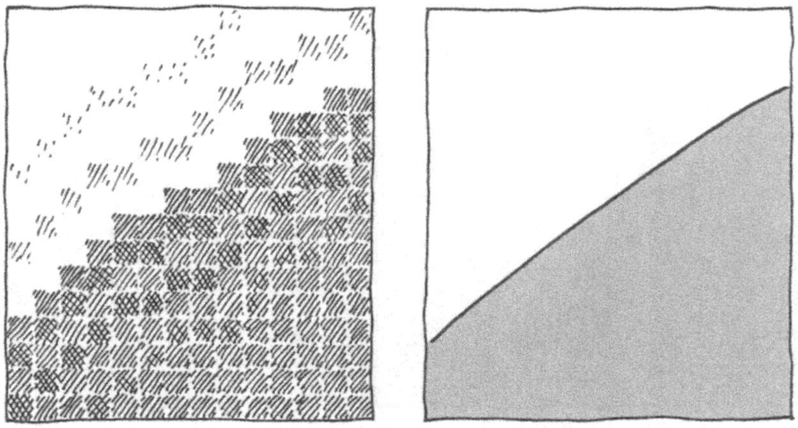

Fig. 1. Aliasing effect

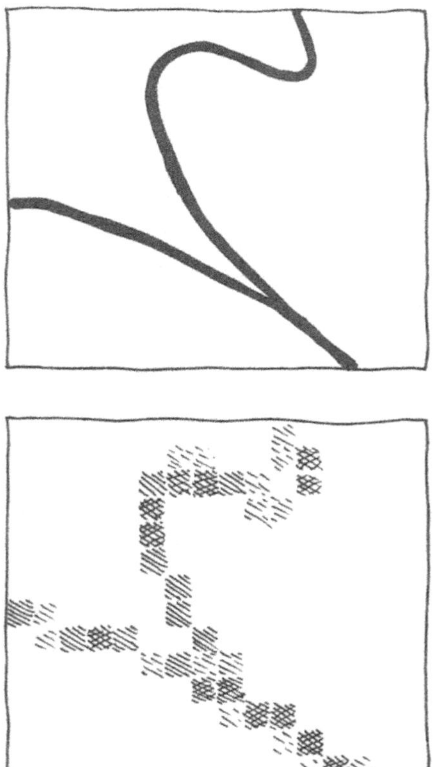

Fig. 2. Staircase-edge effect

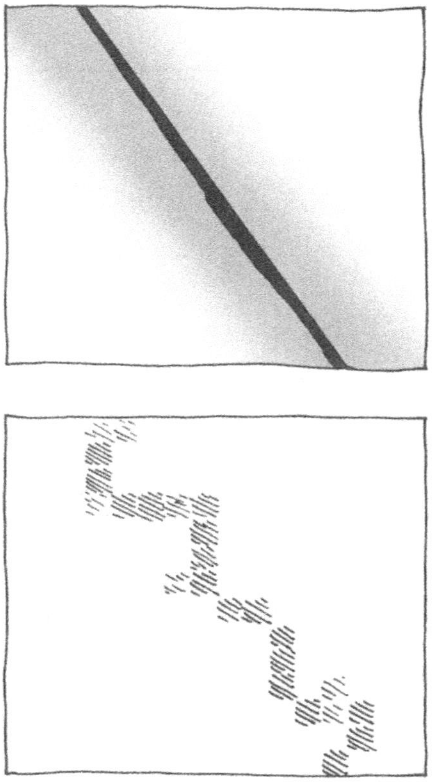

Fig. 3. Motion distortion

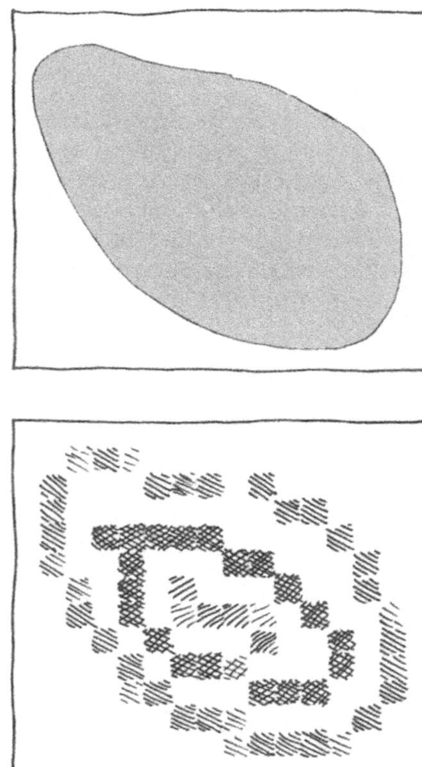

Fig. 4. Contouring effect

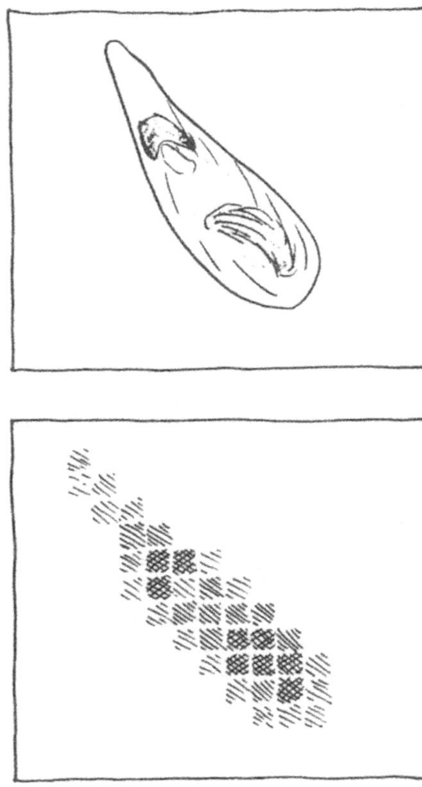

Fig. 5. Pixeling effect

version step the two scans are out of phase, the image will exhibit artificially low frequency components (Fig. 1). In optics, aliasing errors are called moiré effects or moiré patterns.

Staircase-Edge Effects

In case of coarse pixelization, namely at levels easily detectable visually, one gets a jagged pattern for smooth objects' edge representations. Figure 2 illustrates the possible appearance of a smooth vessel.

Motion Distortion: Scanning Action Result

In the situation of pulsatile, periodic motion of an object being scanned over a long time period (with respect to the pulse duration), a periodic distortion will be shown in what should otherwise be a smooth edge. Figure 3 illustrates the diffuse analog and the distorted digital representations of a vessel.

Contouring Effects

When too few, and significantly interspaced, levels of gray are used, large areas smoothly varying in density will exhibit a characteristic blotchiness, recognizable by apparent contour lines delineating the edges of constant-density regions (Fig. 4).

Pixeling Effect: Raster Noise

If the size of the pixels is visually recognizable, one will have this image segmentation noise superimposed on the information (Fig. 5).

The Effects of Processing

An infinite variety of processing effects is possible. Four key effects tend to predominate in medical diagnostic applications, and these will be reviewed here.

Random-Noise Enhancement

When amplifying a low-contrast set of digital data, one will amplify noise which previously was sub-threshold visually; this adds noise to the ultimate image produced for diagnosis (Fig. 6).

Signal Suppression

This effect occurs when one uses various noise-suppression algorithms or spatial filters to do away with the random, spurious noise data which reside with the signal in the image. Typically, an algorithm or filter cannot distinguish between good and bad "bits" of information. Figure 7 illustrates how some detail character may be lost.

False-Signal Development: Mottle Evolution

When using signal-enhancing algorithms, one again may find simultaneous enhancement effects on the spurious background, which then might mimic real signal information. Figure 8 illustrates the appearance of signals which are potential artifacts and thus false.

Subtraction Artifacts

When multiple images are obtained for the purpose of either adding them together or subtracting one from the others, the possibility always looms large that the patient will move in temporally distinct acquisition or that image distortion is inhomogeneous for simultaneously acquired frames. This will usually result in the creation of very strong false signals in the final sum or difference images, making diagnosis quite difficult, if not impossible. Figure 9 illustrates the type of erratic conclusion one might expect from this motion-type artifact.

Conclusions

As pointed out earlier, this review is not an exhaustive listing of the strange situations which might be encountered in the fascinating world of image processing, but it does give one a glimpse into the key effects with which we will all have to be familiar or be capable of recognizing. The literature which exists on the subject tends to be mathematical and thus not easily comprehensible to all; however, if the effort is invested to deal with its theoretical aspects, one may enter the awe-inspiring world of image manipulation, which alters our perception of information.

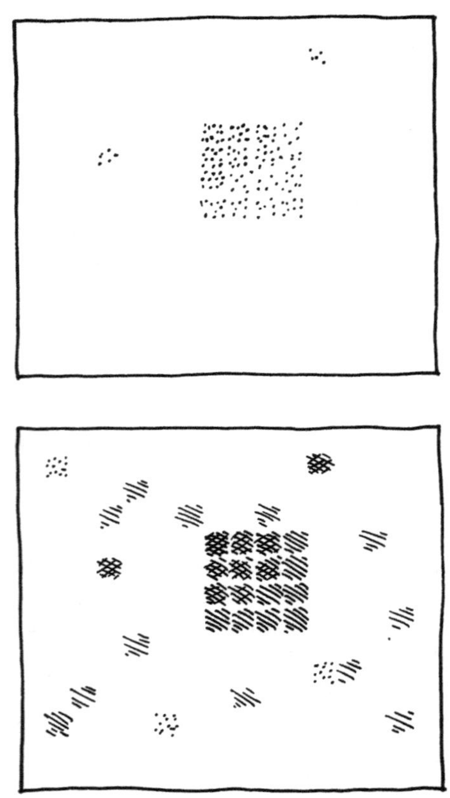

Fig. 6. Random-noise enhancement

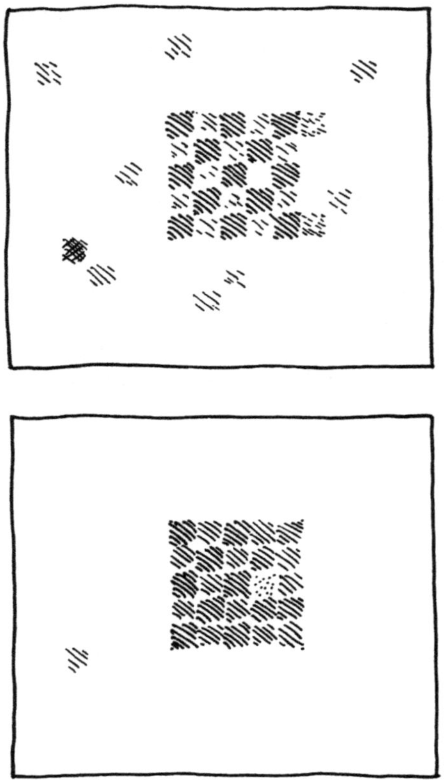

Fig. 7. Signal suppression

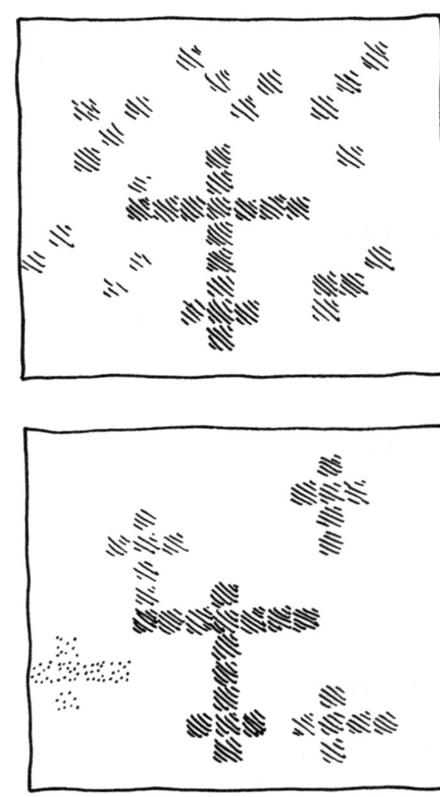

Fig. 8. False-signal development

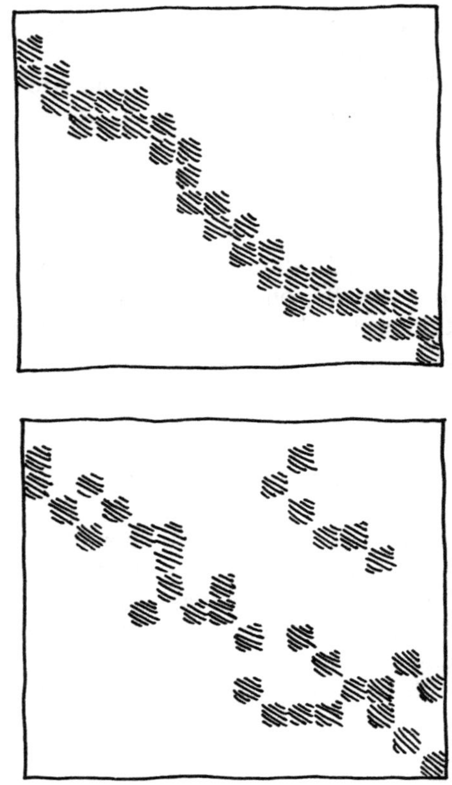

Fig. 9. Subtraction artifact

Of course, after competence is established in the optimum use of the computer for processing our diagnostic images, we will then be faced with having to prove clinical diagnostic efficacy. Here, too, a marvelous little monograph exists to assist the strong-hearted [11].

References

1. Vizy KN (1983) Electronic imaging fundamentals: basic theory. In: Cardiovascular and interventional radiology, vol 6, no 4. Springer, Berlin Heidelberg New York Tokyo, pp 174–182
2. Oppenheim AV, Schafer RW (1975) Digital signal processing. Prentice-Hall, Englewood Cliffs
3. Pratt WK (1970) Digital image processing. Wiley-Interscience, New York
4. Preston K Jr, Onoe M (1976) Digital processing of biomedical images. Plenum, New York
5. Gonzales RC, Wintz P (1982) Digital image processing, 4th edn. Addison-Wesley, Reading MA
6. Image and vision computing (quarterly journal) Butterworth, Guildford
7. Vizy KN (1983) An overview of digital radiography systems. In: Cardiovascular and interventional radiology, vol 6, no 4–6. Springer, Berlin Heidelberg New York Tokyo, pp 296–299
8. Brody WR (1984) Digital radiography. Raven, New York
9. Jensen N (1968) Optical and photographic reconnaissance systems. Wiley, New York
10. Sherr S (1970) Fundamentals of display system design. Wiley-Interscience, New York
11. Evans ALI (1981) The evaluation of medical images. Hilger, Bristol (Medical physics handbooks, vol 10)

Paramagnetic Contrast Media of the Present and the Future

U. Speck and R. Felix

Proton magnetic resonance imaging (MRI) is a sensitive technique capable of visualizing small differences in the composition of soft tissues. The question is, therefore, why we should use contrast media. From a theoretical point of view, at least, there are some reasons why contrast media might be useful in MRI:

- To visualize functions such as excretion, permeability (blood-brain barrier), and perfusion of tissues
- To detect very small lesions due to a contrast-enhanced difference in signal intensity
- To reduce the time necessary to obtain a diagnostic picture and to achieve good contrast resolution and good spatial resolution at the same time

The most advanced contrast medium at this time is GdDTPA (Fig. 1). Gadolinium decreases both T1 and T2 relaxation times due to its strong paramagnetic efficacy. The chelating agent DTPA ensures complete excretion and the detoxification of the gadolinium. The DTPA surrounds the gadolinium ion like a cage. Gadolinium was chosen from a number of paramagnetic ions because of its strong influence on relaxation times, chemical stability, and relatively low toxicity. The use of DTPA as chelating agent resulted in a very stable complex displaying far better tolerance than similar chelates such as EDTA.

Gadolinium injected as chloride in rats is stored in the liver and spleen. Even 7 days after intravenous injection, only a small proportion of the free gadolinium was recovered from urine and faeces. On the other hand, no such disposition of the gadolinium was observed after the injection of the DTPA chelate. The course of the blood level and the excretion of GdDTPA very closely resemble the pharmacokinetics of urographic X-ray contrast media in the rat [1].

The same is true in humans. The half-life of GdDTPA in volunteers was found to be about 2 h. The excretion occurs almost exclusively through the kidneys [2].

In order to be able to start clinical trials, a large number of preclinical studies has been performed, most of them to investigate tolerance of the new contrast material. The most convincing results were obtained during the studies on subacute toxicology in the rat and the dog. In these studies the animals received 16–18 injections, one per day, at three different dose levels. Up to a dosage 10 times the clinical dose, no relevant side effects were observed with regard to hemotology, clinical chemistry, organ function tests, or tissue histology. The results of these studies indicate that GdDTPA offers a sufficient margin of safety and does not have delayed side effects even after repeated administration (Table 1).

The product used in clinical trials is injected intravenously. It is an 0.5 molar solution of GdDTPA dimeglumine. The dosage is equivalent to 0.1 mmol/kg body weight (0.2 ml/kg; about 15 ml per patient). The dose is distinctly lower than with X-ray contrast media (Figs. 1, 2).

Table 1. Subacute tolerance studies on SHL 451A (GdDTPA, dimeglumine); evaluation of clinical, biochemical, hematological, and histological alterations

Species	Daily doses (mmol/kg)	Duration	Number of i.v. injections	Findings at 1 mmol/kg
Rat	1; 2.5; 5	Ca. 4 weeks	16–18	None
Dog	0.25; 1; 2.5	Ca. 4 weeks	16–18	Local reddening of the skin, slight increase in plasma fibrinogen, slight vacuolization of renal tubular cells

Preparation

SH L 451A	Schering AG

Composition

469 g gadolinium-DTPA, dimeglumine 0.13 g DTPA
Water for injection ad 1000 ml

Viscosity	2.9 mPa.s(= cP) at 37 °C
Osmolality	1940 mosm/kg water at 37 °C
pH	6.5 – 7.5

Administration

Intravenous injection

Dose	0.1 mmol/kg body weight = 0.2 ml SH L 451A/kg body weight kidney: 0.05 mmol/kg body weight = 0.1 ml SH L 451A/kg body weight

◂**Fig. 1.** Contrast medium for magnetic resonance imaging

▾ **Fig. 2.** Ganglioglioma II, left hippocampus [6]. **a** Plain CT scan (Sonatom 2). Inhomogeneous hypodense area, enlargement of the left temporal horn. **b** CT scan after administration of contrast medium. Inhomogeneous enhancement in a lobulated tumor located in the left hippocampus. **c** Precontrast MRI scan (SE 800/35). Tumor not directly visible. Slice of MRI scan lower and titled in relation to CT scan. **d** Postcontrast MRI scan. Inhomogeneous increase of signal intensity in the tumor. **e** Precontrast MRI scan (SE 1600/35). No sufficient differentiation between tumor and surrounding tissue. **f** Precontrast MRI scan (SE 1600/70). No sufficient differentiation between tumor and surrounding tissue

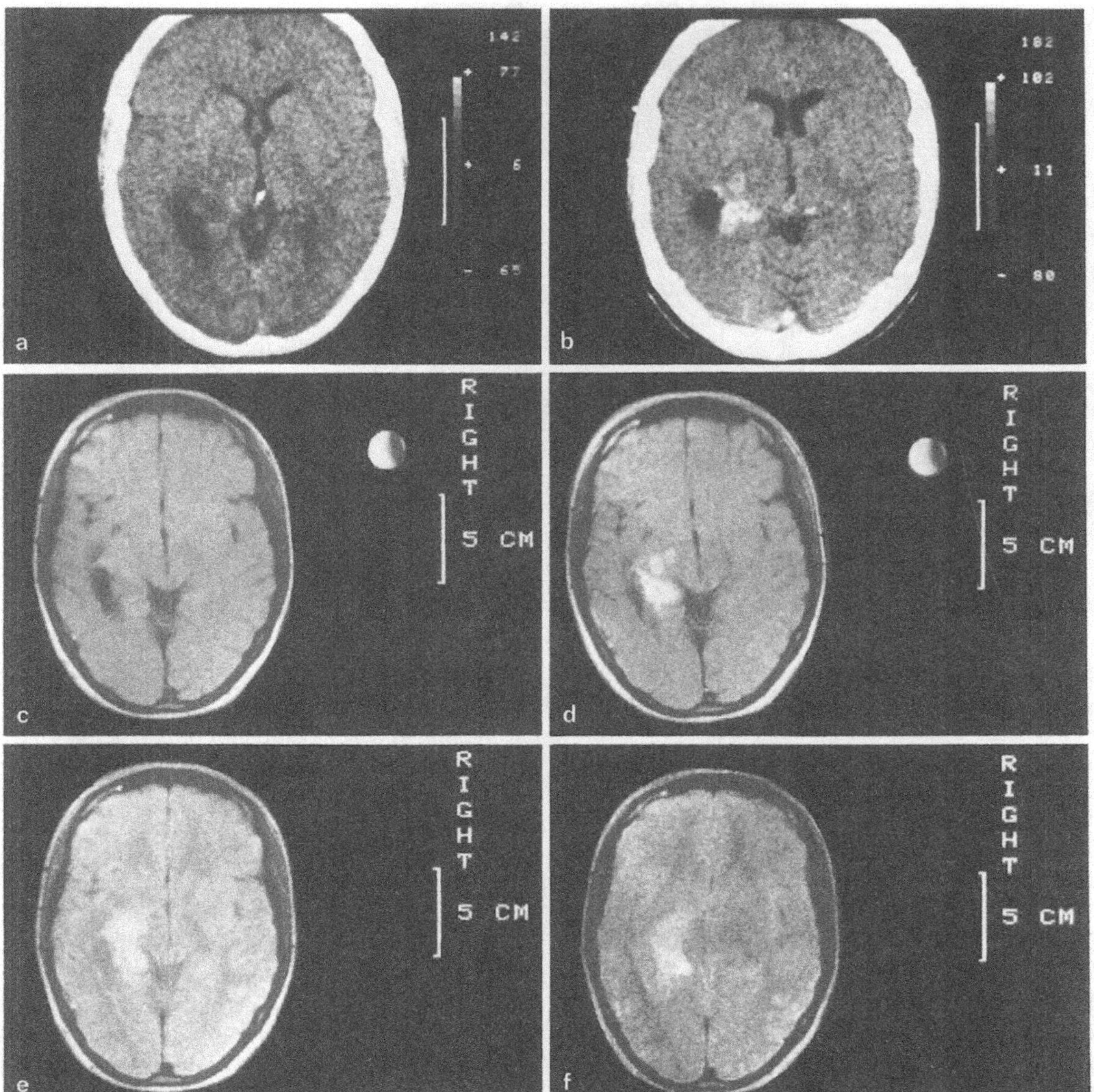

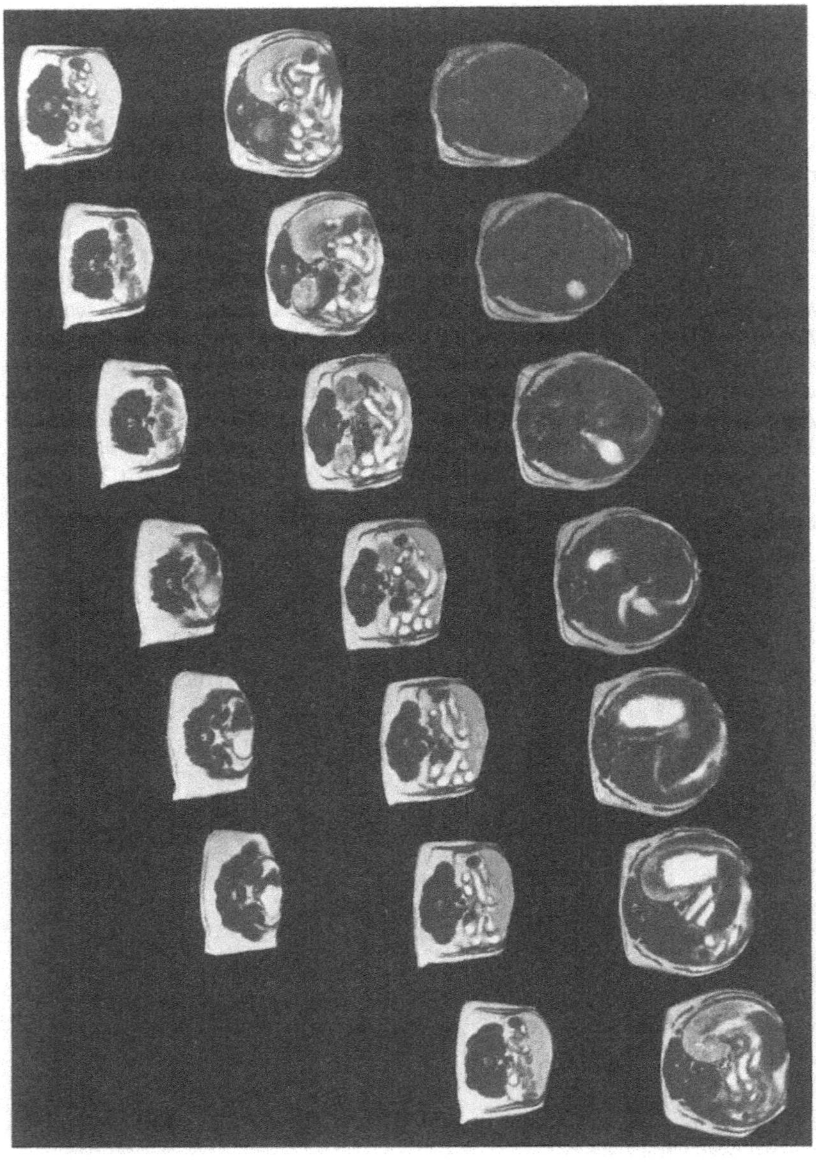

Fig. 3. Multiple slices through a dog following oral administration of a special preparation of GdDTPA

In addition, we are adapting the product for oral use. Figure 3 shows a study in the dog.

Another class of proton MR contrast media is the nitroxide stable free radicals, originally proposed and investigated by R. Brasch from the University of California, San Francisco [3]. Only recently has significant progress been achieved with these compounds. The margin of safety has been improved, and further improvement can be foreseen for the near future.

We expect the following developments in regard to contrast media in MRI:

1. Contrast media like GdDTPA will probably find a place in certain routine applications of MRI.
2. Organ-specific contrast media might be developed, e.g., for the liver and the pancreas.
3. Function-specific contrast media, e.g., to visualize the uptake of glucose or fatty acids, are conceivable.
4. Pathology-specific contrast media might become reality in MRI. The literature [4] already indicates that some success has been achieved with a monoclonal antibody raised against myosin, and the dream is naturally tumor imaging by monoclonal antibodies [5].
5. Finally, one should not forget that MRI offers the capability of visualizing atoms other than hydrogen. Since most of these atoms occur in very low concentration in the organism, the dis-

tribution of the respective contrast medium could be visualized without a background. Furthermore, atoms other than hydrogen could offer the opportunity to separate extracellular from intracellular space, and to measure pH values or temperature of healthy tissue or pathologic lesions within the organs in a totally noninvasive way.

It is not very likely that further developments will be introduced in clinical practice within the next 10 years.

References

1. Weinmann H-J, Brasch RC, Press W-R, Wesbey GE (1984) Characteristics of Gadolinium-DTPA complex: a potential NMR contrast agent. AJR 142:619–624
2. Weinmann H-J, Laniado M, Mützel W (1984) Pharmacokinetics of GdDTPA/Dimeglumine after intravenous injection into healthy volunteers. Physiol Chem Phys Med NMR 16[2]:167–172
3. Brasch RC, Nitecki DE, Brand-Zawadzki M, Enzmann DR, Wesbey GE, Tozer TN, Tuck LD, Cann CE, Fike JR, Sheldon P (1983) Brain nuclear magnetic resonance imaging enhanced by a paramagnetic nitroxide contrast agent: preliminary report. AJR 141:1019–1023
4. Brady TJ, Rosen BR, Gold HK, Khaw BA, Fallon JT, Coldman HR, terPenning BJ, Yasuda T, Haber E (1983) Selective decrease in T_1 relaxation times of infarcted myocardium with the use of a manganese-labeled monoclonal antibody, antimyosin. Society of Magnetic Resonance in Medicine, San Francisco
5. McNamara MT, Ehman RL, Quay SC, Epstein AL, Schmidt H, Brasch RC (1984) Selective alterations of tumor relaxation times using a paramagnetic-labeled monoclonal antibody to Burkitt's lymphoma. Society of Magnetic Resonance in Medicine, New York
6. Claussen C, Laniado M, Kazner E, Schörner W, Felix R (1985) Application of contrast agents in CT and NMR: their potential in imaging of brain tumors. Neuroradiology (in press)

PROBLEMS OF PROGRESS IN RADIOLOGY: SUPPLEMENTARY INFORMATIONS

Variations and Cost Containment in Radiology

W. P. Cockshott

Concern about health care costs is universal. The relative priorities to be accorded to such broad issues as curative vs preventive medicine, the hospital sector vs primary care, and government health service vs the private sector will continue to be discussed for years to come, despite the efforts of health care planners who believe in the exhilarating myth that all problems are soluble. Politics has been defined as the art of the possible, and our discussion on cost containment in radiology should address what is feasible, which is not always synonymous with what is optimal.

What is desirable for a poor developing nation may differ in details from what would be acceptable to an affluent industrial country. Indeed, because the economic pressures are greater in poor countries, their responses may have lessons for those of us operating in richer areas.

I will briefly comment on three aspects that allegedly lead to the high cost of diagnostic imaging: (a) overutilization, (b) the level of capital and operating costs of new technologies, and (c) the high cost of imaging personnel. This classification is simplistic and reductionist, and does not indicate the underlying degree of complexity, but it serves as a basis for discussion.

Overutilization

If we compare the utilization of radiologic services, measured as examinations per 1000 patients, in several countries, we see vast differences, for instance between Ghana and North America (Ghana 20; USA 1000) [1]. What is the optimal usage? I believe it lies between two such extremes. Health indices in Scandinavia and Britain are generally better than those in the USA, yet radiology is used less in these countries. Why? Doubtless governmental financial constraints are of importance. Perhaps there is more selective use of indications for studies. The salaried system may remove economic motivation for a high patient throughput. There is less preventive radiology to avoid litigation. There are few mandatory X-rays (pre-employment, annual check-ups, etc.).

I sent a questionnaire to 41 countries and enquired about the routine projections used to investigate a number of specific clinical problems related to the skeletal system. Representative results are displayed in Figs. 1 – 5. Individual countries are not specifically identified apart from the USA respondents. Comparisons can be made between private clinics and hospital practices.

These examples suggest that in poor countries fewer routine views are taken because of economic factors; in fee-for-service settings, more projections are obtained, and in salaried social health services there is no limitation of views obtained when there is a complex clinical problem, as shown in cervical spine trauma.

We have the knowledge to reduce the number of inappropriate studies. The WHO booklet *A Rational Approach to Radiodiagnostic Investigations* (Technical Report 689) sets out the results of an international study group convened to recommend measures for the productive use of radiology facilities. We have to educate our clinical colleagues and medical students as to the appropriate imaging techniques and the order in which they should be used. Radiology should not be used as a crutch to provide that extra certainty of diagnosis. An increase in likelihood from 80% to 90% is costly: does it help management? How we get this message across and change the behavior of referring doctors is not known. All that is certain is that any strategy will take time, probably a decade.

Equipment

The price of imaging equipment rises faster than inflation. New technologies and added complexity are factors, yet the newer techniques are cost-effective in the overall health care budget

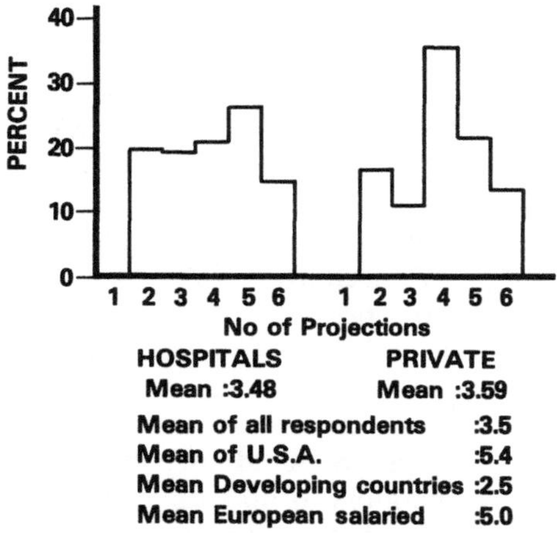

Fig. 1. Utilization of radiologic services in cervical spine trauma

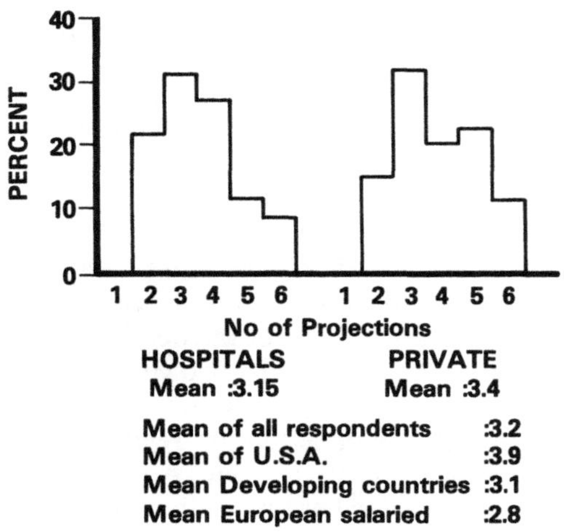

Fig. 2. Utilization of radiologic services in lumbar spine trauma

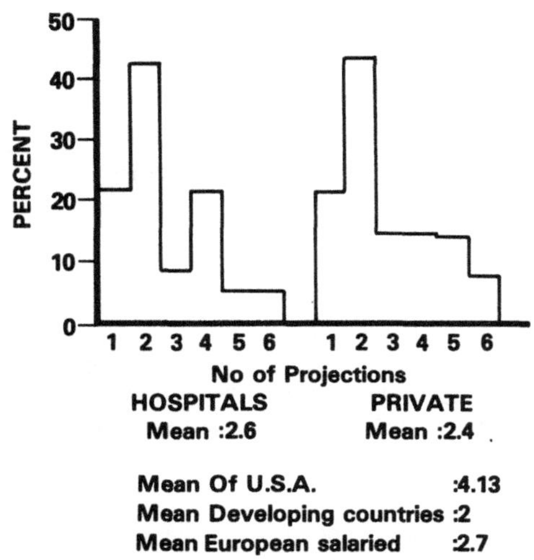

Fig. 3. Utilization of radiologic services in pre-employment back studies

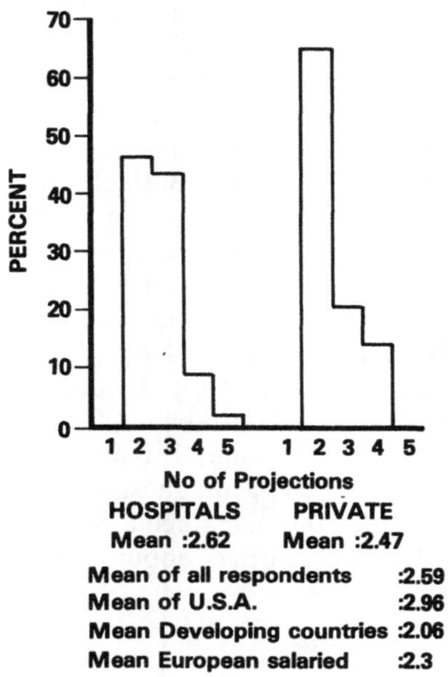

Fig. 4. Utilization of radiologic services in ankle trauma

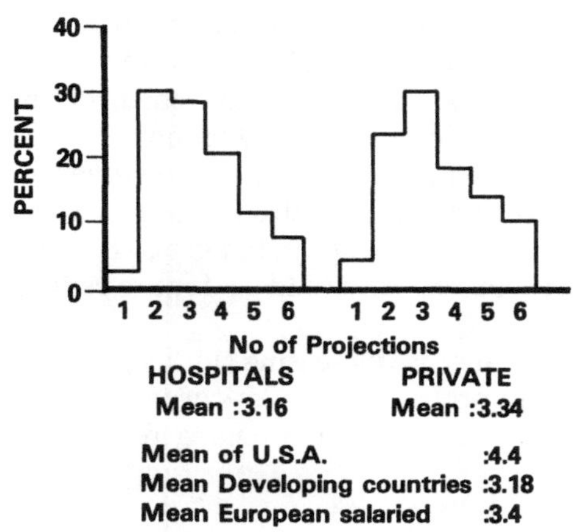

Fig. 5. Utilization of radiologic services in lumbar backache

picture. So in moderation we do need CT scanners, NMR, etc., though proliferation due to commercialization, as has occurred in some areas, is to be decried. In my view it is not particularly high technology that is expensive, but rather the misapplication of the standard state-of-the-art radiography that constitutes 70% of the daily work load. Because of the large volume, savings here can be dramatic and so can help offset the costs of the new technologies.

As I have stated elsewhere, routine equipment is over-engineered and complex without adding to our diagnostic yield [2]. A Volkswagen will transport you as effectively as a Rolls Royce. Do we need all the refinements offered to us?

High-frequency generators have arrived unheralded but constitute a significant technological advance, bringing increased reliability and simplicity at lower costs. The WHO Basic Radiography Service (BRS) concept can be extended beyond the confines of the developing world. Already several Scandinavian governments and other European countries have embraced this concept. WHO is soon to extend its equipment specifications to include fluoroscopy. I question whether we need remote-control tables. Must we all precipitately jump into digital technology without any assurance of extra diagnostic information? Society pays for our armamentarium, so we have a duty to be circumspect about our requirements.

Cost of Personnel

Wages are the highest operational cost in an imaging department, since imaging is unusual in that it is both labor-intensive and capital-intensive. In larger departments, computerization may lead to reduced clerical costs, quite apart from advantages of operational convenience, but generally it results in little cost reduction.

Radiographers and radiologists are expensive. To be sure, both professions require prolonged training, acquisition of skills and judgments, and long hours of work, but can anything be done to reduce such costs?

Technical training is increasing in length and complexity, yet probably only 25% of technicians use the whole range of their imaging repertoire. Do we need to train all to a high level, particularly if the equipment available to them is simple? In some settings, the answer is no. This has been admirably shown in a PAHO/WHO project in Colombia. There, after 10 days training, individuals who had previously never seen an X-ray unit became and remained proficient in the performance of 72 projections. To be sure, BRS units are simple to operate, and the training manual is superbly designed by WHO. This restricted range of radiography would probably cover over 70% of the work of the most sophisticated hospital. Perhaps we should have two levels of technicians – operators to do simple routines and radiographers for more complex studies and for administrative roles. Such a policy, besides leading to economies, has the potential of increasing job satisfaction for both levels. The more highly trained person would be freed from simple repetitive tasks.

Radiologist costs are high in some societies, and training is relatively expensive everywhere. In developing areas with one or less radiologists per 100 000 population, what is to be done?

It seems desirable to initiate shorter training courses which are suited to local equipment and diseases and are held locally, not overseas in Europe or North America. Most of the possible techniques can be taught in an initial two years. WHO and the International Society of Radiology are exploring the possibility of setting up regional centers in, say, Africa, the Pacific, etc. Another way of providing a service where no radiologists exist is to develop a practical booklet to help primary care physicians apply selective interpretation to answer the following questions. Is this a life-threatening emergency needing immediate correction? Can it wait? If so, do I need to send film, the patient, or both to a larger center? Finally, is this a condition for which nothing can be done and the patient can be spared needless strain and expense? Such a booklet is about to be published by the WHO BRS group.

References

1. Cockshott WP (1979) Diagnostic radiology; geography of a high technology. AJR 132:339–344
2. Cockshott WP (1983) Rolls Royces or Compacts? Radiology 148:862

Cost Development in Uroradiology and Neuroradiology

H. Schreyer and E. Tölly

Uroradiology

In the period 1981 – 1983 at the University Clinic of Radiology, Graz, there was a drop of 35% in urographic investigations and renal angiography was down by 30%. On the other hand, we recorded increases of 393% in sonography and 182% in CT (Fig. 1). The changes in frequency of the individual investigation methods may be explained as follows.

Urography

Prior to the introduction of sonography, urography was the method of choice both in cases of unclear abdominal symptoms, to exclude diseases of urinary organs, and also where clinical symptoms pointed to a urinary tract disease. Urography was, moreover, applied routinely in general internal checkups. Today, however, the screening of urinary organs is mainly done by means of sonography. The use of urography has been further reduced by the employment of sonography in investigation of the azotemic patient and in diagnosis of certain retroperitoneal disorders, although the numbers involved are small compared to the above-mentioned routine examinations.

Angiography

The decline in the use of angiography is mainly due to the fact that, with some exceptions, it is not longer utilized for primary investigation of mass lesions.

Sonography

The kidneys are examined sonographically not only alone, but also together with the liver, gallbladder, and pancreas in the course of an abdominal sonogram. The high number of investigations reflects the application of sonography as a screening method.

Computed Tomography

The figures include all abdominal CTs done on account of kidney disease, above all for diagnosing of mass lesions, and also those explorations in which the kidneys were included in the diagnosis because of a disease of adjacent organs.

Costs

The reduction in conventional investigations results in a saving of 37%, but the costs for sonography and CT have increased by 230%, giving a total increase of 33%. However, in this connection we must consider that screening sonography displays a number of organs in the course of one examination, resulting in an additional reduction in the use of other investigation methods, for instance cholecystography and scintigraphy of the liver. A similar situation arises with CT, where several organs are also displayed in one examination, offering more efficient diagnostic possibilities and potentially justifying the increased costs.

Neuroradiology

In cerebral CT an increase of 373% since 1977 has been recorded. B-scan sonography of carotid arteries, carried out since 1981, has increased by 226%. The figure for cerebral angiography remains almost unchanged (Fig. 2). The development of frequency in the different investigation methods is explained as follows.

Angiography

It is of interest to note that the frequency of cerebral angiography has remained almost un-

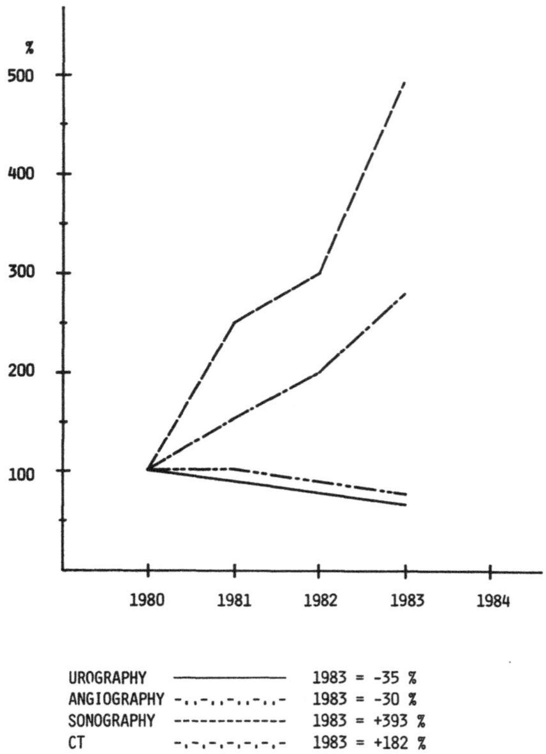

Fig. 1. Frequency of various upper urinary tract investigation methods at the University Clinic of Radiology, Graz (1980–1983)

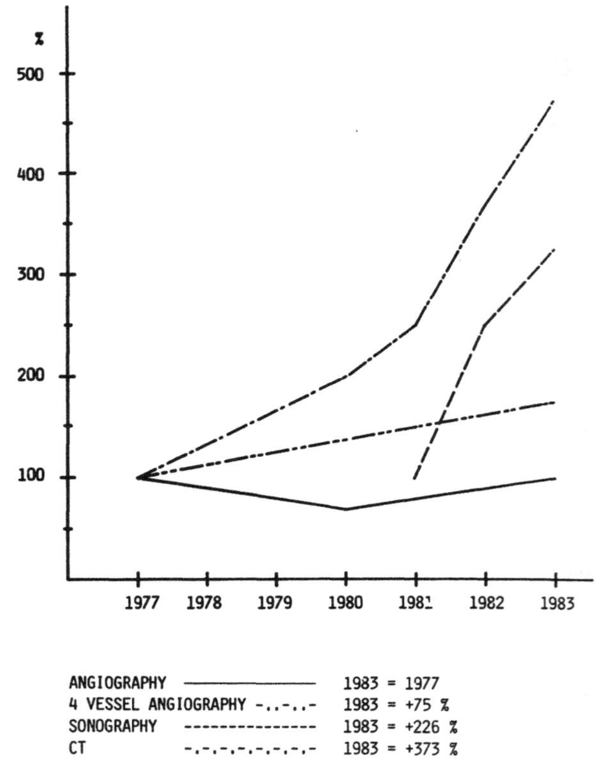

Fig. 2. Frequency of various cerebral and cerebrovascular investigation methods at the University Clinic of Radiology, Graz (1977–1983)

changed. Today, however, the investigation is performed mostly in the form of four-vessel angiography together with thoracic aortography. This has led to greatly increased costs, since formerly in many cases only one vessel was angiographically investigated. However, a certain cost reduction is to be expected from the introduction of DSA.

Sonography

Since the equipment has been available, the number of ultrasonic investigations of the carotid arteries has increased rapidly. This again caused a slight rise in cerebral angiography since by ultrasound clinically asymptomatic arteriosclerotic disease of the cerebral vessels in risk patients can be diagnosed.

Computed Tomography

The diagram shows a steep rise in the frequency of cerebral CTs performed during the last 4 years. The two newly installed scanners, together with an enlargement of the catchment area covered by the clinic, explains the far larger number of patients investigated.

Spinal CT. A special development is offered in spinal diagnostics by the new generation of CT equipment. In our institution CT of the vertebral discs cannot routinely be done as a primary diagnostic procedure, owing to lack of CT capacity. Therefore, so far hardly any reduction in the frequency of myelographies can be observed (on average 950 investigations per year); however an increasing number of spinal CT examinations were carried out in the past 2 years (1983: 167; 1984: 343) partly complementary to myelography using the administered contrast material, partly as a primary investigation.

In total, the results show that the number of examinations rises automatically when noninvasive investigation methods are used. The advantages in imaging of the CNS, bony structures and intervertebral discs, as well as the lack of invasiveness, lead to extensive use of the new imaging modalities.

The Development of Algorithms for Radiologic Procedures: Avoidance of Duplication Through Education of Physicians

A. R. Margulis

With the technological explosion in radiology, the entire diagnostic approach has changed. The pursuit of diagnosis has become less invasive, much more sensitive, yet greatly more specific. This, however, has created problems, as the equipment making these approaches possible is very expensive. A CT scanner costs approximately 1 million dollars in the United States, a magnetic resonance imaging (MRI) unit between 1.5 and 3 million dollars, a digital arteriographic room about 1 million dollars, and a modern ultrasound (US) unit between 100 000 and 300 000 dollars, depending on the degree of automation (Table 1).

Although these instruments have tremendous potential they pose the danger of duplication of tests, with a resulting increase in cost. Devising algorithms that can be modified with experience and are locally applicable according to existing talent and equipment is one of the approaches that reduces or at least contains costs (see Figs. 1–3 for examples). This permits containment of space and personnel and leads to substitution of tests and equipment. Algorithms should not be legislated, as this usually results in illogical decisions in many instances and in resistance to any type of coordination of radiologic tests. It is important to have the cooperation of clinical colleagues, and this can be achieved through education and continuous contact, with daily patient-management conferences.

On a broader scale, costs can be contained if an effort is made to perform tests on an outpatient basis, which eventually should reduce the number of hospitals. The secret of containing costs while performing sophisticated studies with expensive equipment is to (a) avoid duplication, and (b) proceed from broad screening studies based on clinical data to more specific studies, wherever possible with needle biopsy.

The *future directions of MRI* can be summed up as follows: (a) artificial intelligence, (b) echo-planar scanning with high resolution, (c) imaging of elements other than hydrogen, (d) chemical shift imaging, and (e) spectroscopy based on MRI.

Table 1. Cost (in $ 1000s) of advanced radiologic equipment in the USA (1984)

	Equipment costs	Installation costs
Basic CT	600	500
Sophisticated CT	1000	500
Cine CT	1400	500
MRI (0.5 T)	1500	500
MRI (1.0 T)	1800	600
MRI (1.5 T)	2200	1300
Biplane digital angio	900	500
Fluoro + rad. room	500	500
Multipurpose biplane fluoro room with digital	900	500
Ultrasound	120	0
Automated ultrasound	400	50

US or CT (with biopsy)	or	MRI
ERCP	or	PTC
If stone, more likely with sphincterotomy and duct sweeping		If tumor, more likely with drainage and endoprosthesis

(Upper gastrointestinal examination only if hemoccult positive)

Fig. 1. Algorithm for obstructive jaundice (strongly suspected on chemical tests)

Hemoccult positive – double contrast barium enema & upper gastrointestinal examination
Neoplasm stage with CT
Hemoccult negative US or CT with biopsy – (pancreatic mass ERCP)

Fig. 2. Algorithm for upper midabdominal mass

Hemoccult positive – double contrast barium enema
Neoplasm: stage with CT or MRI
Hemoccult negative US or MRI or CT

Fig. 3. Algorithm for pelvic mass

New Advances in Diagnostic Imaging and Their Influence on the Practice of Radiology

J. Lissner and G. Fenzl

Many developments have taken place in X-ray diagnosis since the early days of tomography and the introduction and development of the image intensifier, and many new trends can be discerned.

Ultrasound

Real-time ultrasound has progressed swiftly from a crude imaging tool to a refined modality. Although echography is a relative newcomer to the field of diagnostic imaging, it is already a well-established method. There are now about 12 000 ultrasound units in the FRG, and in 1983 2.8 million examinations were performed by specialists in various disciplines. The many lengthy discussions about the responsibility for the use of this technology finally ended in the practice of investigative ultrasound being opened to a wide variety of medical specialties, none of which has the exclusive right to work in a particular area, as reflected in the recommendations made by the European Federation of Societies for Ultrasound in medicine and biology.

Table 1 shows how the use of ultrasound devices is divided among various specialties in Western Germany. Radiologists take the second place.

In order to obtain authorization for the use of ultrasound, the guidelines issued by the Confederation of Health Insurance Societies of the FRG must be fulfilled. Radiologists have to perform at least 400 examinations. In our department in Großhadern we experienced a continuous growth in the number of ultrasound examinations from 1977 (590 cases) onwards, levelling off in recent years at about 7000 cases. However, in the last 2 years colleagues from other disciplines in our hospital have started carrying out ultrasound examinations, which was earlier seldom the case. This means that the total number of examinations for diagnosis has nevertheless continued to increase.

Table 2 gives a breakdown by organ of the total number of examinations in our department during 1983. The number of special examinations, e.g., of the neonatal skull, thyroid gland, mammary gland, and scrotum, altogether about 800, is quite remarkable.

In summary, one might say that in general practice ultrasound is mainly used for screening the abdominal organs, whereas in hospitals evaluation of blunt traumas, identification of aneurysms of the aorta, and follow-up of kidney and pancreas transplants are of great importance.

Nuclear Medicine

The figures from the Department of Nuclear Medicine in Großhadern reveal some new trends (Table 3).

Even though restricted to a right-to-left comparison of hemispherical cerebral perfusion, computer-assisted radionuclide angiography (CARNA) provides sensitivity of 70% in detecting patients with transient ischemic attacks (TIA) and 96% in patients with completed stroke, and is therefore still used as a screening procedure in patients suspected to have cerebrovascular disease. Despite the increasing use of digital vascular imaging, an increase of 7% in CARNA was observed. Brain scanning has no further relevance in identification of intracranial tumors.

The 25% increase in bone scanning emphasizes the wide acceptance of its importance in the screening and follow-up of patients with malignant tumors.

There has been a continuous decrease in liver and spleen scintigraphy, reflecting the dominant position of CT and ultrasound.

The increase in radiohippurate I-131 renography is due to its importance in monitoring the nephrotoxicity of certain cytostatic therapies. Radiohippurate clearance is the appropriate parameter for assessing tubular nephropathy induced by *cis*-dichlorodiamminoplatinum, being superior to creatinine levels or creatinine clearance values in this respect.

As to perfusion scans of the lung, there has been no change since 1982. Lung perfusion scan is a simple and noninvasive procedure for diagnosing pulmonary embolism, especially useful for patients in intensive care.

The relatively low number of thallium-201 myocardial imaging procedures is due to the enormous expense. All examinations were carried out using the single photon emission computed tomography (SPECT) technique at rest and in an exercise redistribution fashion [7]. In this way transient myocardial ischemia can most be identified elegantly. In addition, using transverse, sagittal, and frontal planes of reconstruction, better anatomic association can be achieved.

First-pass radionuclide angiography followed by gated radionuclide ventriculography was performed at rest and at several stages of exercise to assess changes in parameters such as total and regional ejection fraction, end-systolic volume, end-diastolic volume and cardiac index. The increasing importance of the method is partly due to its use in monitoring the cardiotoxic effect of doxorubicin (Adriblastina).

After the phase of clinical validation of the noninvasive measurement of regional cerebral blood flow by xenon, the indication was restricted to special cases, for instance follow-up after extra-intracranial bypass surgery, which is being performed increasingly often in the Department of Neurosurgery in Grosshadern.

Computed Tomography

In recent years CT has revolutionized radiology. The number of CT units in the FRG has been increasing rapidly (Fig. 1). In 1983 there were 60 head scanners and 301 whole body scanners, in total 361. Of these, 10 head scanners and 113 whole body scanners were in general practice.

At present there are body scanners in nearly all the larger hospitals although there is still a lack of numbers of CT unit's in hospitals.

The number of all kinds of CT investigations in hospitals and in general practice has been increasing during the past years. Looking at the frequency of CT examinations at our University Hospital one can see a great change from 1979 to 1983 (Fig. 2). Above all, examinations of the pelvis and kidneys, the spine, and the heart are increasing.

Heart

There is hardly a diagnostic field in which the clinician finds so many alternative and com-

Table 1. Frequency of ultrasound devices in the FRG (1983)

Gynecologists	60%
Radiologists	35%
Internal specialists	30%
General practitioners	12%
Urologists	3%
Pediatricians	2%
Surgeons	2%

Table 2. Ultrasound examinations carried out in 1983 at the Clinic and Policlinic for Radiology of the University of Munich

Organ	*n*
Upper abdomen and kidneys	6182
Neonatal skull	257
Thyroid gland	249
Testicle	123
Others	52
Total	7020

Table 3. Nuclear medical examinations at the Clinic and Policlinic for Radiology of the University of Munich, 1982–1983

	1982	1983	Difference (%)
1. Cerebral radionuclide angiography with ^{99m}Tc-DTPA	1662	1773	+ 7
2. Bone scans	3098	3869	+25
3. Liver Scans	134	68	−49
4. Spleen scans	60	46	−23
5. Thyroid scans	1244	1195	− 4
6. Thyroid I-131 uptake studies (as test before radio-iodine treatment)	279	320	+15
7. Radiohippurate I-131 renograms	780	1051	+35
8. Perfusion scans of lung	634	622	− 2
9. Thallium-201 myocardial imaging	184	215	+17
10. First-pass radionuclide angiography followed by gated radionuclide ventriculography	230	265	+15
11. Xenon regional cerebral blood flow	396	335	−15

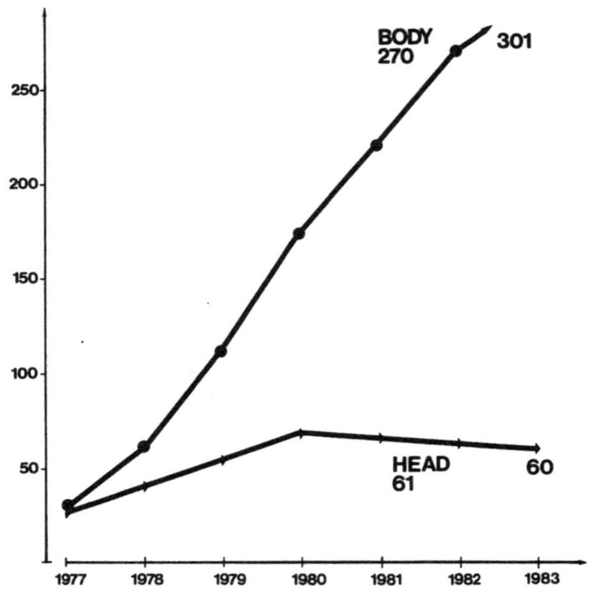

Fig. 1. CT units installed in Federal Republic of Germany

plementary imaging procedures as in cardiac diagnostics. We have reached a stage, particularly in ventricular volume measurements, where the precision of noninvasive angio-CT can compete with angiocardiography [11].

Spine

CT has opened new possibilities in the diagnosis of *spinal diseases* and has led to a new orientation in diagnostic proceeding [4, 5].

During the 3 years from May 1981 to March 1984 we performed 1368 CT examinations of the spine: 447 of the cervical spine, 264 of the thoracic spine, and 657 of the lumbar spine. In 30% of the examinations of the lumbar spine a prolapse was found, in 38% of the thoracic investigations spine metastases were encountered, and in 10% of the investigations of the cervical spine we diagnosed fractures. Intraspinal bleeding, post-traumatic or post-operative, was rarely diagnosed in our case material (1.9% of the cases).

The AP and lateral plain films continue to be the mainstay of radiographic screening in *spinal trauma.* Nevertheless, conventional radiographs underestimate the degree of injury in a significant number of patients (Fig. 3a, b) [1]. For further clarification, CT proved to be the fastest and best method of recognizing the causes and extent of compression of the spinal canal.

CT has reached high accuracy (80%–90%) in the diagnosis of *lumbar prolapse* [4, 5]. In the case of a clear diagnosis it replaces myelography. CT should also be preferred to myelography in suspected *recurrent prolapse.* Location, form, and density are the criteria for distinction between scar and prolapse on CT.

Percutaneous Transluminal Arteriography

PTA certainly serves a good purpose in respect to reducing the risk of operation. In our department PTA is performed about 200 times a year in stenosis and occlusion of pelvic and leg arteries.

Table 4 shows the changes of the clinical stage, according to the Fontaine classification, before PTA and up to 2 years after PTA [13]. Three years after PTA the flow capacity of pelvic arteries is about 84% and that of femoropopliteal arteries is about 70%.

We have performed PTA of stenosed kidney arteries in 200 patients since 1978. At present the frequency is about 35 patients per year. About 35% of the patients are cured, in about 40% blood pressure is decreased, and in about 25% blood pressure is unchanged after a follow-up of 18 months.

PTA is also used in patients with transplanted kidneys.

The complication rate can now be stated to be about 5%. Only 2% of patients have needed operative treatment of the renal artery.

Digital Subtraction Angiography

Digital subtraction angiography (DSA) is a new imaging method which has become well established and is now available in major departments, mainly being performed after transvenous contrast medium injection in the region of the carotids, the renal arteries, the aorta, and also the larger vessels of the extremities (Table 5) [2, 12].

There are many new advances in the field of digital radiography. We performed studies with a prototype of an electronic examination unit for overall digital X-ray diagnostics (Imatron, Siemens) with a special X-ray TV installation [8, 10]. This unit has a signal-to-noise ratio of 6000:1 and produces digital angiographic images with high spatial resolution and a wide range of enhancement.

Our unit is universal, since it allows not only digital angiography with and without subtraction

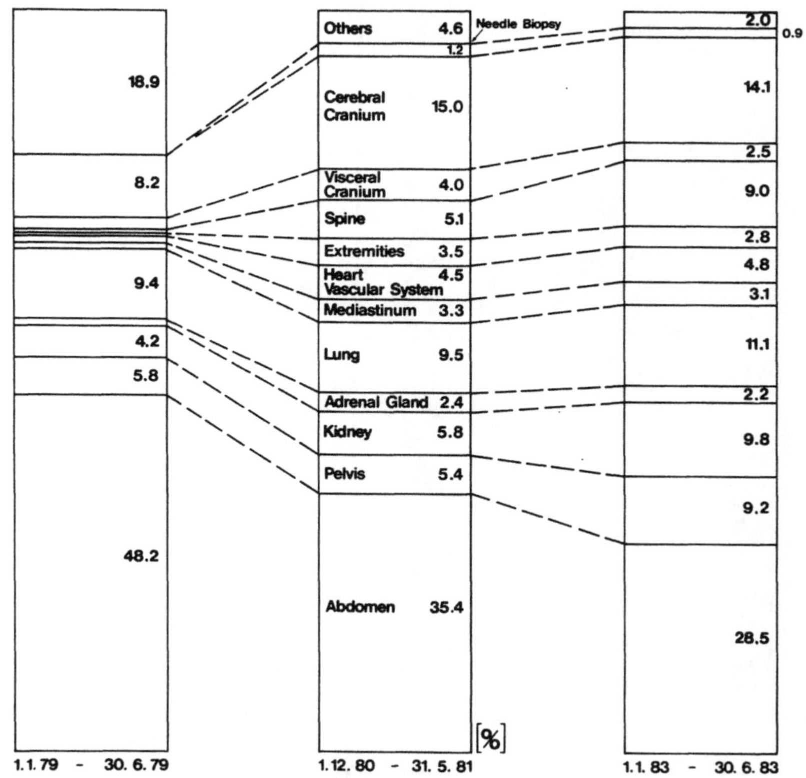

Fig. 2. Frequency of CT investigations (%) during first half-years of 1979, 1981, and 1983 at Clinic for Radiology of University of Munich

Table 4. PTA: Changes of clinical stage (aorta, common iliac artery, and external artery ($n = 65$))

Stage (Fontaine)	I	IIa	IIb	III	IV
Before PTA	0	22	39	1	3
After PTA (3–24 month)	36	19	7	1	2

Table 5. Relative distribution of DSA examinations at the Clinic and Policlinic for Radiology of the University of Munich (June 1982 to January 1984)

Region	n	%
Carotids	1053	48
Renal arteries	508	23.3
Transplanted renal arteries	83	3.9
Upper extremity	87	3.9
Lower extremity	146	6.8
Aorta and pelvic arteries	191	8.7
Heart and pulmonary arteries	11	0.6
Others (digital subtraction phlebography, arterial DSA)	97	4.8
Total	2176	100

technique, but also spot filming with high spatial resolution and, for the first time, high-contrast resolution. This new technique seems to be a breakthrough.

Regarding the image quality of the electronic image, with a matrix of 1024 pixels, the following proportions are thus achieved: The contrast ratio, or dynamic range, is comparable to or even bigger than that of the direct X-ray film. The resolution is about 3.4 Lp/mm for the 9-cm image intensifier entrance field and about 1.8 Lp/mm for the full-size 27-cm image intensifier entrance field. By improving the video intensifier, a signal-to-noise ratio can be achieved for these electronic images which is several times higher than 1000:1. (The signal-to-noise ratio of good TV cameras is about 1000:1.)

Figure 4a, b gives an example of an electronic image with and without digital filtration. One can achieve even better image quality with the help of the electronic image than is possible with the usual 100-mm image from the image intensifier. This is because with digital methods, the ever-present loss of detailed contrast of an image intensifier can be rectified as much as possible given the limits of resolution of the system.

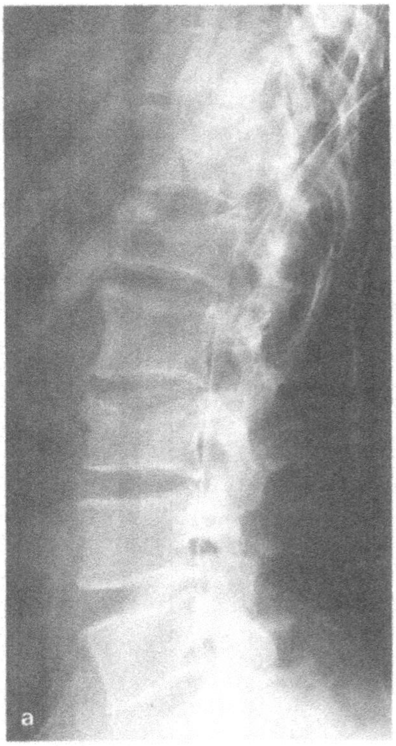

Fig. 3. **a** Compression fracture of first and third lumbar vertebrae with suspected damage of dorsal edge. **b** CT of same patient: third lumbar vertebrae shows high-grade spinal bony compression with fracture of left vertebral arch

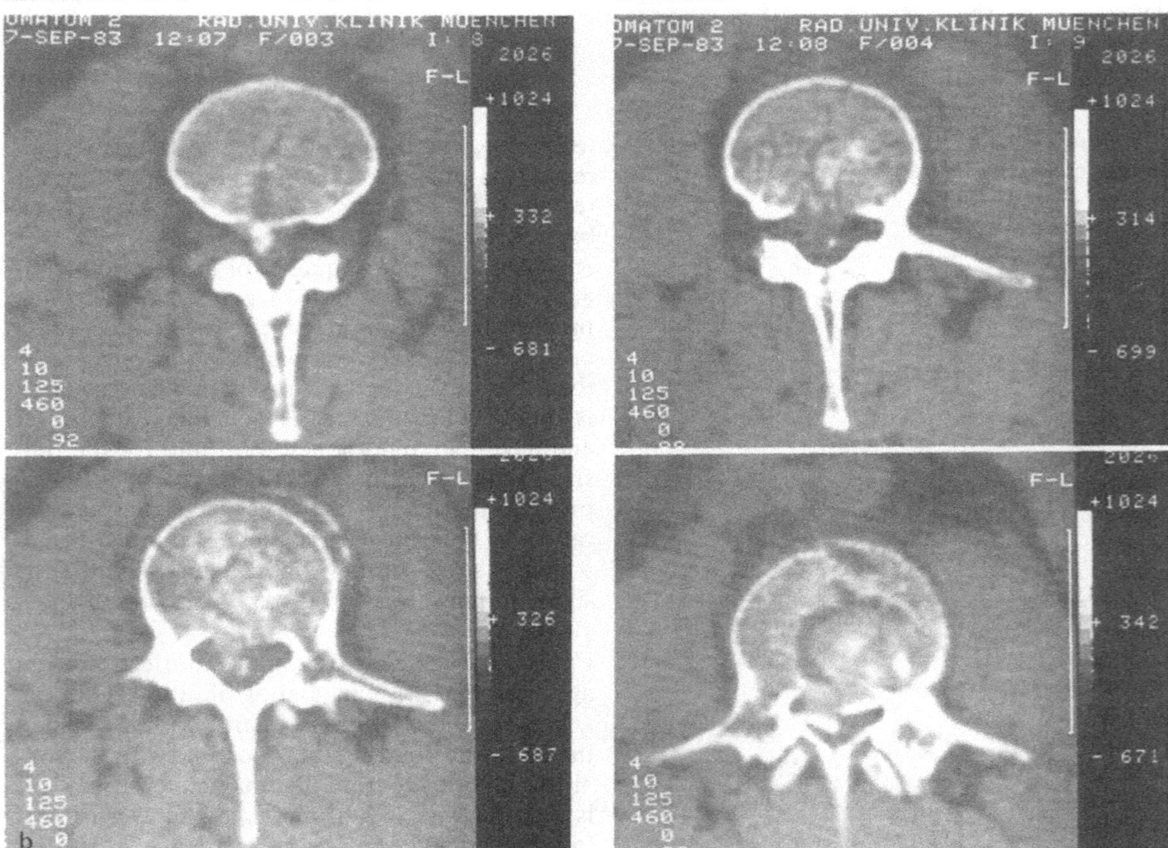

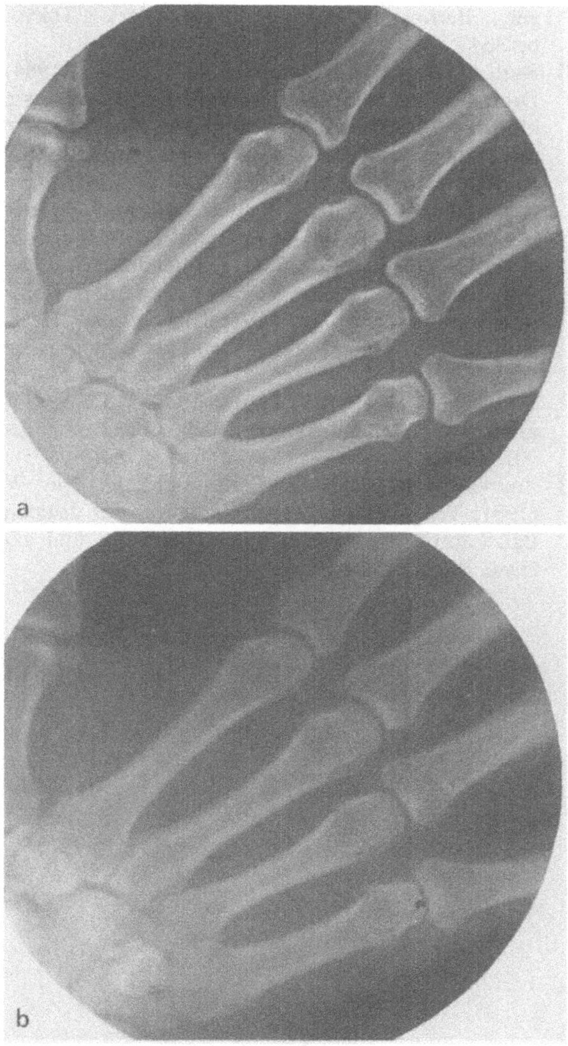

Fig. 4. **a** Hand with digital filtration. **b** Hand without digital filtration

Magnetic Resonance

In the short time that magnetic resonance (MR) imaging has become available, it has created a tremendous uproar and has rapidly emerged as an exciting clinical tool (or toy).

In contrast to CT, MR images depend on four parameters: proton density, longitudinal and transverse relaxation times, and flow. They therefore potentially offer information beyond the capabilities of any other diagnostic imaging method. Furthermore imaging is possible in any desired plane without repositioning of the patient. The possibility of obtaining multiple slices simultaneously holds out the hope of achieving acquisition times per slice similar to those for CT in the near future [3].

It becomes more and more apparent that MR will be the imaging modality of choice for examination of the pelvis [9], particularly in the study of diseases of the prostate, the urinary bladder, the seminal vesicles, and the uterus. One of the great advantages is the availability of direct coronal and sagittal imaging, which improves the diagnosis of the extension of neoplasms.

We think that MR will also become the procedure of choice in the examination of the heart. In comparison to CT there is a significant improvement in the imaging of anatomic details within the chambers of the heart. Another advantage is differentiation between solid tissue and flowing blood without the administration of contrast agents [6]. The imaging of the central nervous system is one of the most striking features of MR. Gray and white matter can be clearly differentiated with the inversion recovery technique, and multiple projections improve diagnosis, especially for small lesions [9]. The absence of bone artifacts and the possibility of midsagittal imaging improve diagnosis of the posterior fossa and the spinal cord.

It is very difficult to judge what influence the various methods discussed here may have on diagnostic radiology in the future. Quantitatively, conventional methods have not been very much affected so far. Obviously the new methods have to be regarded as additional aids for diagnosis and treatment, as CT has already proved to be. We cannot yet venture any opinion as to which of them will stand the test of time and become the most helpful for the patient, but we must support all modern developments: without, however, forgetting that "all that glisters is not gold."

References

1. Brant-Zawadzki M, Miller EM, Federle MP (1981) CT in the evaluation of spine trauma. AJR 136:369
2. Buonocore E, Meany TF, Borkowski GP, Pavlicek W, Gollagher J (1981) DSA of the abdominal aorta and renal arteries. Radiology 139:281
3. Crooks L, Arokawa M, Hoenninger J, Watts J, McRee R, Kaufman L, Davis PL, Margulis AR, De Groot J (1982) Nuclear magnetic resonance whole-body imager operation at 3.5 K Gauss. Radiology 143:169–174
4. Fenzl G, Rath M, Steinhoff M, Matzen KA (1984) Neuorientierung des radiologisch diagnostischen Vorgehens bei Erkrankungen im Bereich der Wirbelsäule durch die spinale Computertomographie. Digitale Bilddiagnostik 4:79–85

5. Haughton VM, Williams AL (1982) Computed tomography of the spine. Mosby, St. Louis
6. Herfkens RJ, Higgins ChB, Hricak M, Lipton MJ, Crooks LE, Lonzer P, Botvinick E, Brundage B, Sheldon PHE, Kaufman L (1983) Nuclear magnetic resonance of the cardiovascular system: normal and pathologic findings. Radiology 147:749–759
7. Kirsch C-M, Doliwa R, Buell U, Roedler D (1983) Detection of severe coronary heart disease with Tl-201: comparison of resting single photon emission tomography with invasive arteriography. J Nucleic Med 24:761–767
8. Lissner J, Rath M, Rienmüller R, Haendle J (1983) Digital radiography: clinical experience with a prototype unit for combined high-quality digital radiographs and digital angiography with and without subtraction technique. Paper presented at the 69th scientific assembly of the radiological society of north america, Chicago, nov 1983
9. Margulis AR (1983) Nuclear magnetic resonance with a 3.5-KG superconducting imager. In: Heuck FHW, Donner MW (eds) Radiology today 2. Springer, Berlin Heidelberg New York Tokyo, pp 334–335
10. Rath M, Lissner J, Rienmüller R, Haendle J (1984) Digitale Radiographie. Gerätetechnik und erste klinische Ergebnisse der digitalen Angiographie mit einem elektronischen Universalarbeitsplatz. ROFO 140, 3:243–250
11. Rienmüller R, Lissner J, Kment A, Bohn J, Strauer BE, Hellwig D, Erdmann E, Cyron J, Steinbeck G, Höss D, Höfling B (1981) Das endodiastolische Volumen des linken Ventrikels in der Computertomographie im Vergleich zur Herzkatheterventrikulographie. Computertomographie 1:62–67
12. Seyferth W, Morhoff P, Zeitler E (1982) DSA: diagnostischer Stellenwert und Risiko. Electromedica 502:60–68
13. Zorn-Bopp M, Ingrisch A, Miltaschk H, Frey W (1981) Transluminale Gefäßdilatation der distalen Bauchaorta, der Arteria iliaca communis und externa. ROFO 134:471

Promotion of Radiology in Nonindustrialized Countries

W. A. Fuchs

Medical radiology is an example of "expensive high-technology medicine". This puts our specialty in a critical position when the public and governments are concerned about the cost of medical care and its socio-economic impact.

Analyzing the present global situation of radiologic services, there is a great discrepancy throughout the world between the developing and the industrialized countries. This fact is clearly reflected in 1980 WHO figures. In industrialized countries one X-ray machine is available for 1500 – 10 000 inhabitants, there is one diagnostic radiologist per 10 000 – 30 000 people, one radiographer per 5000 people and 300 to over 1000 radiologic examinations are performed per 1000 population.

In developing countries the figures are as follows: One X-ray machine per 30 000 – 50 000 population, one diagnostic radiologist per 50 000 – 100 000, one radiographer per 10 000 – 20 000, and 150 – 300 radiologic examinations per 1000 population. In other words, radiologic services are 3 – 5 times less available than in industrialized countries.

In the least developed countries the level of radiologic services is appalling: One X-ray machine is available for 50 000 to 1 million people, one diagnostic radiologist for 100 000 to 2 million, one radiographer for 50 – 200 000, and the number of radiologic examinations is less than 10 – 100 per 1000 population. The availability of radiologic services in these least developed countries is about 100 times less than in the industrialized countries.

This enormous gap is increasing today not only in terms of the ratio between machines and personnel per 1000 population but also in terms of the quality of services offered, the efficacy of such services, the modernization of equipment, and the updating of training. More than three-quarters of the world population is at present covered by radiologic services at an unsatisfactory level, and this situation must be improved.

Constraints

Analyzing the existing radiologic services in the developing countries, it is obvious that the large majority have the services concentrated in large medical institutions in urban areas, leaving the majority of the rural and periurban population underserved. This population is obliged to travel long distances to get an X-ray, spending time, money, and energy which are not offset by the benefit obtained.

The radiologic services at regional and university hospitals, the so-called general purposes and specialized services, are overburdened with investigations, the majority of which are of a basic nature. At most of these hospitals between 90% – 95% of the examinations are plain films examinations and only 5% – 10% need fluroscopy and/or contrast media. The departments are equipped with high-output machines, often provided with image intensifiers and other expensive attachments, and are staffed by the best-qualified radiologists and radiographers of the country, but most of the investigations performed could be undertaken with much simpler and less costly machines and by less skilled personnel.

In terms of health economics, opting to spend a high percentage of the radiodiagnostic services budget on equipment, staff, and recurrent expenditure at the university hospital levels produces a much higher expenditure per examination than choosing to perform a great number of basic radiologic examinations at the community front-line hospital level.

A major constraint which should be considered is the storage, retrieval, and circulation of the radiodiagnostic information in the overcrowded services. Similar consideration should be given to the quality of diagnostic work by the radiologist, who has to examine the radiographs of more than 50 – 60 patients every day and report on each.

Another important constraint is the technical performance of X-ray machines which were not specially designed for conditions such as adverse climate (heat, high humidity or dryness, dust), heavy fluctuations of voltage and frequency, high impedance, and lack of systematic maintenance and regular checks. Particularly sensitive parts of the equipment and annexes, such as image intensifiers, microswitches and relays, intensifying screens, and automatic processors, are under the continuous influence of the factors mentioned, especially the absence of routine maintenance. It is obvious that the life span of a machine in developing countries depends greatly on its sensitivity to these factors and that a more sophisticated machine is more prone to frequent breakdowns. Very few radiologic services in developing countries have more than 60% – 80% of the available equipment in working condition at any given time.

One of the factors which makes the maintenance and repair of equipment extremely difficult is the lack of a supply policy at the level of health authorities. Equipment purchased and donated to countries originates from too many different manufacturers and it is almost impossible to keep a reasonable stock of spare parts.

Chemicals and film supply constitutes another important constraint for a great number of developing countries. The continuous rise in film prices and the difficulties in getting the films supplied continuously throughout the year to avoid excessively long storage in unsuitable conditions are critical problems faced by many countries, resulting in the use of films with a high background fog which therefore produce poor-quality radiographs.

Basic Radiologic Equipment

Since the problem of equipment maintenance is a major constraint for radiologic services in developing countries, the World Health Organisation and the International Society of Radiology have together developed a basic radiologic system (BRS). The BRS has a simple design which makes it very easy to use and is independent of constantly available external power sources and of local maintenance service.

The BRS can, with very few exceptions, handle all types of radiologic procedures which do not require fluoroscopy, tomography, or rapid serial film changing. The BRS is especially designed to handle chest radiography and bone examinations, including radiographs of the skull, with good results, except for a few projections with angulated beam or extremely narrow collimation of the X-ray beam. Abdominal surveys and urography can be performed. Examinations which are possible with the BRS unit constitute 90% – 95% of all radiologic investigations needed in a developing country or in an outpatient service of any country. The examination unit must be simple and should combine the functions of a Bucky table, a vertical Bucky, using a single X-ray tube in a fixed geometry, and an X-ray generator which can function independent of a reliable power line and of advanced local maintenance. The generator has to have an output of at least 10 kW at 100 kV for 1 s and a kV range of 55 – 120 kV.

Medium frequency invertor generator technology makes the BRS available at reasonable cost. Recent high technology may thus be adapted to the needs of basic radiologic services.

Implementation of the BRS project on a large scale is planned by the WHO/ISR working group, with the aim of having the BRS adopted by 60 – 70 countries by 1990.

Radiologic Manpower

The competing demands between preventive and curative health care on a small budget mean that radiologic facilities tend to be very limited.

In order to cover the basic needs for medical radiology, each central referral hospital has to have one qualified staff radiologist. For a teaching hospital performing 100 000 investigations, a minimum of two to five consulting staff radiologists should be available. The extreme shortage of trained radiographers is analogous to that of radiologists. Trained nonradiologist medical doctors play an important role to provide radiologic services. In the front-line community hospitals the BRS X-ray units are run by nonradiologist doctors and by operators trained in basic radiologic techniques.

Training of Radiologists

To cover the basic needs of manpower for radiologic services there is obviously a lack of training centers geared to provide systematic guidance, instruction, and experience for radiologists and radiographers in training. The training and experience received in a Western country is often irrelevant and out of the context of the requirements of the home country. It is better to provide basic training in a home environment. What is needed at present is to build up regional training centers in adequately staffed departments where an intake of doctors from neighbouring countries can be taken and trained systematically. In order to realize this goal, the WHO and the ISR are collaborating in the development of such centers in Kenya and Cameroon, which should be the first steps in covering the African continent. Training centers in South-East Asia and the South Pacific are being created for the countries of those regions.

The training of a specialist radiologist should extend over a 3-year period spent in the WHO/ISR regional training center, where systematic teaching will take place with graded experience and supervision provided. The syllabus indicates only the general scope and character of the course. The first part can be covered adequately in 6 months practical departmental apprenticeship and includes radiologic anatomy, basic principles of radiation physics and apparatus construction, radiation hazards and protection methods, the principles of ultrasound, radiographic techniques, darkroom procedure, and radiologic techniques, including the use of contrast media. The teaching of clinical radiology includes radiologic diagnosis as applied to the various systems of the body in normal and pathological states with particular emphasis on the skeletal system, chest disease, the gastrointestinal system, uroradiology, and pediatric radiology. It is essential that the trainee radiologist should learn how to undertake radiographic procedures. Assessment of the trainee will be made by examination at the end of the 1st year and again at the end of the 3rd year.

A candidate for training in radiology must have undergone full medical training and hold a medical degree recognized and registrable in the country proposing him. The candidate should have spent at least 1 year in hospital clinical practice after qualification.

The hospital selected as a radiologic training center will be a university hospital. Ideally, all disciplines of medicine should be represented. There should be at least two, and preferably more, full-time or almost full-time specialist radiologists on the staff. It is important that these radiologists act as auxiliary teachers, supporting the WHO/ISR tutor.

To maintain credibility and to raise funds in the future, mainly from national radiologic societies, the Teaching Centers must become a success. The program has to be supported by the regional WHO authorities and the "host" government who will agree to admit citizens of adjacent countries as trainees. A wide participation network of countries of that particular region must be ensured. The training program must, of course, be acceptable to participating countries and must not disturb the local status quo to any great extent. Although different in content, the quality standard of training must match with international standards.

The obvious task of the radiologists trained in these centers would be to teach nonradiologist doctors how to handle the BRS equipment and to ensure the quality of essential diagnostic radiology.

Finances

The finance available from the ISR is very limited. Ten percent of the registration fee for the International Congress of Radiology, which takes place every 4 years, is allotted to promotion of radiologic services in developing countries. In addition, there is very limited direct financial support from WHO. However, this seed money may attract financial contributions from national radiological societies of industrialized countries and from other sources. National radiological societies should be encouraged to contribute radiologic manpower for teaching purposes at their own expense and to make cash donations for the running costs of the training centers. They should also be encouraged to donate both teaching material and equipment.

The task is a formidable one, and the requirements are increasing exponentially. For instance, the appalling shortage of diagnostic radiologists on the African continent needs immediate remedy: at present only about 20 radiologists are working in the whole of Africa south of the Sahara.

Appeal for Support and Contributions

The pledge made by the WHO at Alma-Ata in 1978 to support a global effort to ensure "Health for All by the Year 2000" represents a most optimistic goal. In this context the role of radiology is certainly very limited, since preventive health care, agriculture, planning, housing, education, and sanitation have the greatest bearing on health. However, the radiologic community must become aware of the global demand for social and economic justice for people who have less privileges than others.

Every medical specialty must set new priorities, work out new institutional and professional relations, and design new teaching and research structures in order to challenge the immense problems of health care in developing countries and to turn these concepts into practice. The WHO/ISR projects are a modest beginning. They may seem unimportant in the global concept of "Health for All by the Year 2000", but however small the contribution of the radiologic community to this most ambitious global goal might be, it does serve multiple purposes: to teach optimization of radiology, to share experience in feasible approaches under difficult circumstances, to find technically correct solutions, and to identify the fundamental needs and the role of radiologic services in meeting them.

Subject Index

www.ingramcontent.com/pod-product-compliance
Lightning Source LLC
Chambersburg PA
CBHW061209240926
51846CB00006B/1159
* 9 7 8 3 6 4 2 6 9 7 3 9 5 *